MASTERING MEDICAL TERMINOLOGY

By Verlee E. Gross

Former Instructor of Medical Terminology
Adult Education Division
Los Angeles City Schools

REVISED
SIXTH EDITION

Anatomical Illustrations
by Verlee E. Gross

Illustrations of Surgical Instruments reprinted with permission of
The Lawton Company Inc., New York, N.Y.

Library of Congress Catalog Card Number 78-85804

Standard Book Number 0-912256-01-X

Published by Halls of Ivy Press, 13050 Raymer Street, North Hollywood, California 91605, Phone (213) 875-3050

PRINTED IN U.S.A.

CONTENTS

PREFACE

A new educational frontier has opened with a rapid burst of need. It is the need for a working knowledge of medical terminology in a variety of medical and paramedical office positions. This current burst of interest is the result of constantly expanding paper work caused by increased population, more national attention to the improvement of health, and ever increasing medical and hospital insurance coverage.

Employers -- doctors, hospitals, medical insurance companies, federal, state and local health services -- are discovering that applicants with "experience" are not readily available. Therefore, education must take over to prepare a larger number of potential employees for all medical and paramedical positions.

All courses for these jobs start with the language of medicine. A deeper understanding of medical terms adds new meaning and more efficiency to the work produced by the employee.

In order to learn the whys and wherefores of medical terminology and to cope with its vast coverage the medical terms must be reduced to their component parts and each of these elements translated into English. This was the purpose of the first textbook "The Structure of Medical Terms."

"Mastering Medical Terminology" goes one step further. Now, medical terms are placed in their proper context in the body's anatomical systems. To follow the practice of the first textbook, English translations are again given in the text as well as pronunciations. Footnotes have been added wherever possible to add a spark of interest, some historical highlights and also various oddities in terminology to make the study of medical terms more interesting.

Medical terminology as it occurs in the body's many anatomical systems is the main concern of this textbook. Most of the stress is placed, therefore, on medical terms, their use, spelling, English translation and pronunciation. In the process of learning these four important areas of medical terms it is also intended that a knowledge of the structure of each anatomical system, some of the more common diseases, anomalies and surgeries will also be acquired.

WHAT YOU SHOULD KNOW ABOUT THIS TEXTBOOK

TRANSLATION OF TERMS INTO ENGLISH--why it is such an important part of the textbook.

1. To bring about a better understanding of terminology by showing a relationship which we can see in English. This takes the mystery out of the word components.

2. To facilitate the spelling of medical terms. The ability to recognize the terms through translation of the word components makes the words much easier to spell. It is the secret of learning medical terms.

3. To prove how interesting and fascinating the study of the language of medicine can be when the terms are broken down and it is discovered how people, many eons ago, labeled the parts of the body and their related problems and treatments.

PRONUNCIATION--why it, too, is so important.

1. To remove the embarrassment and fears most people have when they attempt to pronounce medical terms.

2. To provide an aid to those foreign born students who have a language problem.

3. To bring out into the open the wide divergence in pronunciation of certain medical terms. When unknown this can be very confusing and embarrassing to medical and paramedical employees.

4. To make the initial acquaintance with medical terminology into a more binding and lasting relationship.

REPETITION--how it applies to this text material.

1. To use the terms as often as possible in their related areas of the body and through this consistent redundance become aware of the terms with less effort.

2. To make the terms appear natural in their element so that students eventually accept their presence in the material without any struggle. In other words, the presence of medical terms becomes as natural as any of our English words.

3. To have the terms brought constantly to the students' attention, not only to make the terms familiar but through this consistently visual reminder, to promote better spelling.

ILLUSTRATIONS--why they are used so extensively.

1. To clarify specific medical terms and make them easier to understand and remember.

2. To provide visual aids for the orientation of anatomy of the various anatomical systems. These drawings are designed to acquaint the students with a basic knowledge of anatomy and the relationship of organs in each of the systems. After all, this is a textbook dealing with words and not the treatment of the patient.

SUFFIXES--why they are listed separately.

1. To reduce redundant translation because the number of suffixes is fairly well established and they occur over and over again.

2. To enable students to learn the suffixes more quickly.

PRONUNCIATION FROM PHONETICS GIVEN IN TEXT

1. The strongest accented syllable is given in capital letters, for example: RĒ-nal, bī-LAT-er-al.
2. If there is a secondary accent it will be noted by a double quote mark ("), for example: glom-er"ū-lō-ne-FRĪ-tis.
3. If there are several secondary accents, as may occur in very long terms, all of these secondary accents will be noted by the double quote mark ("), for example: sal-ping"gō-ō"oo-fōr-EK-tō-mē.
4. The secondary accent (") has some degree of emphasis but is not as strongly accented as the syllables noted in capital letters which are often called the heaviest accent.
5. Pronunciation of vowels is as follows:

   Where vowels are pronounced with a long sound this is signified by a line above the vowel. Therefore, these vowels would be pronounced as follows:

   ā as in māke, ē as in bē, ī as in īvy, ō as in pōle, ū as in pūre

   Unless otherwise shown in the phonetics any vowels not so marked will be pronounced with the short sound as follows:

   i as in bit and sip, e as in met and bet, o as in not, u as in bud

   Additional phonetics are as follows:

   a as in father is written ah and the diphthong oi is written oy

The principle followed for pronunciation is to present the actual, current use rather than what is supposed to be correct. There is no implication intended that these pronunciations given are the ONLY ONES used. This would be impossible as there has been (and probably always will be) a strong degree of conflict between doctors and dictionaries and also between doctors and doctors as regards pronunciation of medical terms. Because medical and paramedical personnel will have more contact with doctors' pronunciations it is felt these pronunciations should be used. However, optional pronunciations (as from the dictionaries) appear in the footnotes.

ALPHABETICAL LIST OF SUFFIXES

Medical terms have the habit of using the same suffixes[1] over and over again. The following is an alphabetical listing of the most common suffixes used. It will be necessary to refer to this listing to complete the English translation of medical terms used in the text.

SUFFIX	ENGLISH TRANSLATION
-able	capable of (adjective)[2]
-ago	disease
-agra	seizure (as of gout), catching, rough
-al	pertaining to (adj.)
-algia	pain
-alis	pertaining to (adj.)
-ar	pertaining to (adj.)
-ary	one who, or that which (adj.)
-asis, -asia	condition or state of
-ate	possessing or characterized by (adj.)
-ation,-ion,-tion	act or state of
-atresia	without opening
-cele	hernia, protrusion, swelling, tumor
-cid(e), -cis	cut, kill
-cleisis	closure
-clysis	injection
-cytosis	condition of cell
-desis	binding, fixation
-dynia	pain
-ectasia,-ectasis	stretching, dilatation
-ectomy	cut out, remove, excision
-emia	condition of blood
-esis	condition or state of
-facient, -fact	make
-ferent	bear, carry
-form	shape, form
-fug(e)	avoid
-glia	glue
-gram, -graph	scratch, write, record
-ia	condition or state of
-ible	capable of (adj.)
-ic, -icus	pertaining to or connected with (adj.)
-ician, -ist	physician, one who practices
-itis	inflammation
-ive	having power to (adj.)
-ize	to treat by a special method
-lepsy	seizure
-logy, -logical	study or science of
-lysis	solution, loosening, dissolve
-ode, -oid	resemble, like, form
-ol	oil
-oma	tumor
-ory	place or thing where (adj.)
-ose	to be full of (adj.)
-osis, -osia	condition or state of
-ous	to be full of (adj.)
-pellent	to drive
-pexy	fixation
-phobia	fear
-phrenia	the diaphragm, the mind
-physis	nature, to grow
-plasia	formation
-plasty	mold, shape, form (plastic surgery)
-plegia, -plexy	stroke, paralysis
-pnea	to breathe
-rrhage, -rrhagia	to burst forth
-rrhaphy	to suture
-rrhea	flow, discharge
-scope, -scopic, -scopy	to observe, to look at, to view
-some	the body
-stomy	to make an artificial opening
-stringent	to draw tight, compress, bind, to cause pain
-thymia	thymus gland, mind, soul, emotions
-tocia	birth
-tome	a cutting instrument
-tomy	cutting into, incision
-trophy, -trophic	nourishment
-tropia	turn, react
-uria	urine, condition of urine

1. *The correct plural of suffix is "suffices." The modern trend is to "suffixes."*
2. *Wherever the suffix is an adjective ending the word adjective will be abbreviated to "adj."*

ACKNOWLEDGEMENTS

When so many do so much to make the publication of a textbook possible, it takes more than verbal appreciation to express an author's gratitude.

To the following my sincerest thanks for their moral, spiritual and physical support:

> to my mother and brother, John, who took over so many of my household and business chores, respectively, thus adding the extra hours needed to write and illustrate this book;
>
> to Marilyn "Winkie" Takahashi, who took so many hours of her spare time after teaching, for her help not only in research but in the proofreading of the text matter. Proofreading is a monotonous, tiring job and one which requires someone well skilled in medical terminology. "Winkie" not only qualifies in this area but is a very exacting proofreader;
>
> to the many surgeons who understood my desire to keep the surgical procedures as basic and routine as possible and who took their valuable time to read and edit the surgical portion of the material;
>
> to my good friends in the medical profession who were most generous in loaning their valuable medical texts. Without their help it would have been impossible to research the vast amount of material which has been accumulated over the past 17 years.

In gratitude to these members of the medical profession for their unselfish help, I have deleted suggested treatments for diseases, etc. (with the exception of surgical procedures). Treatments are constantly changing through continued research and the introduction of new medications. In addition, not all doctors agree on the same method of treatment for certain conditions. The material in this textbook is concerned with medical terminology and not the care and treatment of the patient. These belong in the realm of the doctor and the nurse.

Verlee E. Gross
North Hollywood, Calif.
May, 1969

Knowledge is the goose that lays the golden eggs.

\- Ira Wolfert

CHAPTER I
INTRODUCTION

Ana/tomy[1] [up] (ah-NAT-ō-mē) and physio/logy [nature] (fiz-ē-OL-ō-jē) along with other classes of organized knowledge concerning living matter are divisions of the great science bio/logy [life] (bī-OL-ō-jē).

Anatomy belongs to that group of bio/logic/al (bī-ō-LOJ-i-kal) sciences known as morpho/logy [form] (mōr-FOL-ō-jē).

Gross anatomy is the science of macro/scop/ic [large] (mak-rō-SKOP-ik) structure or that which can be seen with the naked eye.

Patho/logic/al [disease] (path-ō-LOJ-i-kal) anatomy has to do with diseased structures -- cells, tissues, organs.

Histo/logy [tissue] (his-TOL-ō-jē) stresses minute or micro/scop/ic [small] (mī-krō-SKOP-ic) structures or structures that can only be seen with the aid of a micro/scope (MĪ-krō-skōp).

Physiology is the science of function and activity. It shows what cells, tissues and organs do individually, in relation to each other, and in the integrated behavior of the organism as a unit.

Embryo/logy [full of life] (em-brē-OL-ō-jē) is the science of growth from the cell stage to the adult but frequently is restricted to mean the period of growth and development before birth.

The cell is the structural and physio/logic/al (fiz"ē-ō-LOJ-i-kal), as well as the developmental, unit of the body. Groups of cells with more or less inter/ [between] cell/ular [room] (in-ter-SEL-ū-lar) material make up tissues. The type of tissue is determined by the type of specialized cell of which it is composed. For example: bone tissue from bone cells, muscle tissue from muscle cells, nerve tissue from nerve cells, etc.

Two or more tissues associated in performing some special function make up

1. Refer to the alphabetical SUFFIX LIST just ahead of this page for translation of all commonly used suffixes.

an organ. For example: bones from bone tissue, muscles from muscle tissue, nerves from nerve tissue, etc. The organs are arranged into systems. A system is an arrangement of organs closely allied to each other and concerned with the same functions. The following are the systems of the body with their functions:

1. The SKELETAL SYSTEM consists of the bones of the body and the connective tissue which binds them together. The main functions are support, protection and motion.

2. The MUSCULAR SYSTEM consists of the striped muscles (<u>bi/ceps</u> *two head* [BĪ-seps] muscle), the unstriped muscles (the muscle coats of the stomach), and the cardiac muscle tissue. The main function of the Muscular System is to cause movement by contracting.

3. The NERVOUS SYSTEM consists of the brain, spinal cord, <u>ganglia</u> *knot* (GANG-glē-ah), nerve fibers and the sensory and motor terminals. It is a network for the transmission of outgoing and incoming impulses -- much as a telephone switch-board -- and it also contains centers for sensation, emotion and for thinking.

4. The VASCULAR or CIRCULATORY SYSTEM consists of the heart, the blood vessels and blood, the <u>lymph</u> *water* (limf) vessels and lymph. The main function is to distribute the body fluids steadily to all cells.

5. The ENDOCRINE SYSTEM or the system of the ductless glands includes the <u>thyr/oid</u> *shield* (THĪ-royd) gland, the <u>para/thyr/oids</u> *beyond* (par-ah-THĪ-royds), <u>thymus</u> *spirit, mind* (THĪ-mus), <u>ad/ren/als</u> *near kidney*[1] (ad-RĒ-nals), <u>pituit/ary</u> *mucus, phlegm* (pi-TŪ-i-tār-ē) body, <u>pine/al</u> *pine cone* (PIN-ē-al) body, and portions of the glands with ducts such as the islands of <u>Langerhans</u> (LANG-er-hanz) in the <u>pan/creas</u> *all flesh* (PAN-krē-as), portions of the <u>ovaries</u> *egg bearer* (Ō-vah-rēz) and <u>testes</u> *testicle* (TES-tēz), as well as the liver. The organs of this system contribute to the body fluids specific substances which affect the activity of cells.

6. The RESPIRATORY SYSTEM consists of the nose, <u>pharynx</u> *throat* (FAR-inks), <u>larynx</u> (LAR-inks), <u>trachea</u> *rough* (TRĀ-kē-ah), <u>bronchi</u> *windpipe* (BRONG-kī) and lungs. The main func-

1. Although an adjective, this word in the plural is often used as a noun.

tions are to provide oxy/gen (sour, sharp / produce) (OK-si-jen) and get rid of excess carbon (coal, charcoal) (KAR-bon) di/oxide (two sharp, sour) (dī-OK-sīd).

7. The DIGESTIVE or GASTRO-INTESTINAL SYSTEM consists of the aliment/ary (to nourish) (al-i-MEN-tah-rē) canal and the accessory glands (the saliv/ary (saliva) [SAL-i-var-ē]), the pancreas, the liver and gall (GAWL) bladder. The main functions are to receive, digest and absorb food and eliminate some wastes.

8. The EXCRETORY SYSTEM[1] consists of the urin/ary (urine) (Ū-ri-ner-ē) organs, the kidneys, ureters (urinary canal) (UR-i-ters)[2], bladder, urethra (canal leading from bladder) (ū-RĒ-thrah) and also the respiratory and digestive systems and the skin. The main function is to eliminate the waste products that result from cell activity.

9. The REPRODUCTIVE SYSTEM consists of the testes, semin/al (seed) (SEM-i-nal) ducts, seminal ves/icles (bladder / small) (VES-i-kals), penis (Latin) (PĒ-nis), urethra, pro/state (before / to stand) (PROS-tāt) and bulbo-/urethr/al (bulb / urethra) (bul"bō-ū-RĒ-thral) glands in the male; the ovaries, uter/ine (womb)[3] (Ū-ter-in) tubes, uterus (womb) (Ū-ter-us), vagina (sheath) (vah-JĪ-nah) and vulva (wrapper or covering) (VUL-vah) in the female.

The SENSES are not essentially considered a system although each has a physiological function in the body. They cover TOUCH (skin and appendages); TASTE (the tongue); SMELL (the nose); HEARING (the ear); and SIGHT (the eye).

1. The EXCRETORY SYSTEM as it refers to the urinary organs and the REPRODUCTIVE SYSTEM are commonly classified as the GENITO-URINARY SYSTEM.

2. Optional pronunciation ū-RĒ-ters.

3. Optional pronunciation Ū-ter-īne

Dors/al [back] (DŌR-sal) or posterior [in back of] (POS-tir-ē-er) refers to the side containing the backbone.

Ventr/al [belly] (VEN-tral) or anterior [in front of] (an-TĒ-rē-er) is for the opposite side (abdomin/al [belly] [ab-DOM-i-nal] side).

The head end is spoken of as crani/al [skull] (KRĀ-nē-al) or superior [above] (sū-PĒ-rē-er) (also as cephal/ad [head toward] [SEF-ah-lad]).

The opposite end is spoken of as caud/al [tail] (KAW-dal) or inferior [below] (in-FĒ-rē-er).

A part above another part is described as superior to it and a part below another part is said to be inferior.

The sagitt/al [arrow, straight] (SAJ-i-tal) plane divides the body into right and left sides. It is also referred to as the mid-sagittal plane.

A coron/al [crown] (kō-RŌ-nal) or front/al [forehead] (FRON-tal) plane divides the body into front and back or front and dorsal parts.

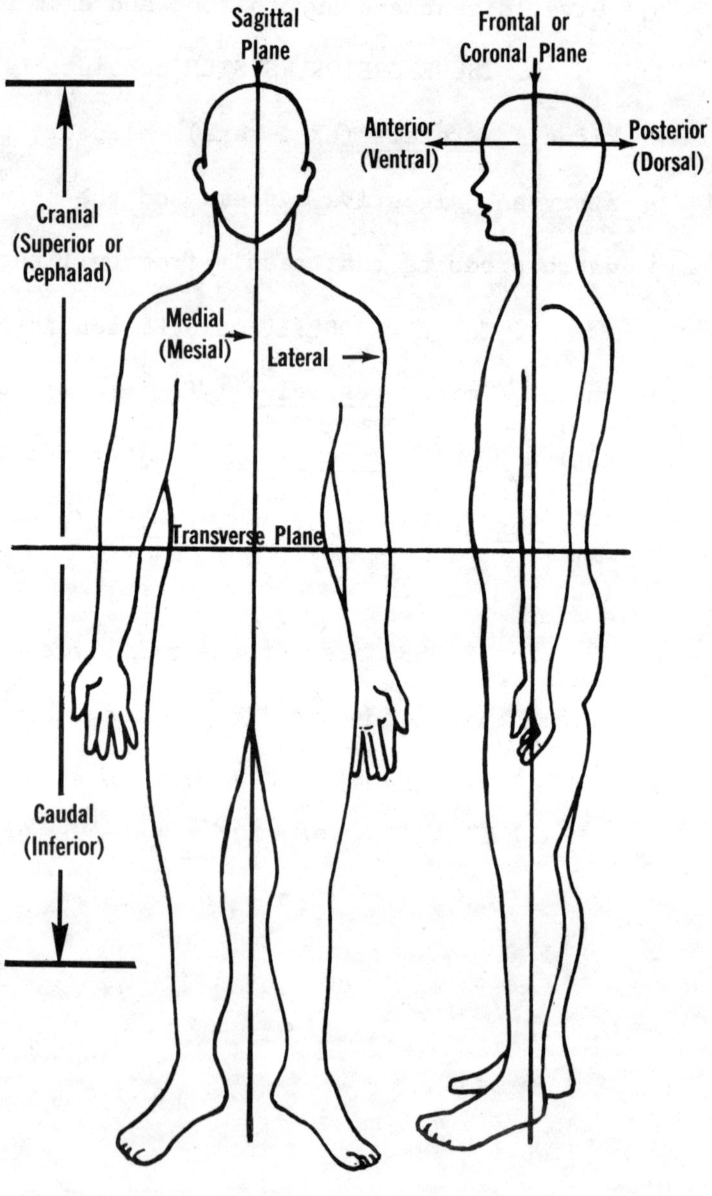

A trans/verse [across to turn] (trans-VERS) plane divides the body into cranial and caudal parts.

Those parts nearest the mid-sagittal plane are medi/al[1] [middle] (MĒ-dē-al); those farthest from this plane are later/al [side] (LAT-er-al).

Intern/al [inside] (in-TER-nal) and extern/al [outside of] (eks-TER-nal) are used almost entirely

1. Also known as mesi/al (MĒ-sē-al)

for describing the walls of cavities or of hollow viscera [organ (plural of viscus)] (VIS-er-ah).

Proxim/al [nearest] (PROK-si-mal) is used to describe a position nearer the central portion of the body or point of origin; the wrist is proximal to the hand.

Dist/al [farthest] (DIS-tal) is used to describe a position distant or farthest away from the center of the body or point of attachment; the foot is distal to the ankle.

Inter/mediate [between middle] (in-ter-MĒ-dē-at) means between two other structures; the intermediate cutane/ous [skin] (kyo͞o-TĀ-nē-us) nerve is between the medial and lateral nerves.

Pariet/al [wall] (pah-RĪ-i-tal) is used to describe the walls enclosing the body cavity or surrounding organs.

Viscer/al (VIS-er-al) is applied to the organs within the body cavity.

Peri/phery [around to bear] (peh-RIF-er-ē) and peri/pher/al (peh-RIF-er-al) mean away from the center; the outside or surface of a body or an organ.

Deep is used to denote away from the surface; the humerus [shoulder] (HYO͞O-mer-us) is in the depth of the arm.

Superfici/al (sū-per-FISH-al) denotes near the surface; superficial fascia [band] (FASH-ē-ah) lies just under the skin.

SURFACE MARKINGS OF BONES

The surfaces of bones present various projections, depressions, or perforations. The projections and depressions may be articular in nature (forming joints), or they may mark the attachments of muscles, tendons or ligaments. The perforations may serve as passageways for blood vessels, nerves, etc.

Projections are designated, according to their size and form as:

Type of Projection	Description
tuber/osity (tū-ber-OS-i-tē) or *node condition* trochanter[1] (trō-KAN-ter) *runner*	rough, large
tuber/cle (TŪ-ber-kl) *node small*	blunt, small
spine	pointed, slender
condyle (KON-dīl) *knuckle*	enlargement at an articular extremity
epi/condyle (ep-i-KON-dīl) *on, upon*	projection above the condyle
head	enlarged, rounded articular end of long bones separated from the shaft by a narrow part, the neck
facet *face*	flat, articular surface
line	slight ridge
crest	narrow, prominent ridge
process (PROS-es) *progress*	used for any marked prominence

Depressions are known by the terms:

fovea (FŌ-vē-ah) *pit*	shallow
fossa (FOS-ah) *ditch*	deep
sulcus (SUL-kus) *trench*	groove
incisura (in-si-SŪ-rah) *incision, cut*	notch

Perforations receive such names as

foramen (fō-RĀ-men) *opening*	hole or orifice for passage of vessels
canal	tubular passage, also called a meatus[2]
fissure (FISH-ur) *to split*	narrow, cleftlike

Sinus (SĪ-nus) and antrum (AN-trum) apply to cavities within certain bones.
hollow — *cavity*

1. The ball on which the hip bone turns in the socket.

2. Meatus (mē-Ā-tus) means "passage".

Sutures are prepared from two types of material which make them either absorbable or non-absorbable.

Absorbable sutures are those which are absorbed or digested by the body cells and fluids during and after healing processes and do not have to be removed. Some of the types used are:

Surgical gut (catgut) which is really sheepgut. Plain surgical gut has not been treated in any manner to alter its rate of being digested by body tissues and fluids. Chromic surgical gut has the same origin as plain, but is chromic/ized [chromium, to treat] (KRŌ-mi-sīzd) or made tissue-resistant by means of a tanning process.

Fascia lata [band, broad] (FASH-ē-ah LAH-tah) are strips or sheets taken from the fibr/ous [fiber] (FĪ-brus) tissue which covers the thigh. Living fasci/al (FASH-ē-al) transplants are prepared in the operating room by the surgeon as needed from narrow strips from the apo/neur/osis [from, sinew (tendon)] (ap"o-nū-RŌ-sis) of the external oblique muscle. Living grafts are also taken from the fascia lata, or the lateral portions of the thigh muscles by the use of the fascial "stripper."

Non-absorbable sutures are those which the cells and fluids cannot absorb or digest. When used as skin sutures, non-absorbable sutures are removed after the wound has healed. When buried in tissues, they are not removed but remain as foreign bodies. Usually they become en/cysted [in, sac] (en-SIST-ed) and cause no trouble. Several of the types used are:

Cotton comes in a variety of sizes consisting of 80 to 100 plain cotton, quilting cotton, No. 30 crochet cotton, No. 20 and 40 cotton, No. 10 mercerized crochet cotton. Their uses range from lig/ation [tie, bind] (lī-GĀ-shun) sutures to tension sutures.

Silk is inexpensive, well tolerated by body tissues and practically devoid of foreign materials unless dyed or treated. It normally becomes en/capsul- [in, capsule] ated (en-KAP-sū-lāt-ed) and remains permanently in the tissues.

Metal wire comes in various gauges and metals and is used primarily in ortho/pedic (or-thō-PĒ-dik) surgery.

normal, straight   child

Silkworm gut is "unborn" silk obtained from the caterpillar of the silkworm.

Artificial silkworm gut is natural silk, twisted and encased in a non-absorbable smooth coating of gelatin or other protein substance.

Nylon is a synthetic, protein-like material. It and other new synthetic sutures are replacing many of the non-absorbable sutures because they are strong, elastic and water-resistant.

Metal clips are known as Michel (me-SHEL) clips after the Frenchman who developed them. They are used in ap/proximating (ah-PROK-si-māt-ing) skin edges. Cushing clips, named for the late Dr. Harvey Cushing, are used in brain surgery. Unlike the removable Michel clips, they are left in the tissues. Tantalum (TAN-tah-lum) clips are also used in brain surgery.

toward nearest

Tantalum wire is bio/log/ically (bī-ō-LOJ-ik-al-ē) inert, non-irritating and possesses high tensile strength. It resists corrosion and chemical attack by body cells and fluids. It remains in the body permanently.

The gauge of the suture is determined by the area and the purpose for which it will be used. Most suture materials start at 6-0 which is the finest. Other gauges are 5-0, 4-0, 000 (triple 0), 00 (double 0), 0, 1, 2, 3, 4, 5. Some suture materials are designated as fine, coarse and medium.

<u>apposition</u> (ap-ō-ZISH-un)--suturing that includes only the skin.

<u>approximate</u> (ah-PROK-si-māt)--to bring together

<u>approximation</u> (ah-PROK-si-mā-shun)--the bringing together of tissues in layers (like tissues meeting tissues) to close a wound.

<u>blanket</u>--a continuous suture with the needle passed over the suture material at each stitch.

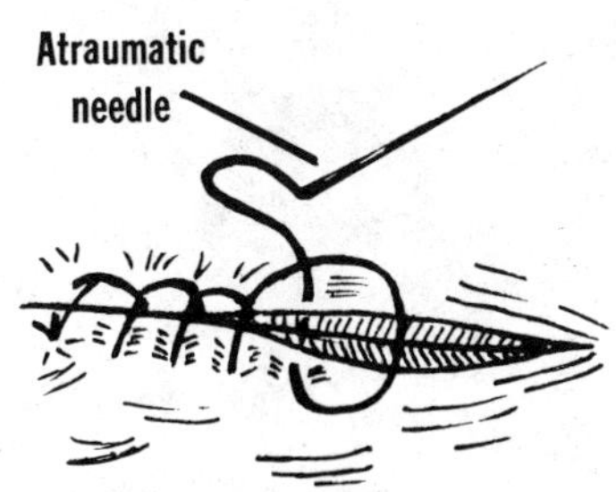

Blanket or Continuous Locked Suture

<u>bolster</u>--a suture, the ends of which are passed over pads of gauze or rubber tubing in order to lessen the tension on the skin.

<u>buried</u>--a suture placed completely under the skin.

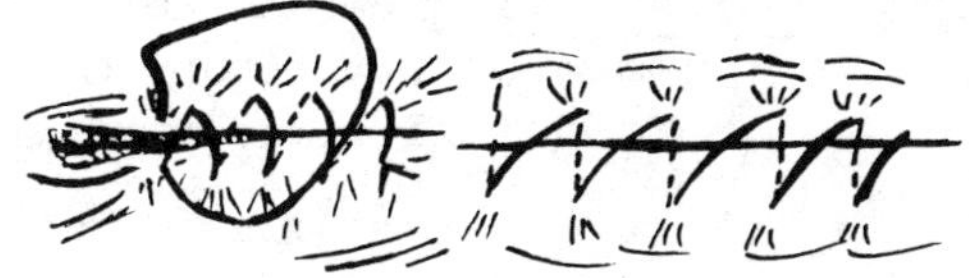

Continuous Over and Over Closing Sutures (2 methods)

<u>button</u>--a suture passed through button-like disks to prevent the thread from cutting.

<u>coaptation</u> (kō-ap-TĀ-shun)--an apposition suture

<u>Connell's</u>--1. an intestinal suture for end-to-end <u>anastomosis</u> (ah-nas-tō-MŌ-sis) 2. a mattress suture

<u>continuous</u>--a "running" type of stitch in which the surgeon ties the first and last stitches only.

<u>dry</u>--a suture in which the stitches are made through two strips of adhesive tape applied along each edge of the wound.

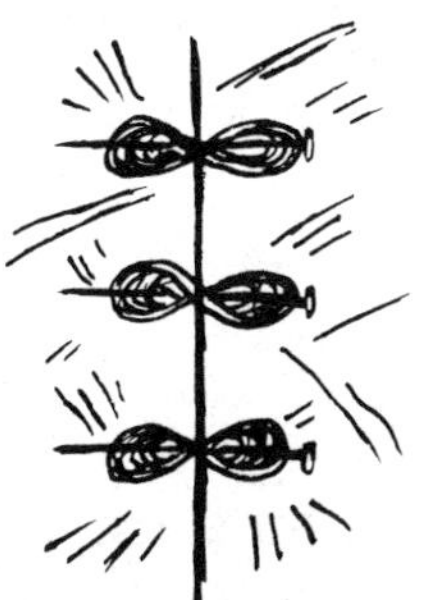

Figure-of-eight Sutures around pins

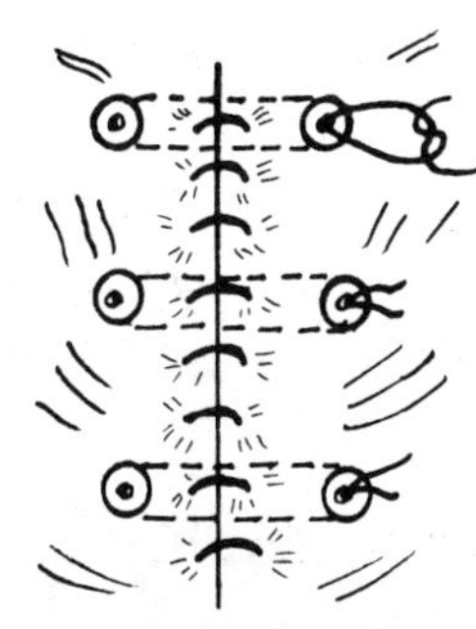

Continuous Suture with perforated buttons to support tension suture

<u>figure-of-eight</u>--a suture in which a pin is passed through the lips of the wound at right angles to the line of incision. The thread is passed over the ends of the pin in the form of a figure 8. Also known as twisted or harelip suture.

<u>implanted</u>--a suture made by passing pins into the flesh parallel to the wound. The pins are drawn together with threads, thus closing the lips of the wound.

<u>interrupted</u>--a type of suture in which the surgeon ties each stitch separately.

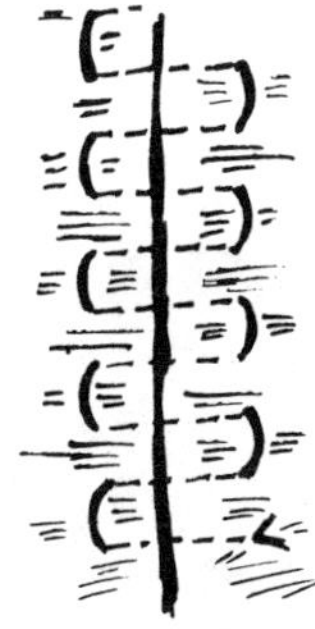

Continuous Mattress Suture

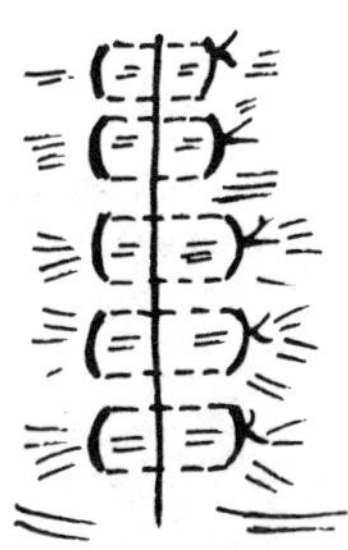

Interrupted Mattress Suture

<u>Lembert</u>--a suture for the stomach and intestines

<u>ligate</u> (LĪ-gāt)--refers to the ligating or tying off of blood vessels or other tissues.

Interrupted Skin Sutures

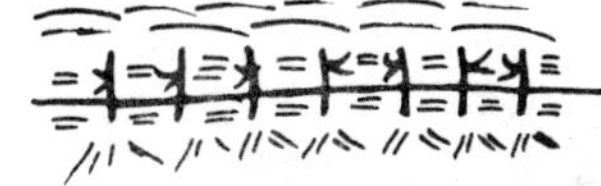

<u>mattress</u>--a suture that is applied back and forth through both edges of a wound.

*As these terms are alphabetized and do not require English translations they will not be included in the index at the end of the chapter.

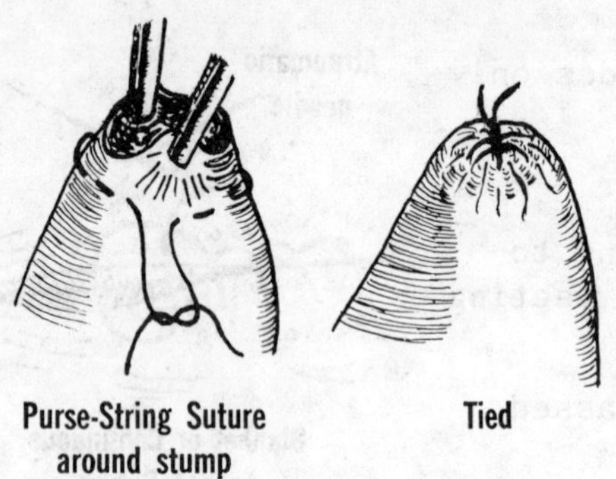

Purse-String Suture around stump

Tied

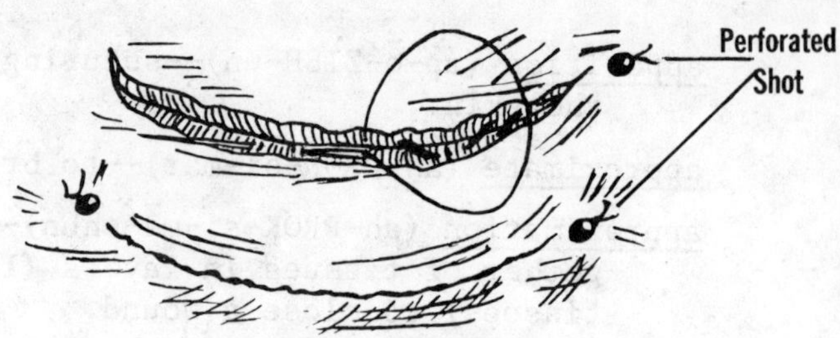

Subcuticular Suture for closing of skin incision

purse string--a continuous stitch passed in and out through the skin encircling the wound. When the ends are pulled together and tied the tissues are drawn together as a drawstring closes the mouth of a bag.

quilted--a continuous mattress suture in which each stitch is tied as soon as formed and the next stitch is passed in the opposite direction.

shotted--a suture in which the two ends are fastened by passing them through a split shot which is then compressed.

stick tie--a suture drawn through a small Mayo needle. Used to tie off bleeders.

subcuticular (sub-kū-TIK-ū-lar)--a continuous buried suture concealed by the epidermis (ep-i-DER-mis). Also known as Halsted's suture.

superficial--one which is made through the skin only, or which does not include any deep tissue.

suture--to sew or unite body tissues.

suture-ligature--a suture with a needle used to tie off large vessels embedded in fatty tissue or muscle; also prevents the ligature from slipping.

tension or stay--sutures placed at a short distance from primary suture line. Designed to relieve tension on primary suture line.

uninterrupted--a continuous suture

During wound healing three tissues are regenerated: epi/thelium[1] [on, upon / nipple] (ep-i-THĒ-lē-um), fibrous tissue and blood cells. These three tissues comprise the scar or cicatrix (SIK-ah-triks)[2].

Every bit of deep tissue wounded or destroyed during the process of healing is replaced by generating fibrous tissue. Thus, infection and necr/osis [death] (nē-KRŌ-sis) increase the amount of scarring. Terms used in the healing process include re/strati/fic/ation [again / layer / to make] (rē"strat-i-fi-KĀ-shun), kerat/iniz/ation [horny / to treat] (ker-at"in-i-ZĀ-shun), fibro/plasia [fiber] (fī-brō-PLĀ-zē-ah), epi/thel/iz/ation (ep-i-thē-li-ZĀ-shun), gran/ul/ation [grain / small] (gran-ū-LĀ-shun) and bacterio/stasis [bacteria / stoppage] (bak-tē-rē-ō-STĀ-sis).

Ex/udative [out / sweat] (EKS-ū-dah-tiv) phase: during the days immediately following wounding, the exudative phase of healing occurs. During it, hemo/rrhage [blood] (HEM-ō-rej) is arrested, fibrin (FĪ-brin) deposited, bacteri/al (bak-TĒ-rē-al) infection resisted, dead tissue liquified and foreign bodies sloughed [to cast off] (sluf'd).

Contraction occurs simultaneously with the regeneration of tissue. It is a powerful force for closing wounds resulting from the inward movement of the surrounding healthy tissues.

Wound infection is caused by 1. dead tissue, 2. foreign bodies and 3. bacteria.

The function of sutures is to hold the edges of a wound together until healing occurs.

Debridement[3] (dah-bred-MAW) is the cutting away of crushed tissues after injury to prevent local infection of a wound.

Chemo/therapy[4] [chemical / treatment] (kē-mō-THER-ah-pē) of wounds is treatment with anti/biotics[5] [against / life] (an"te-bī-OT-iks). It aids in the healing of wounds by preventing infection from becoming established, by preventing spread of infection from the wound and by hastening the resolution of the localized established infection.

1. A term applied originally to the thin skin covering the nipples and the papillary layer of the border of the lips.
2. Optional pronunciation (sik-Ā-triks)
3. The term debridement may also be pronounced (dā-brēd-MON). The word is not derived from "debris."It comes from the French "brides", the English "bridles" and, therefore, implies unbridling, the removal of a barrier to free drainage.
4. Optional pronunciation (kem"ō-THER-ah-pē)
5. Antibiotic is basically an adjective but modern usage tends to make it a noun.

A/vulsion *(away / to pull)* (ah-VUL-shun)[1] is the condition in which there is a tearing away of a part as in the separation of wound edges.

Dehiscence *(to gape)* (dē-HIS-ens) is the process of splitting; for example, the splitting open of a wound.

E/ventr/ation *(out of / belly)* (ē-ven-TRĀ-shun) is a protrusion of omentum[2] (ō-MEN-tum) and/or intestine through an opening in the abdominal wall; disembowelment.

E/viscer/ation *(out of / organ)* (ē-vis-er-Ā-shun) is a protrusion of abdominal viscera; disembowelment.

1. Optional pronunciation (ā-VUL-shun)

2. The greater omentum hangs in front of the intestines like an "apron". It is a continuation of the peritoneum.

TYPES OF SURGICAL INSTRUMENTS*

applicator--a slender rod of wood or flexible metal, on one end of which is attached a pledget of cotton or other substance for making local applications to the nose or any other accessible surface.

aspirator--an apparatus used for removing by suction the fluids or gases from a cavity.

bag--a sac or pouch of water-proof material which may be inflated for use inside a body cavity.

basket--a device used for removal of calculi.

bistoury (BIS-too-rē)--a long, narrow surgical knife, straight or curved, used for incising abscesses, opening up sinuses, fistulas, etc.

bougie (boo-ZHĒ)--a slender cylinder for introduction into the urethra or a large one for the rectum or some other orifice.

bur or burr--a dental tool with teeth or blades for excavating cavities.

cannula (KAN-ū-lah) (Latin diminutive of canna [KAN-nah] meaning "reed")--a tube for insertion into the body, its lumen being usually occupied by a trocar during the act of insertion.

catheter (KATH-i-ter)--a tubular surgical instrument for withdrawing fluids from a cavity of the body, especially one for introduction into the bladder through the urethra for the withdrawal of urine.

cephalotribe (SEF-ah-lō-trīb)--an instrument used for crushing the fetal head to facilitate delivery.

chisel--an instrument primarily used to remove bone in pieces or chips.

clamp--a surgical device for effecting compression. Some types are bulldog, coarctation (kō-ark-TĀ-shun), hemorrhoidal (hem-ō-ROY-dal), incontinence, pedicle.

colp/eurynter (kōl"pū-RIN-ter)--a bag introduced empty into the vagina and then filled with water; used for dilating the canal.

compresser--a surgical instrument for making compression upon a part.

curette or curet (kū-RET)--a kind of scraper or spoon for removing growths or other matter from the walls of cavities.

depressor--an instrument used to hold certain areas out of the way for better visibility and a larger operating field.

dilator--an appliance used in enlarging an orifice or canal by stretching.

dissector (dis-SEK-ter)--an instrument used in dissection of tissues.

drain--an appliance or substance that affords a channel of exit or discharge from a wound.

drill--an instrument for making holes in hard substances, such as bones or teeth.

dressing--the application of various materials for protecting a wound; also any material so applied.

electrode--an instrument with a point or surface from which to discharge current into the body of a patient.

*As these terms are alphabetized they will not be included in the index at the end of the chapter.

elevator--an instrument for lifting a depressed part or for removing roots of teeth.

erysiphake (er-IS-i-fāk)--an instrument for removal of the lens in cataract by suction.

evacuator--an instrument for compelling an evacuation, as of the bowels or bladder, or for removing fluid or small particles from a cavity.

everter--an instrument used to evert an overlying or overhanging part.

expressor--an instrument used for squeezing or pushing out of a part.

extractor--an instrument used for drawing out, pulling or extracting.

file--an instrument used for smoothing.

filiform (FIL-i-form)--an extremely slender bougie.

forceps (FOR-seps)--an instrument with two blades and handles for pulling, grasping or compressing. Types include alligator, bulldog, hemostat (HĒ-mō-stat), rongeur (rawn-ZHER), punch, tenaculum (te-NAK-u-lum), transfer.

gouge (gowj)--a hollow chisel used in cutting and removing bone.

hemostat--a forceps used for checking hemorrhage.

hook--a curved instrument used for traction or for holding.

irrigator--an appliance for performing irrigation.

knife--a cutting instrument of various shapes and sizes for surgeons' and dissectors' use.

lithotrite (LITH-ō-trīt)--an instrument for crushing stones.

loop--an oval or circle of metal or thin wire used to remove objects from body cavities; sometimes electrified permitting cutting.

loupe (lo͞op)--a convex lens for magnifying or for concentrating light upon an object.

mesh--metallic material used for reinforcement.

needle--a sharp instrument for sewing or puncturing.

nipper--a tool which cuts metallic material.

perforator--an instrument for perforation of the head in craniotomy (krā-nē-OT-ō-mē).

pessary (PES-ah-rē)--an instrument placed in the vagina to support the uterus.

pin--a long slender metal rod for the fixation of the ends of fractured bones.

plate--a piece of metal used for reinforcement of fractures.

probe--a slender, flexible instrument designed for introduction into a wound or cavity for purposes of exploration.

prosthesis (PROS-thē-sis)--the replacement of an absent part by an artificial one, such as an eye, leg or denture.

punch--an instrument for perforating, indenting or for cutting out a disk of material.

rasp--a roughly serrated instrument for filing (usually on bone).

raspatory (RAS-pah-tō-rē)--a file or rasp for surgeons' use; a xyster (ZIS-ter).

resector--an instrument designed to remove tissue from cavities inside the body.

retainer--an appliance which holds something in place.

retractor--an instrument for drawing back the edges of a wound.

rongeur forceps--a sharp biting forceps for gouging away bone.

saw--an instrument having an edge of sharp, toothlike projections; used for cutting bone.

scalpel--a small, straight knife, usually with a convex edge.

scoop--a cutting instrument with two opposed blades.

scope--an instrument designed for observation of the body cavities. Some of the scopes used are: ā'noscope, an'troscope, bron'choscope, cul'do-scope, cys'toscope, en'doscope, esoph'agoscope, gas'troscope, gō'nioscope, hys'teroscope, laryn'goscope, mēat'oscope, na"sopharyn'goscope, ophthal'moscope, ō'toscope, panen'doscope, perito'nēoscope, proc"tosigmoi'doscope, proc'toscope, rec'toscope, ret'inoscope, sigmoi'doscope, sken'eoscope, sphinc'teroscope, steth'oscope, tel'escope, thorac'oscope, trā"chēobron'cho-ēsoph'agoscope, ūre'throscope.

screws--appliances used for fixation of ends of fractured bones.

separator--a device for effecting a separation.

serrefin (sār-FĒN)--a small spring forceps for compressing bleeding vessels.

snare--a wire loop or noose for removing polypi (POL-i-pī) and tumors, being placed around them and tightened so as to either cut them off at the base or tear them out by the roots.

sound--an instrument to be introduced into a cavity to detect a foreign body or to dilate a stricture.

spatula--a flat, blunt, knifelike instrument.

speculum--an appliance for opening to view a passage or cavity of the body.

splint--a rigid or flexible appliance for the fixation of displaced or movable parts.

sponge--various materials which are sterilized and used as absorbents.

spoon--a metallic instrument with an oval bowl placed on a handle (brain, gall bladder, pituitary).

spreader--an instrument which spreads obstacles to provide a better operating field.

stripper--1. a flexible wire instrument used for removing veins and nerves; 2. a knife-like instrument used to remove fascia and periosteum.

syringe--an instrument for injecting liquids into any vessel or cavity.

tenaculum--a hooklike forceps for seizing and holding parts.

tome--an instrument for cutting. Various types are ad'enotome, cap'sulotome, con'chotome, cos'totome, cys'totome, der'matome, elec'trotome, ker'atome, leu'kotome, mi'crotome, os'teotome, perios'teotome, pre'putome, ra'chi-otome, scler'otome, ten'otome, thorac'otome, tonsillec'tome, trach'el-otome, tur'binotome, ure'throtome, vac'utome.

tongs--a two-pronged instrument to furnish traction on various parts of the body.

tourniquet (TOOR-ne-ket)--an instrument for the compression of a blood vessel for the purpose of controlling the circulation and preventing the access of blood to a part.

trephine (trē-FĪN)--a crown saw for removing a circular disk of bone, chiefly from the skull, or for removing a disk of tissue from the cornea or sclera.

trocar (TRŌ-kar)--a sharp pointed instrument used with a cannula for tapping or piercing a cavity wall in paracentesis (par"ah-sen-TĒ-sis) and other procedures.

tube, tubing--an elongated hollow cylindrical instrument (rectal, drainage, endotracheal [en-dō-TRĀ-kē-al], penrose, polyethylene, suction, vitallium [vī-TAL-lē-um]).

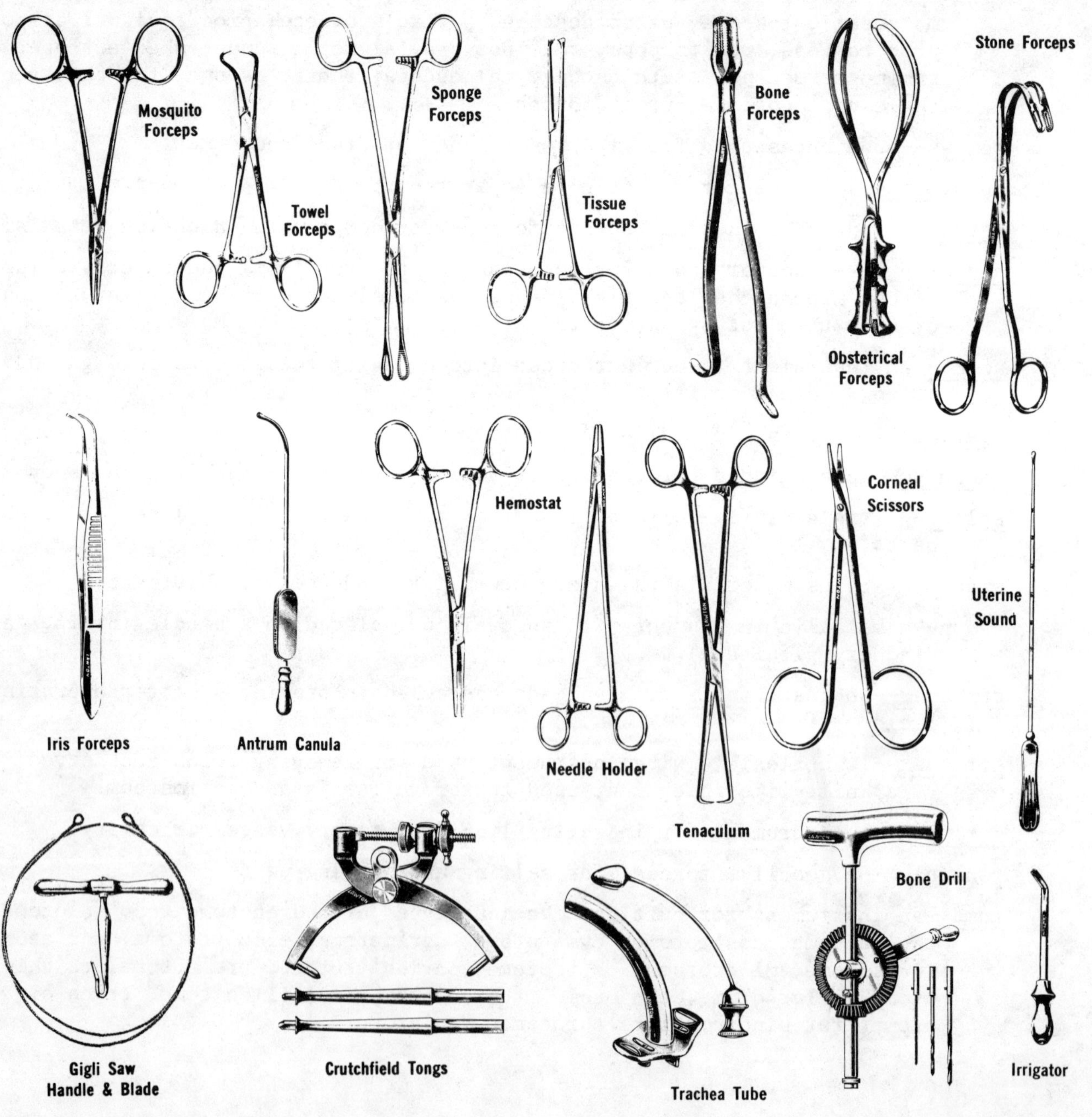

TYPES OF SURGICAL INSTRUMENTS

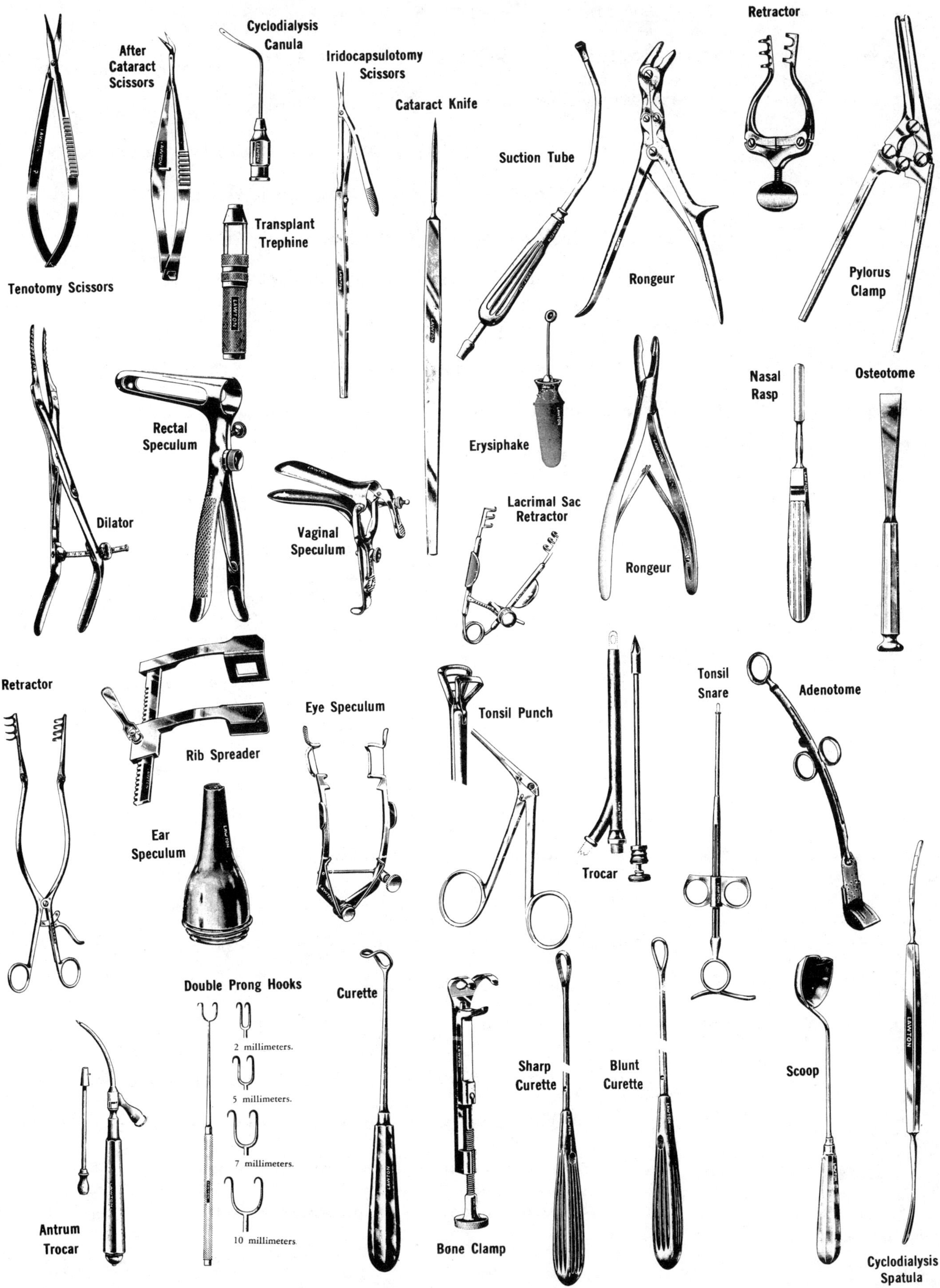
Tenotomy Scissors
After Cataract Scissors
Cyclodialysis Canula
Transplant Trephine
Iridocapsulotomy Scissors
Cataract Knife
Suction Tube
Rongeur
Retractor
Pylorus Clamp
Dilator
Rectal Speculum
Vaginal Speculum
Erysiphake
Lacrimal Sac Retractor
Rongeur
Nasal Rasp
Osteotome
Retractor
Rib Spreader
Ear Speculum
Eye Speculum
Tonsil Punch
Trocar
Tonsil Snare
Adenotome
Double Prong Hooks
2 millimeters.
5 millimeters.
7 millimeters.
10 millimeters.
Antrum Trocar
Curette
Bone Clamp
Sharp Curette
Blunt Curette
Scoop
Cyclodialysis Spatula

ANESTHESIA AGENTS

The ideal an/esthes/ia (an-es-THĒ-zhē-ah) agent:
without feeling

1. For the patient, the agent should act rapidly and be pleasant, and the recovery period should be free of discomfort.
2. The surgeon would like the agent to be non-explosive, produce complete muscular relaxation, and not increase bleeding.
3. The an/esthet/ist (ah-NES-the-tist) would like the an/esthet/ic (an-es-THET-ik) to have a wide margin of safety, to leave the body unaltered, to be potent but yet allow a high percent of oxygen to be used and not be explosive.

Stages of anesthesia produced by volatile and gaseous anesthetics:

Stage 1. An/alges/ia (an-al-JĒ-zē-ah): The first and the lightest stage of anesthesia. Loss of the sense of pain (within limits) without the loss of consciousness or the sense of touch.
without pain

Stage 2. Delirium (de-LIR-ē-um): Called the "fiery hoop" stage by anesthetists. It is at this stage that dreams occur, that people become violent and irrational, and that heart failure may develop.
"off the track"

Stage 3. Surgical Anesthesia: The stage under which operations are ordinarily performed. This stage is subdivided into four planes.

a. The First Plane -- muscle tone is unchanged and eyeball movements continue when the lids are raised. The pupils react to light.

b. The Second Plane -- smaller muscles throughout the body lose their tone and ocular movements cease. The pupils are centrally fixed.

c. The Third Plane -- muscular relaxation throughout

the body includes large muscles. The corne/al (horny) (kōr-NĒ-al) reflexes are abolished. Respiration becomes diaphragmat/ic (dī"ah-frag-MAT-ik).

d. The Fourth Plane -- the relaxation of large muscles and loss of reflexes are complete. The pupils are widely dilated. Diaphragmatic activity is decreased.

Stage 4. Re/spirat/ory (to breathe)[1] (res-PĪ-rah-tō-rē) paralysis followed by shock and death (also called stage of tox/icity (poison condition) (toks-IS-i-tē): that stage beyond surgical anesthesia at which respiration stops. The blood pressure drops rapidly.

Types of anesthetic agents:

Volatile substances administered by inhalation:

Liquids: chloroform (KLŌ-rō-form), ēther, ethyl chloride, avertin (ah-VER-tin), fluothane (FLOO-ō-thān) which is non-flammable, trichloroethylene (trī-klō-rō-ETH-i-lēn) known as Trilene (trī-LĒN), vinyl ether (VĪ-nil Ē-ther) also known as Vinethene (VIN-i-thēn), penthrane (PEN-thrān) which is non-flammable.

Gases: cyclopropane (sī-klō-PRŌ-pān), ethylene (ETH-i-lēn), nitrous oxide (NĪ-trus OK-sīd)

Nonvolatile substances administered intra/venously (into vein) (in-trah-VĒ-nus-lē) or rect/ally (rectum) (REK-tah-lē):

Very fast acting barbiturates (bar-BIT-ū-rats): hexobarbital (hek"sō-BAR-be-tal), thiamylal (thī-AM-i-lal) also known as Surital (SOOR-i-tal), thiopental (thī-ō-PEN-tal) more commonly known as Pentothal (PEN-tō-thal) and Nembutal (NEM-bū-tal).

1. Optional pronunciation RES-pi-rah-tō-rē

Derivatives of ethyl alcohol: tribromoethanol (trī-brō-mō-ETH-ah-nōl) also known as Avertin.

Topical [place] (TOP-i-kal) anesthetics: novocaine (NŌ-vō-kān), cocaine (KŌ-kān), xylocaine (ZĪ-lō-kān), procaine (PRŌ-kān).

Methods of administering anesthetics:

General anesthesia (complete loss of consciousness, freedom from physical pain, muscular relaxation):

1. ENDO/TRACHE/AL [within trachea] (en"dō-TRĀ-kē-al): introduction of a catheter into the trachea for the purpose of introducing the anesthetic mixture directly into the lungs. This may be done by oral or nasal in/tub/ation [in tube] (in-tū-BĀ-shun). The catheter is then attached to an inhaler. This method is very popular because it permits a patent [open] (PĀ-tent) airway, the aspiration of secretions, the use of positive pressure, controlled breathing and adequate ventilation. As a mechanical respirator it is used to assist breathing or it can do the breathing for the patient.
2. INHALATION: produced by the inhalation of vaporized liquids or gases. The various methods used to induce anesthesia include the open, closed or semiclosed techniques.
3. INTRAVENOUS: used to induce basal [base] (BĀ-sal) narcosis [numbness] (nar-KŌ-sis) (a state of unconsciousness which lacks sufficient depth to permit major surgery). This is often supplemented by inhalation anesthesia (nitrous oxide) and the administration of curare[1] (kyōō-RAH-rē) for muscle relaxation.
4. RECTAL: the introduction of pentothal, avertin and ether (rarely used now) into the rectum to produce basal anesthesia. It induces a hypnot/ic [sleep] (hip-NOT-ik) stage and partially abolishes the reflexes.

Local and regional anesthesia (absence of sensation and pain in a part of

1. Optional pronunciation kur-AH-rē

the body but consciousness is retained.

1. CAUDAL or SACR/AL (sacrum) (SĀ-kral) block (also known as saddle block): introduction of the anesthetic solution directly into the sacral canal. If regulated it will only affect a certain area of the lower body -- to "sit in a saddle."
2. CONDUCTION: includes various forms of local anesthesia: direct nerve block, epi/dur/al (dura) (ep-i-DŪ-ral) block, spinal anesthesia and infiltration anesthesia.
3. EPIDURAL or PARA/VERTEBR/AL (beside vertebra) (par-ah-VER-te-bral) block: spinal nerves blocked as they pass through the epidural space.
4. INFILTRATION: injection of a dilute anesthetic agent under the skin to an/esthet/ize (without feeling) (an-ES-the-tīz) the nerve endings and nerve fibers.
5. NERVE AND FIELD BLOCK: insensibility of a local area achieved by:
   a. direct nerve block -- injection of an anesthetic solution into easily accessible nerves, as those of the extremities.
   b. field block -- anesthetic solution deposited into the nerve at the point of its terminal branches.
6. SPINAL: anesthesia produced by the injection of a local anesthetic solution into the sub/arachn/oid (below (spider)) (sub-ah-RAK-noyd) space of the lumbar region to block the roots of the spinal nerves. Procaine and xylocaine are frequently used.
7. SURFACE or TOPICAL: direct application of an anesthetic drug to a mucous membrane to produce insensibility of the nerve endings. Cocaine may be used as a surface anesthetic.

analeptics [a repairing] (an-ah-LEP-tiks) -- stimulants of the central nervous system. For example: coramine (KŌ-rah-min), caffein (KAF-ē-in) and metrazol (MET-rah-zōl).

anti/narcot/ic [against] (an"te-nar-KOT-ik) drugs -- used to reverse action of narcotics. Drug used is Nalline (NAL-lin).

hyper/ventil/ation [above, wind] (hī-per-ven-ti-LĀ-shun) -- excessive respiration causing an abnormal loss of carbon dioxide from the blood.

hypo/tensive [below, to stretch] (hī-pō-TEN-siv) anesthesia -- deliberately induced stage of hypotension to reduce blood loss during surgery. One drug used is Arfonad (AR-fon-ad).

hypo/therm/ia [temperature] (hī-pō-THER-mē-ah) -- refrigeration anesthesia. Cooling only after patient is under anesthesia.

hyp/ox/ia [oxygen] (hī-POK-sē-ah) also known as an/ox/ia [lack] (an-OK-sē-ah) -- a reduction of oxygen supply to the body tissues.

lid reflex -- tapping of the eyelid to evoke its immediate closure; it is a guide to determine the depth of anesthesia.

inhalation therapy -- administration of inhalant gases such as oxygen, helium (HĒ-lē-um) or carbon dioxide to relieve oxygen want or stimulate respiration.

muscle relaxants -- these are drugs that block the passage of motor impulses. Common drugs of this class are curare and anectine (an-EK-tin). Anectine has the advantage of short duration of action and is used in a slow drip. Curare is used at intervals in single shots.

pre/medic/ation [before, medicine] (pre"med-i-KĀ-shun) -- the use of opium (Ō-pē-um) derivatives, barbiturates and drugs from the bella/donna[1] (bel-ah-DON-ah) group prior to administration of anesthesia.

vaso/con/strictors [vessel, together, to draw tight] (vas"ō-kon-STRIK-tors) -- drugs causing a constriction of the blood vessels. They are used with local anesthetics to prevent the anesthetic being carried away from the site of injection.

Intermittent Positive Pressure Breathing (IPPB) -- used often after surgery to prevent lung complications.

1. Means "beautiful lady" in Italian. Is also called "the deadly nightshade." It is a poisonous alkaloid. Atropine is obtained from this plant.

POSITIONS

Used In Surgery and Examination

Head Raised Fowler

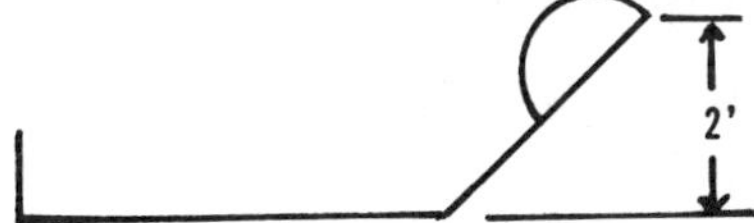

for better drainage after abdominal surgery

Lithotomy (Dorsosacral)

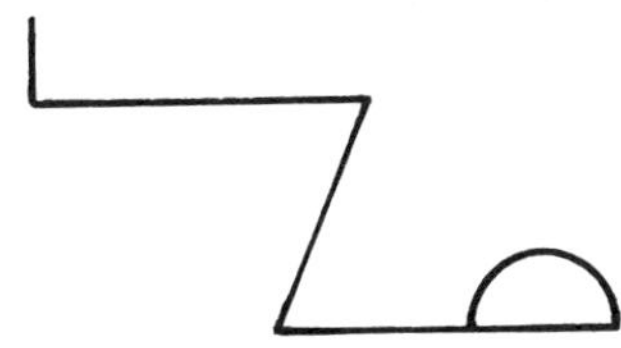

for pelvic examinations and surgery

High Pelvic Trendelenburg

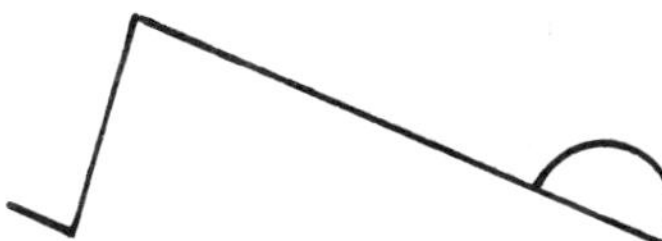

for pelvic surgery

Elliott

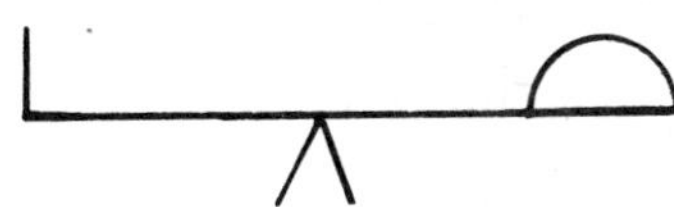

for abdominal section, gall bladder surgery

Right or Left Lateral

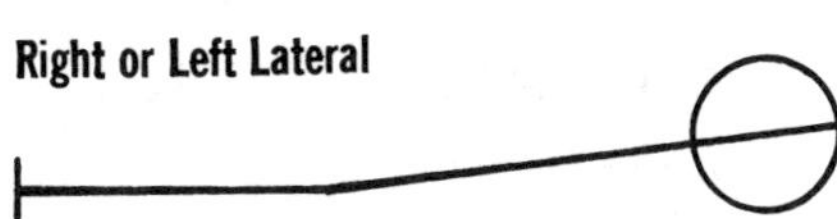

for vaginal examinations

Dorsal

Prone

Jack-knife

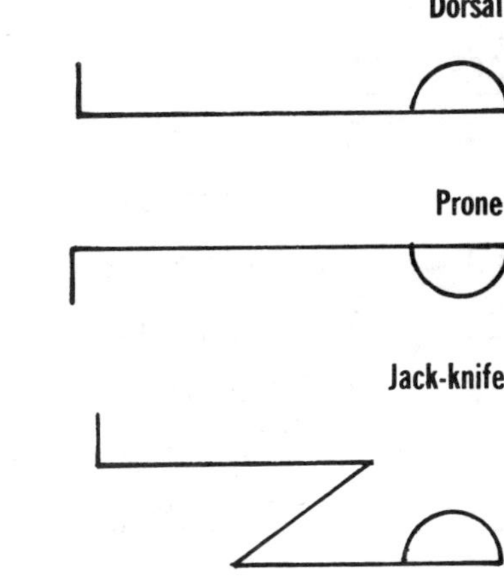

for passing urethral sound

Vertical

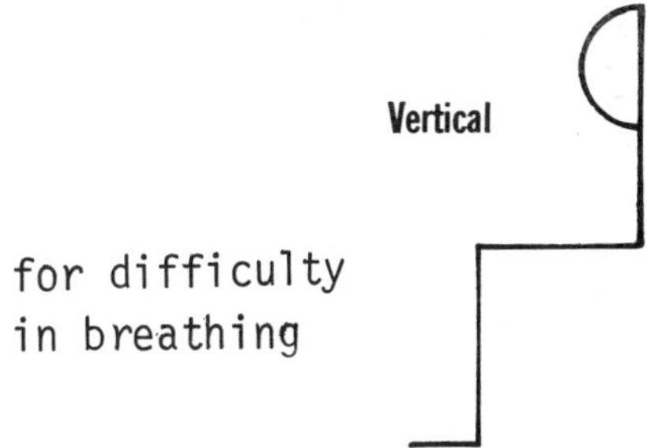

for difficulty in breathing

Head Lowered Scultetus

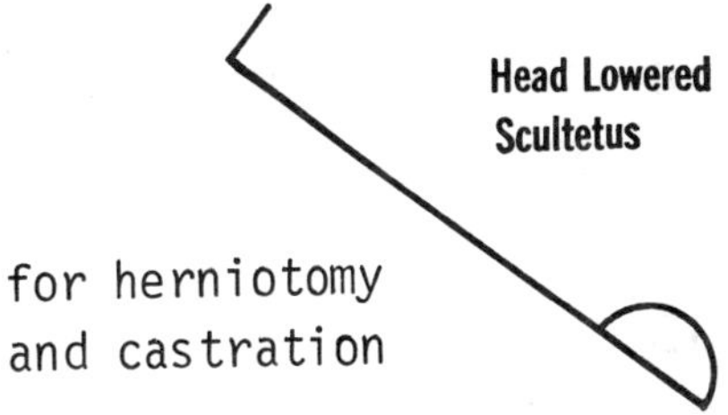

for herniotomy and castration

Edebohls

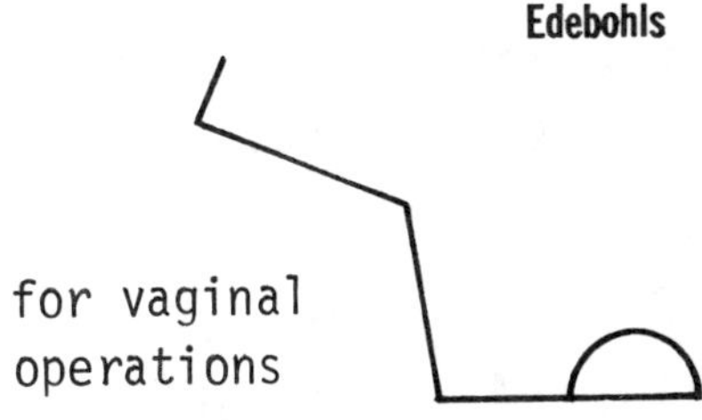

for vaginal operations

Dorsal Elevated

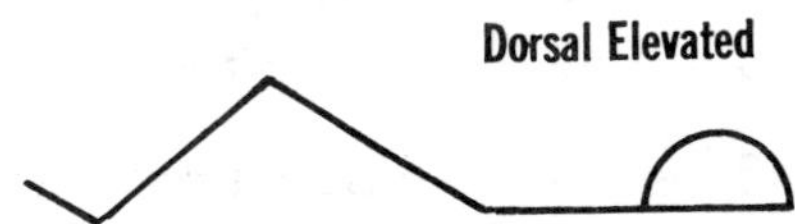

for vaginal examinations, application of obstetrical forceps

INDEX
CHAPTER I

CHAPTER II
THE SKELETAL SYSTEM

The skull, which rests upon the spinal column, is divided into the cranium [skull] (KRĀ-nē-um) and the face. It consists of 21 bones closely joined together and one bone, the lower jaw or mandible [a jaw] (MAN-di-bl), which is freely movable. The three bones or oss/icles [bone, small] (OS-sik-ls) of the middle ear may also be added.

BONES OF THE SKULL

The top of the skull is formed by the front/al [forehead] (FRON-tal) bone, the two pariet/al [wall] (pah-RĪ-i-tal) bones and the occipit/al [back of head] (ok-SIP-i-tal) bone.

The frontal bone forms the forehead, the upper part of the orbits [circle] (OR-bits) and a part of the nas/al [nose] (NĀ-zal) cavity. The arch which is formed by the frontal bone over the eye sockets is known as the supra/orbit/al [above] (sū-prah-OR-bi-tal) margin or ridge. Just above these ridges are hollow spaces called the frontal sinuses [hollow] (SĪ-nu-sez). These sinuses or antra [cavity] (AN-trah) are filled with air and open into the nose. In the upper and outer angle of each of the orbits are two shallow depressions called lacrim/al [tear] (LAK-re-mal) fossae [ditch] (FOS-ē) for the lacrimal glands which secrete the tears.

The right and left parietal bones form the upper portion of the sides of the skull. They meet in the midline at the sagitt/al [arrow] (SAJ-i-tal) suture.

The occipital bone forms the back and a large part of the base of the skull.

The right and left tempor/al [temple, time] (TEM-po-ral) bones form part of the lateral wall and base of the skull. They are composed of the squama [scale] (SKWĀ-mah), the petrous [stone] (PET-rus), the mast/oid [breast] (MAS-toyd) and tympan/ic [drum] (tim-PAN-ik) parts, and the styl/oid [stake, pole] (STĪ-loyd) process.

The sphen/oid [wedge] (SFĒ-noyd) bone, which binds the cranial bones together, is at the anterior part of the base of the skull. It is composed of a body, two great and two small wings extending from the sides of the body and two pteryg/oid [wing]

THE SKELETON

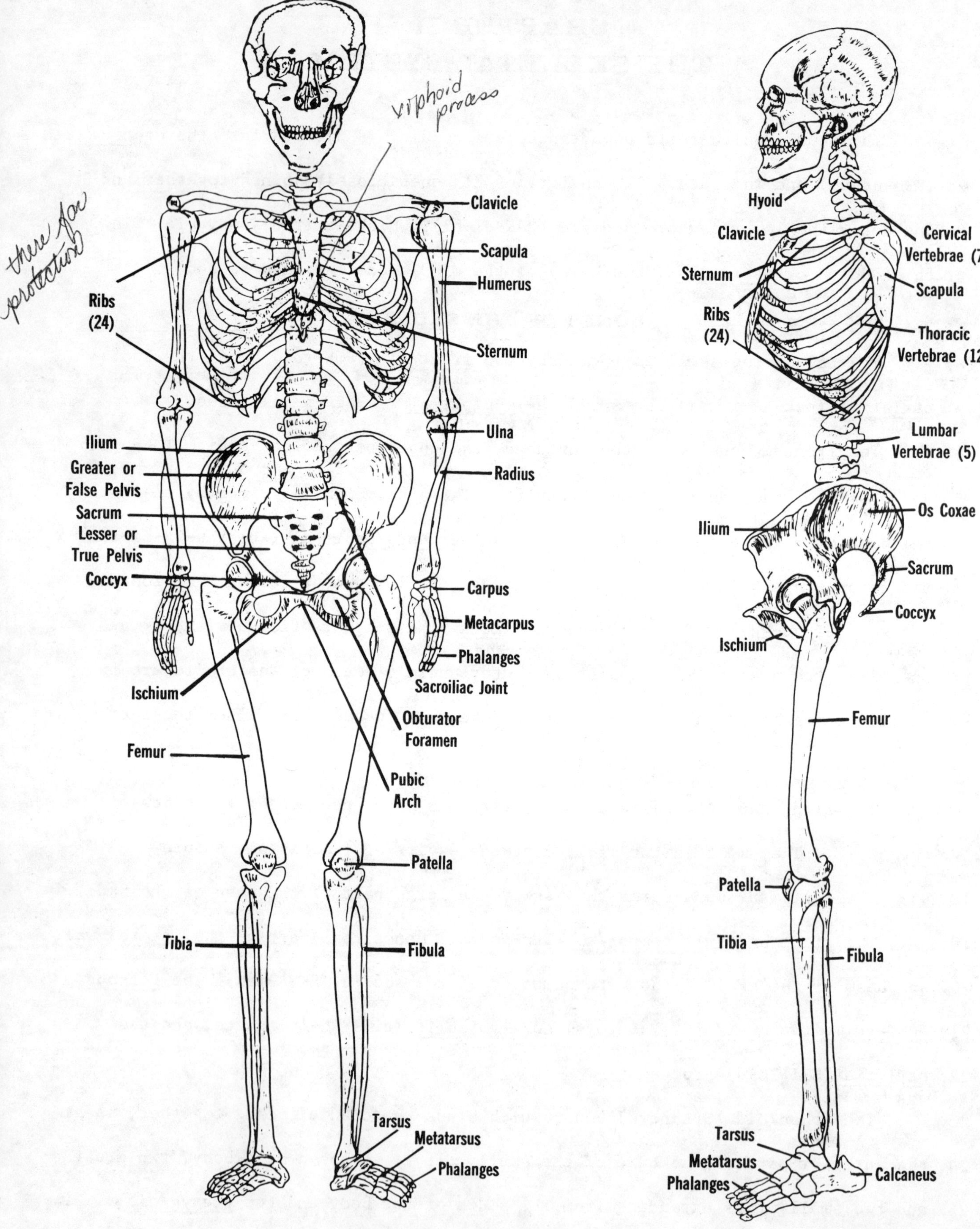
xiphoid process
there for protection
Clavicle
Scapula
Humerus
Ribs (24)
Sternum
Ulna
Ilium
Greater or False Pelvis
Radius
Sacrum
Lesser or True Pelvis
Coccyx
Carpus
Metacarpus
Phalanges
Ischium
Sacroiliac Joint
Obturator Foramen
Femur
Pubic Arch
Patella
Tibia
Fibula
Tarsus
Metatarsus
Phalanges
Hyoid
Clavicle
Cervical Vertebrae (7)
Sternum
Scapula
Ribs (24)
Thoracic Vertebrae (12)
Lumbar Vertebrae (5)
Ilium
Os Coxae
Sacrum
Coccyx
Ischium
Femur
Patella
Tibia
Fibula
Tarsus
Metatarsus
Phalanges
Calcaneus

(TER-i-goyd) processes projecting downward. The sphenoid bone somewhat resembles a butterfly with its two pairs of outspread wings. It contains cavities known as sphen/oid/al (sfē-NOYD-al) sinuses which communicate with the naso/pharynx (nā-zō-FAR-inks).

The ethm/oid [sieve] (ETH-moyd) bone lies in front of the sphenoid between the eyes and forms part of the nasal roof. It is a very light cancell/ous [a lattice] (KAN-sel-us) bone. The ethmoid bone is composed of a horizontal or cribri/form [sieve] (KRIB-re-form) plate, a perpendicular plate and two lateral masses or labyrinths [a maze] (LAB-i-rinths).

The nasal bones are two small flat bones which form the bridge of the nose. The lower part of the nose is formed by the nasal cartilages [gristle] (KAR-ti-lij-ez).

The lacrimal bones are thin scale-like bones about the size of a fingernail. Each lacrimal bone helps to form the side wall of the nasal cavity.

The nasal conchae [shell] (KONG-kē) or turbinated [shaped like a top] (TUR-bi-nā-ted) bones are shell-like scrolls of bone which project into the nasal cavity from the outer wall of each nostril. *circulate air in nasal cavity or create turbulence*

The vomer [ploughshare] (VŌ-mer), a single bone, forms the posterior part of the nasal septum.

The zygomat/ic [yoke] (zī-gō-MAT-ik) or malar [cheek] (MĀ-lar) bones form the cheeks. They also form part of the outer wall and floor of the orbits.

The palatine [palate] (PAL-ah-tīn) bones form the posterior portion of the hard palate and part of the lateral wall of the posterior nasal opening.

The upper jaw is formed by the right and left maxillae [jawbone] (mak-SIL-ē) or upper jaw bones, also known as the superior maxill/ary (MAK-se-lār-ē) bones. Each maxilla (mak-SIL-ah) forms the floor of the corresponding orbit and lateral wall of the lower part of the nasal cavity.

The mandible is the bone of the lower jaw. It is the strongest and largest bone in the face. It consists of a horseshoe shaped body and two perpendicular portions, the rami [a branch] (RĀ-mī). The alveol/ar [cavity] (al-VĒ-ō-lar) border of the body has

BONES OF THE SKULL

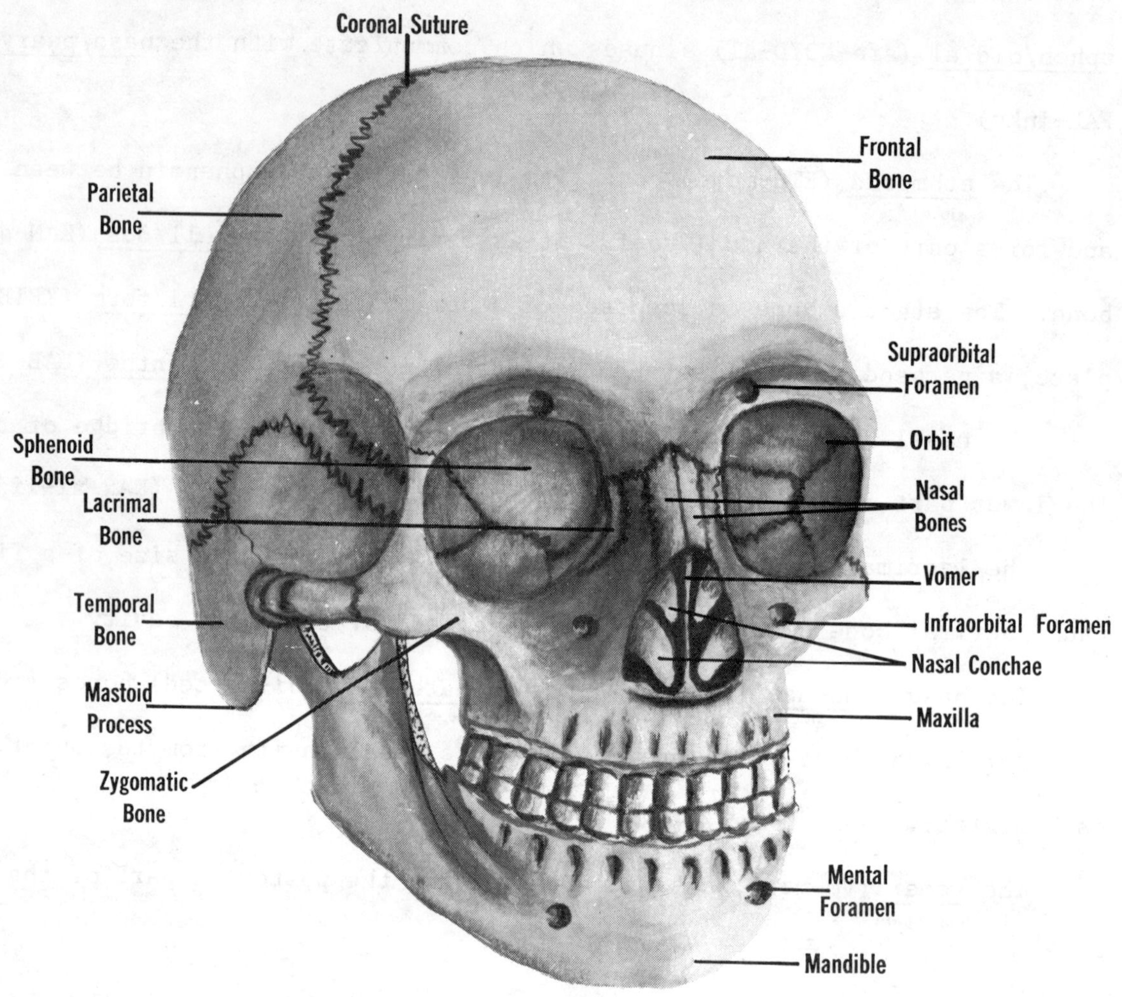

Coronal Suture
Frontal Bone
Parietal Bone
Supraorbital Foramen
Orbit
Sphenoid Bone
Lacrimal Bone
Nasal Bones
Vomer
Temporal Bone
Infraorbital Foramen
Nasal Conchae
Mastoid Process
Maxilla
Zygomatic Bone
Mental Foramen
Mandible

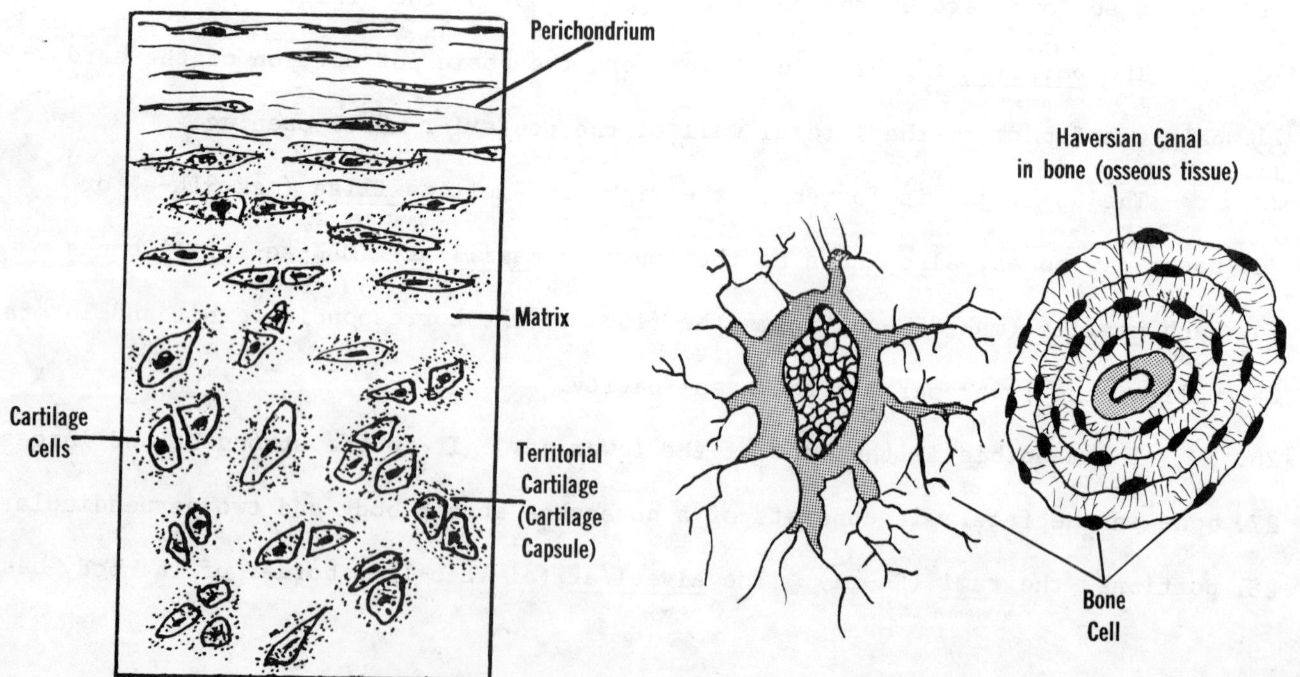

Hyaline Cartilage
Perichondrium
Matrix
Cartilage Cells
Territorial Cartilage (Cartilage Capsule)
Haversian Canal in bone (osseous tissue)
Bone Cell

cavities for the teeth.

The hy/oid [letter 'U'] (HĪ-oyd) bone is a slender, horseshoe shaped bone found below the mandible. It consists of a central portion called the body and two projections, the greater and lesser cornua [horn] (KOR-nū-ah). It may be felt in the neck just above the larynge/al [larynx] (lah-RIN-jē-al) prominence or Adam's apple. The hyoid bone supports the tongue and gives attachment to some of the tongue's numerous muscles.

The bones or ossicles of the middle ear are three tiny bones called the hammer (malleus [mal-LĒ-us]), anvil (incus [ING-kus]) and stirrup (stapes [STĀ-pēz]). They are named from their shapes.

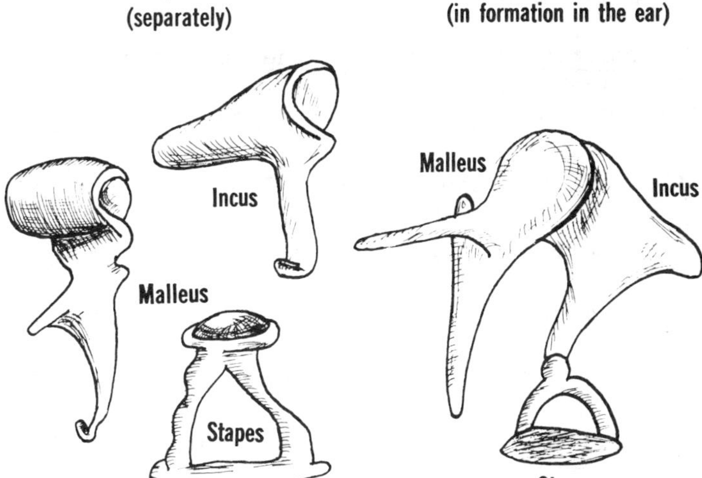

BONES OF THE TRUNK

The trunk of the body is formed of the vertebrae [to turn] (VER-te-brē), the sternum [the chest] (STER-num) and the ribs.

The vertebrae differ in size and shape but in general their structure is similar. Seen from above they consist of a body from which two short, thick processes called ped/icles [foot small] (PED-i-kels) project backward, one on each side. These pedicles join the laminae [thin plate] (LAM-i-nē)(which

LUMBAR VERTEBRA
(as seen from above)

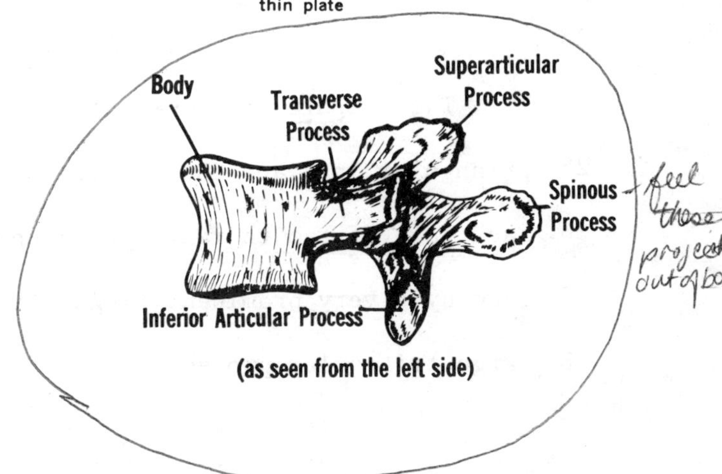

(as seen from the left side)

unite posteriorly) and form the vertebr/al (VER-te-bral) or neur/al [nerve] (NŪ-ral) arch. This arch encloses the spinal foramen [opening] (fō-RĀ-men). Each vertebra (VER-te-brah) has seven processes. The vertebrae which compose the vertebral column are divided as follows: seven cervic/al [neck] (SER-ve-kal), twelve thorac/ic [chest] (thō-RAS-ik), five lumbar [loin] (LUM-bar), five sacr/al [sacrum] (SĀ-kral) and four coccyge/al [coccyx] (kok-SIJ-ē-al). The vertebrae in the sacral and coccygeal regions are firmly united in the adult to form two bones. The five sacral vertebrae form the sacrum [sacred] (SĀ-krum) and the four coccygeal bones form the terminal bone or coccyx [a cuckoo] (KOK-siks). Because of this joining the adult has 26 vertebrae.

The thorax [chest] (THŌ-raks) is a cone-shaped, bony cage. It is formed by the sternum and cost/al [rib] (KOS-tal) cartilages in front, the ribs on each side, and the bodies of the thoracic vertebrae behind.

The sternum or breast bone is a flat, narrow bone (shaped somewhat like a blunt dagger), and is about six inches long. It forms the chest wall in the medi/an [middle adj.] (MĒ-dē-an) line in front. The sternum consists of an upper portion, the manubrium [handle] (man-Ū-brē-um), a middle portion, the body or gladiolus [little sword (L)] (glah-DĪ-ō-lus), and an inferior portion, the ensi/form [sword (L)] (EN-se-form) or xiph/oid [sword (G)] (ZĪ-foyd)

There are 12 pairs of ribs attached behind to the 12 thoracic vertebrae. In front the upper 10 ribs are attached either directly or indirectly to the sternum or breast bone by means of costal cartilages. The spaces between the ribs are known as inter/cost/al [between] (in-ter-KOS-tal) spaces.

BONES OF THE UPPER EXTREMITIES

The scapula [shoulder blade] (SKAP-ū-lah) or shoulder blade is a large, flat bone. It is triangular in shape and is placed between the second and seventh ribs on the back part of the thorax. It is unevenly divided on its dors/al [back] (DOR-sal) surface by a very prominent ridge, the spine of the scapula, which ends in a large triangular projection called the acro/mion [tip shoulder] (ah-KRŌ-mē-on) process. This process articulates with the clavicle. Below the acromion process is a shallow socket, the glen/oid[1] (*socket*) (GLEN-oyd) cavity. The head of the humerus (*shoulder*) (HYO͞O-mer-es) fits into this cavity.

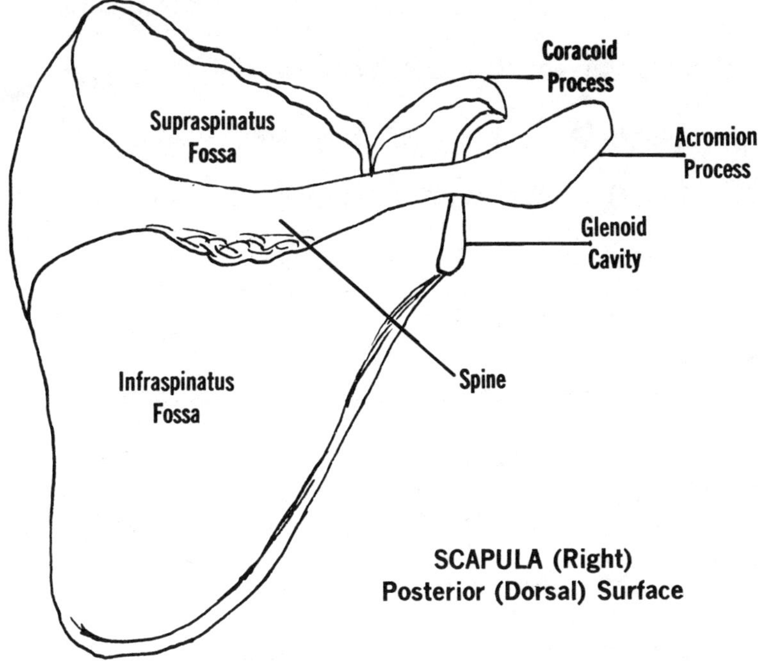

SCAPULA (Right)
Posterior (Dorsal) Surface

The clav/icle (*key small*) (KLAV-i-kl) or collar bone is a long, curved, slender bone which lies in the root of the neck between the upper end of the sternum and the acromion. It has two extremities, the acromi/al (*acromion*) (ah-KRŌ-mē-al) and stern/al (*sternum*) (STER-nal) and a corac/oid (*crow's beak*) (KŌR-ah-koyd) tuber/osity (*node condition*) (to͞o-be-ROS-i-tē).

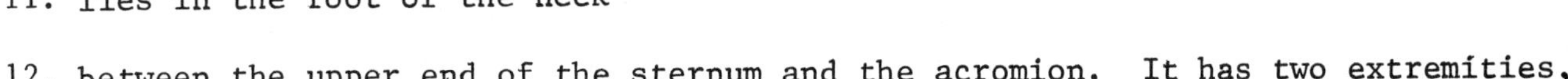

The humerus is the bone of the upper arm. It is the largest and longest bone in the upper limb. The upper end of the humerus has a thick rounded head joined to a shaft by a constricted neck. This head has two eminences (*projections*) (EM-i-nen-ses) called the greater and lesser tuber/cles (*node small*) (TO͞O-ber-kls). Between these tubercles is the inter/tuberc/ul/ar (*between node small*) (in"ter-to͞o-BER-kū-lar) groove. The ana/tomic/al (*up to cut*)

HUMERUS (Right)

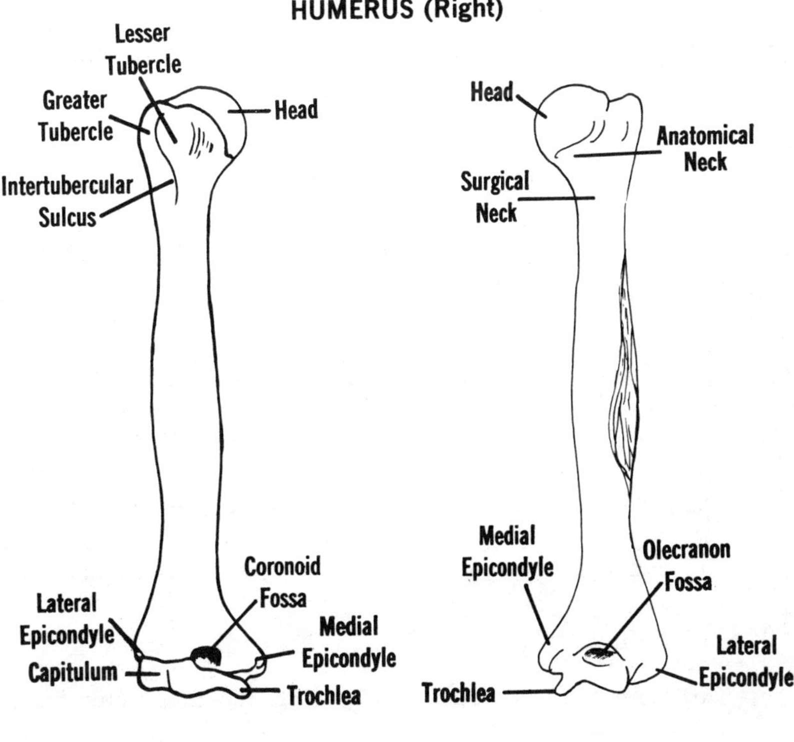

Anterior View　　Posterior View

1. Optional pronunciation GLĒ-noyd

(an-ah-TOM-i-kl) neck is the constricted portion above the tubercles and the surg/ic/al *handwork* (SER-ji-kl) neck is the portion below the tubercles. Because this latter portion of the humerus is so often fractured it is known as the surgical neck. The head of the humerus articulates with the glenoid cavity of the scapula. The lower extremity of the humerus ends in an articular surface. A ridge divides this part of the humerus into a lateral

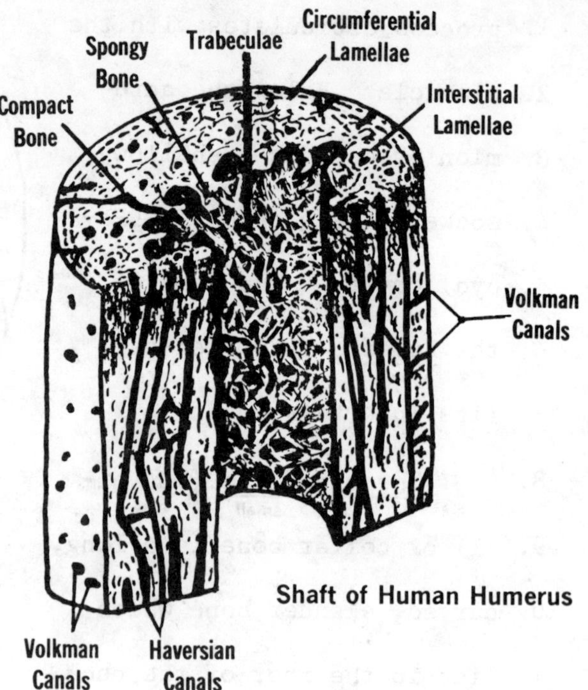

Shaft of Human Humerus

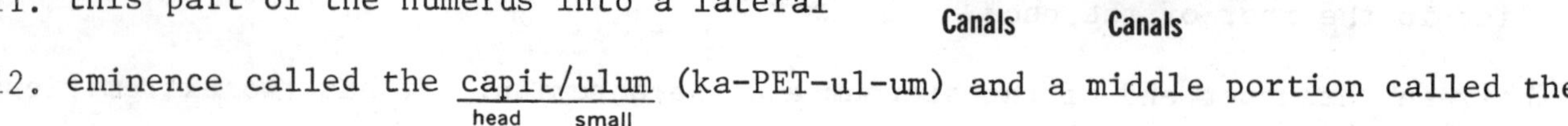

eminence called the capit/ulum *head small* (ka-PET-ul-um) and a middle portion called the trochlea *pulley* (TRŌ-klē-ah). The capitulum articulates with the depression on the head of the radius *rod, ray* (RĀ-dē-us) and the trochlea articulates with the ulna *elbow* (UL-nah). Above these surfaces are projections called epi/condyles *on, upon knuckle* (ep-i-KON-dīls).

The radius is the shorter of the two bones of the forearm. It lies on the outer or thumb side. The distal end of the radius is much larger than the upper end and has a fine tip on the thumb side called the styloid process. At its lower end the radius articulates with two bones of the wrist, the scaph/oid *boat* (SKAF-oyd) and the lun/ate *moon* (LŌŌ-nāt). There is also an articulation with the head of the ulna.

The ulna or elbow bone is the longer of the two bones of the forearm. It is on the medial side (little finger side) and is parallel with the radius. The upper end of the ulna has two large, beaklike projections and two concave cavities. The largest projection forms the prominence of the elbow and is called the olecranon *head or point of elbow* (ō-LEK-rah-non) process. The smaller projection is called the coron/oid *crow* (KŌR-ō-noyd) process. The trochlea of the humerus fits into the cavity, the semi/lun/ar *half moon* (sem"i-LŌŌ-ner) notch or greater sigm/oid *letter "S"* (SIG-moyd) which is formed by these two processes.

The carpus [wrist] (KAR-pes) or wrist joint is composed of eight bones arranged in two rows and closely welded together. However, the arrangement of their ligaments permits a certain amount of motion. These eight small bones are known as:

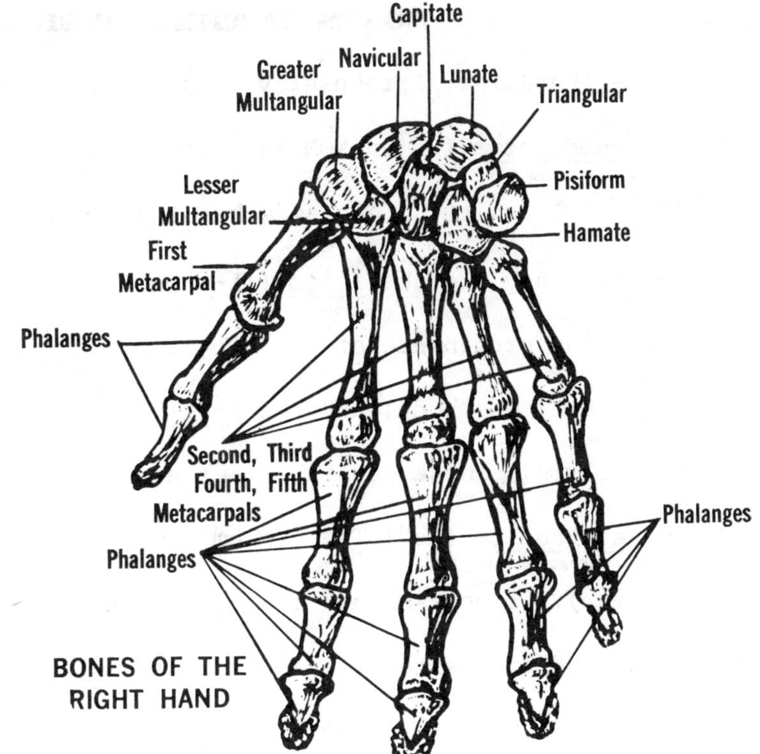

BONES OF THE RIGHT HAND

Proxim/al [nearest] (PROK-se-mal) or upper row:

1. navic/ul/ar [ship small] (nah-VIK-ye-lar) or scaphoid
2. lunate or semilunar
3. triangular or cunei/form [wedge] (kyo͞o-NĒ-i-form)
4. pisi/form [pea] (PĪ-si-form)

Distal or lower row:

5. greater mult/angul/ar [many angle] (mul-TANG-gū-lar) or trapezium [table, counter] (trah-PĒ-zē-ahm)
6. lesser multangular or trapez/oid [table, counter] (TRAP-i-zoyd)
7. capitate [head] (KAP-i-tāt) or os magnum [bone great] (os MAG-num)
8. hamate [hooked] (HAM-āt) or unci/form [hooked] (UN-se-form)

The meta/carpus [beyond wrist] (met-ah-KAR-pes), body of the hand, is formed by five bones. These bones articulate at their bases with the second row of carp/al [wrist] (KAR-pal) bones and with each other. The heads of the metacarpals articulate with the bases of the first row of phalanges [a line of soldiers] (fah-LAN-jēz). The phalanges are the bones of the fingers. There are 14 phalanges in each hand, three for each finger and two for the thumb.

BONES OF THE LOWER EXTREMITIES

The large, irregularly shaped hip bones, known as os [bone] coxae [hip joint] (os KOK-sē) or os innominatum [nameless] (os in-NOM-in-ā-tum) form the sides and front wall of the pelv/ic [pelvis] (PEL-vik) cavity. Each side has three separate parts which are united in the adult. They are the ilium [groin] (IL-ē-em), the upper broad and expanded portion which forms the prominence of the hip; the ischium [hip, haunch] (IS-kē-em), the lowest and strongest portion of the bone; and the pubis [the genitals] (PYŌŌ-bis) which helps to form the front of the pelvis. These portions meet and ankylose [stiffened] (ANG-ke-lōs) to form a deep socket, the acetabulum [a vinegar cruet] (as"i-TAB-ye-lem), for the reception of the head of the femur [thigh] (FĒ-mer). Processes are formed by the projection of the crest of the ilium in front and are called the anterior superior ili/ac [groin] (IL-ē-ak) spine and the anterior inferior iliac spine. The obturator [to occlude, stop up] (OB-tōō-rā-ter) foramen is the largest foramen in the skeleton and is situated between the ischium and the pubis. The sym/ [together] physis [to grow] (SIM-fi-sis) pubis is the articulation formed by the two pubic bones in front.

The femur or thigh bone is the longest and strongest bone in the skeleton. The upper extremity of the femur consists of a rounded head joined to the shaft by a constricted neck and of two projections called the greater and lesser trochanters [runner] (trō-KAN-ters). The head articulates with the acetabulum. The lower extremity of the femur is larger than the upper and is divided into two large projections or condyles [knuckle] (KON-dīls). The condyles are called lateral and medial and the intervening notch which divides them is called the inter/condyl/oid [between] (in-ter-KON-dil-oyd) fossa [ditch] (FOS-ah). The lower end of the femur articulates with the tibia [shin bone] (TIB-ē-ah) and the

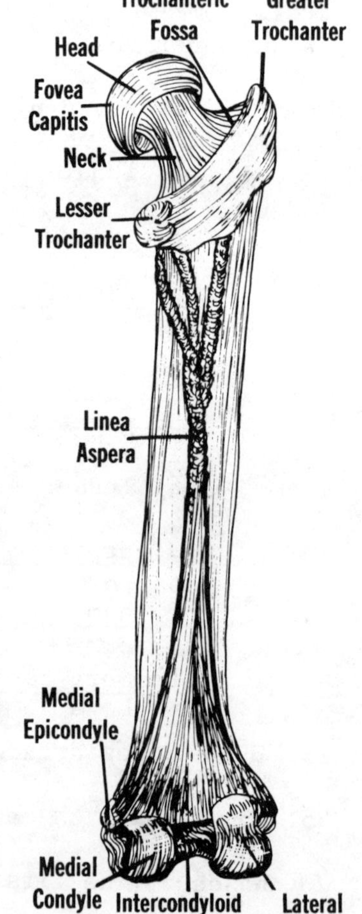

FEMUR

patella *[pan (kneepan)]* (pah-TEL-lah) or kneecap. The patella is a sesam/oid *[an Eastern plant]* (SES-ah-moyd) bone, small, flat and triangular in shape, placed in front of the knee joint which it serves to protect.

The tibia or shin bone is situated in the front and medial side of the leg. The upper extremity of the tibia is large and expanded into two lateral prominences with a sharp projection called the intercondyloid eminence. The lateral prominences are called the medial and lateral condyles. The upper extremity of the tibia is much larger than the lower extremity which is prolonged downward on its median side into a strong process, the medial malleolus *[hammer]* (mah-LĒ-ah-les), thus forming the inner projection of the ankle. At this same lower extremity is the surface for articulation with the talus *[ankle]* (TĀ-les) where the ankle joint is formed.

VERTICAL SECTION OF A LONG BONE

The fibula *[buckle]* (FIB-yo͞o-lah) or calf bone is situated on the lateral side of the tibia, parallel with it. The fibula is smaller than the tibia. In proportion to its length the fibula is the most slender of all the long bones. The upper extremity consists of an irregular quadr/ate *[four]* (KWOD-rāt) head by means of which it articulates with the tibia. However, this articulation is excluded from the knee joint. The lower extremity prolongs downward into a pointed process, the lateral malleolus, which forms the outer ankle bone.

The tarsus *[a flat surface]* (TAR-ses) is made up of seven tars/al *[tarsus]* (TAR-sal) bones which are called the calcaneus *[heel]* (kal-KĀ-nē-es), talus, cub/oid *[cube]* (KYO͞O-boyd), navicular, first, second and third cuneiforms. The tarsal bones are larger and more irregularly shaped than the carpal bones. The longest and strongest of the tarsal bones is the calcaneus or heel bone.

The meta/tarsus *[beyond / flat surface]* (met-ah-TAR-ses) or sole and instep of the foot is formed by five bones which closely resemble the metacarpal bones of the hand. Each bone articulates with the tarsal bones at one extremity and at the other with the first row of phalanges. The tarsal and <u>meta/tars/al</u> (met-ah-TAR-sal) bones are so arranged that they form two distinct arches: the one running from the heel to the toes on the inner or medial side of the foot is called the longitudinal arch and the other, which runs across the foot in the metatarsal region, is called the transverse arch.

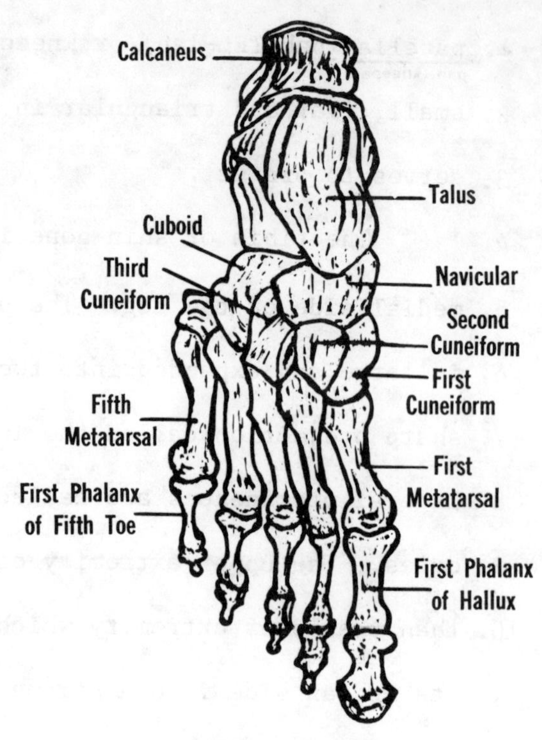

BONES OF THE RIGHT FOOT

The phalanges, both in number and general arrangement, resemble those in the hand. There are two phalanges in the great toe and three in each of the other toes.

JOINTS

Wherever two bones glide over one another, articulations permitting movement arise. They are known as joints. If a person sustains a fracture where the fragments do not unite but continue to rub against each other, a typical, even though imperfect joint is produced. This is called a "false joint" <u>pseudo/</u> (*false*) <u>arthr/osis</u> (*joint*)[1] (sū"dō-ar-THRŌ-sis).

The cartilages surrounding the joints (forming what is called a joint capsule) secrete a whitish fluid something like raw egg white in consistency. This is the <u>syn/ovi/al</u> (*with*, *egg*)[2] (si-NŌ-vē-al) fluid, which, like oil in a machine, reduces friction between the articulating surfaces and helps the smooth functioning of the joint. In addition, the capsule of the joint also possesses certain small sacs containing a clear <u>visc/id</u> (*bird lime*) (VIS-id) fluid. These structures are called

1. Also spelled pseud/arthr/osis (sū-dar-THRŌ-sis)
2. A word invented by Paracelcus (1493-1541), whose greatest contribution to medicine was in pharmacology.

JOINTS and ARTICULATIONS

1. SYNARTHROSES
(Immovable Joints)

Lambdoidal Suture

Sagittal Suture

Coronal Suture

Bones of the Cranium

2. AMPHIARTHROSES
(Slightly Movable Joints)

Symphysis (Male Pelvis)

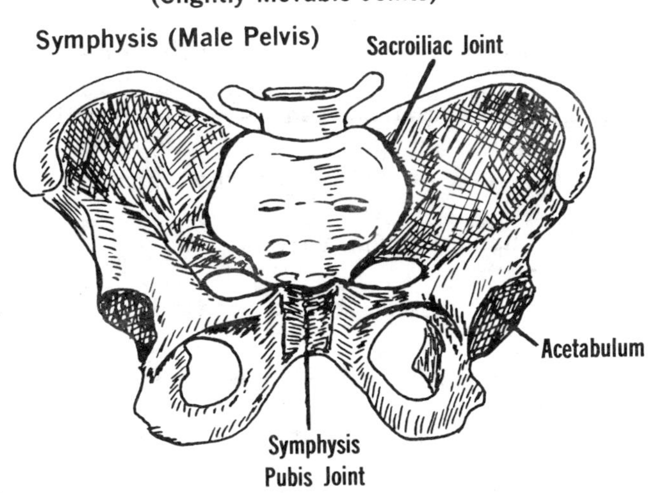

SYNDESMOSIS

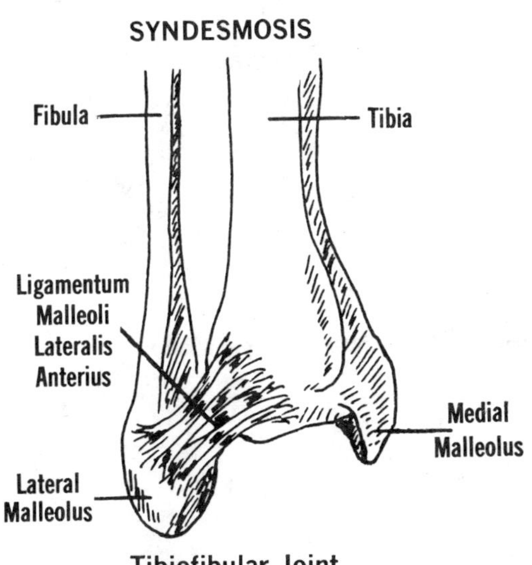

Tibiofibular Joint

3. DIARTHROSES
(Freely Movable Joints)

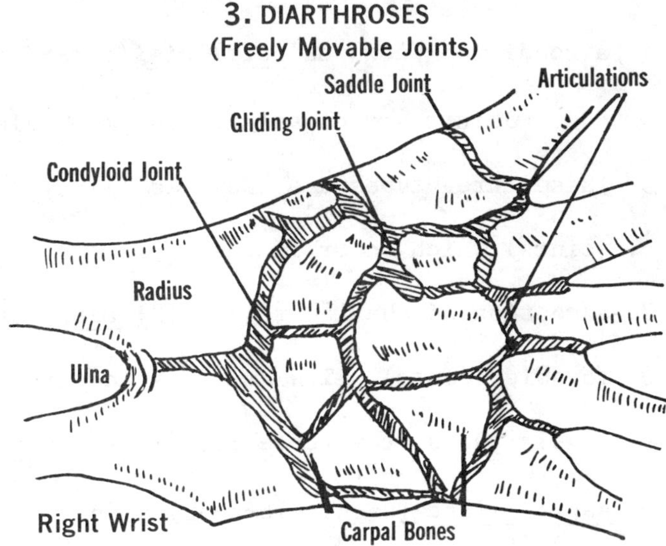

Condyloid, Gliding and Saddle Joints

Hinge Joint

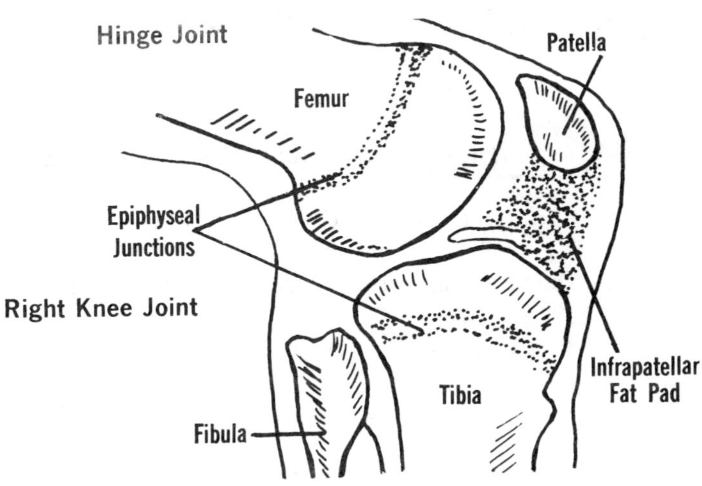

Ball-and-Socket Joint

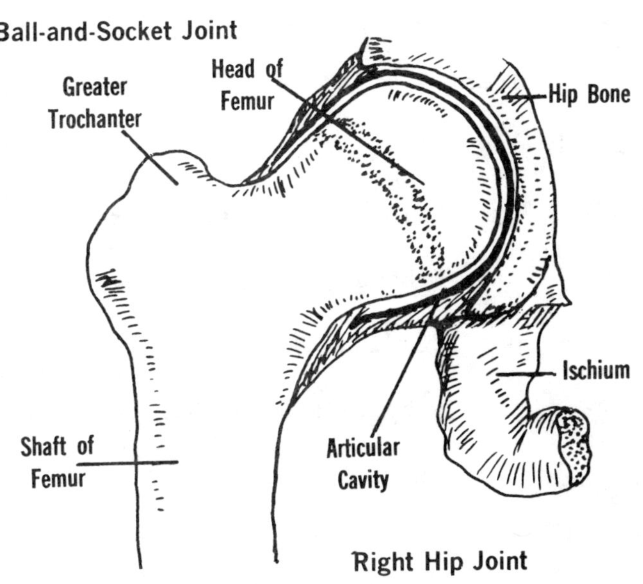

Right Hip Joint

muc/ous (MYŌŌ-kus) bursae [a purse] (BUR-sē). The bursae pad the joint like water-cushions. If the bursae are chronically irritated they become thickened. This results in a condition known as burs/itis (bur-SĪ-tis).

Joints are classified as immovable, slightly movable and freely movable. These three types are known as (1) syn/arthroses [together joints] (sin-ar-THRŌ-sēz) (immovable joints) which occur in the bones of the cranium and the facial bones with the exception of the lower jaw; (2) amphi/arthroses [double joint] (am"fē-ar-THRŌ-sēz) (slightly) movable joints) which are divided into (a) the symphysis occurring in the symphysis pubis, the vertebrae (inter/vertebr/al [between vertebrae] [in-ter-VER-te-bral] disks), the sacro/ili/ac [sacrum ilium] (sa-krō-IL-ē-ak) joint; and (b) syn/desmosis [together to bind] (sin-dez-MŌ-sis) found in the tibio/fibul/ar [tibia fibula] (tib-ē-ō-FIB-ū-lar) joint; (3) di/arthroses [through joint] (dī-ar-THRŌ-sēz) (freely movable joints) of which there are six types: (a) gliding joints found in the wrist, ankle and articular processes of the vertebrae; (b) hinge joints occurring in the elbow, knee, ankle and phalanges; (c) condyl/oid [knuckle] (KON-de-loyd) joints found in the wrist; (d) saddle joints of the thumb; (e) pivot joints found in the attachment of the hand to the radius; and (f) ball-and-socket joints occurring where the head of the femur articulates with the acetabulum of the hip (hip joint) and the head of the humerus articulates in the glenoid cavity of the scapula (the shoulder joint).

Joint movements are of vital importance in various types of reports of accidental injuries. The more important and frequently used movements are as follows:

FLEXION: Movement that reduces the angle between the bones, as in bending the arm at the elbow.

EXTENSION: Movement that increases the angle between bones and is thus opposite to flexion.

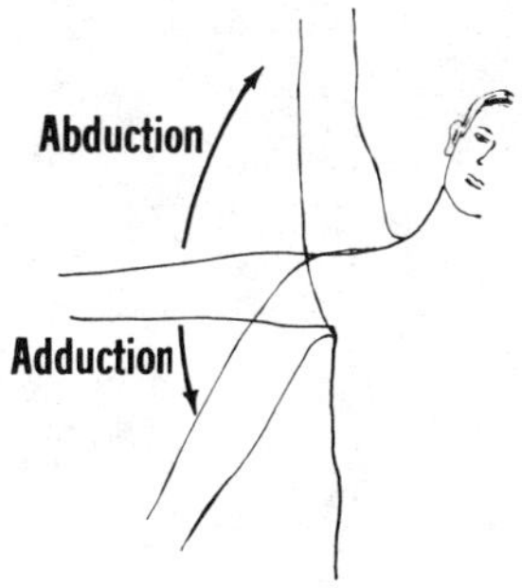

Abduction

Adduction

ABDUCTION: Movement away from the midline of the body as in sidewise movement of the leg or raising the arm.

ADDUCTION: Movement toward the midline of the body, the opposite of abduction.

SUPINATION: Clockwise movement of the hand, turning the palm forward.

Supination

PRONATION: Counterclockwise movement of the hand, turning the palm backward.

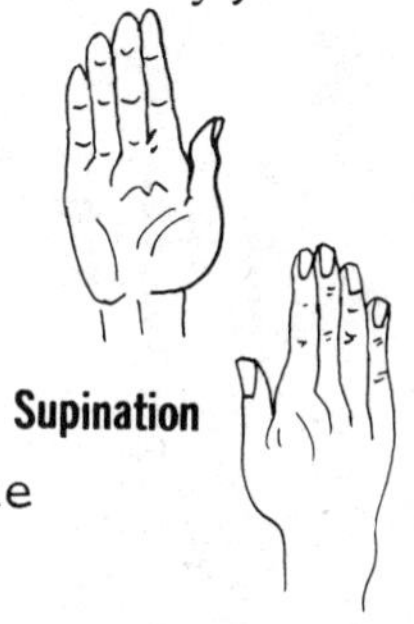

Pronation

CIRCUMDUCTION: Circular movement as in a circular swinging of the arm.

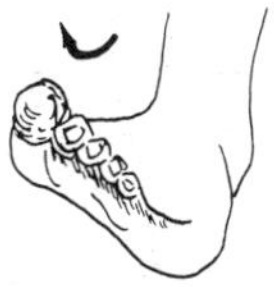

INVERSION: Ankle movement that turns the foot inward.

EVERSION: Ankle movement that turns the foot outward.

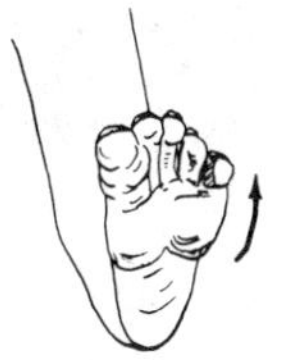

Dorsiflexion and Inversion of foot

Dorsiflexion and Eversion of foot

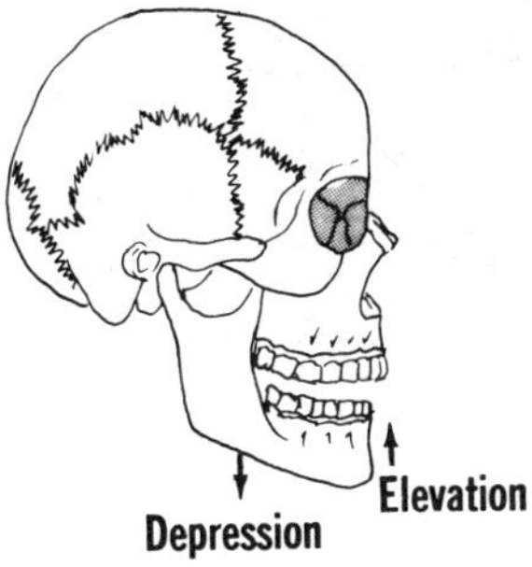

ELEVATION: Movement that raises the bone, muscle or limb (raising lower jaw).

DEPRESSION: Opposite to elevation (dropping lower jaw).

PROTRACTION: Forward movement (pushing lower jaw forward).

Depression

Elevation

RETRACTION: Backward movement (pushing lower jaw back).

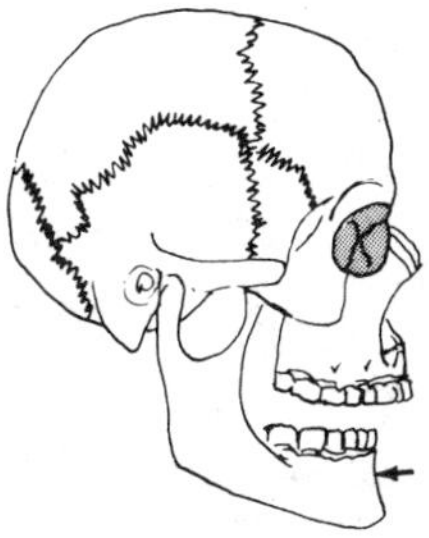

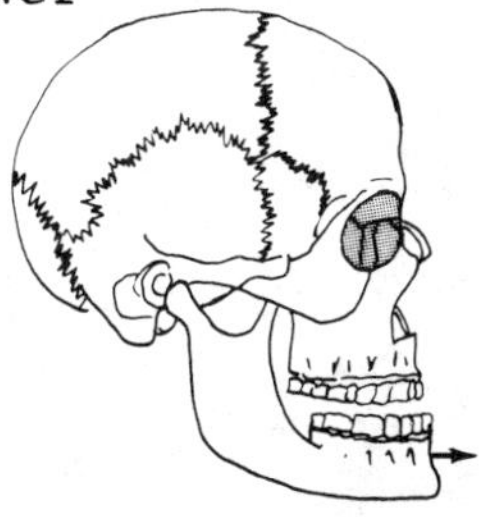

Protraction

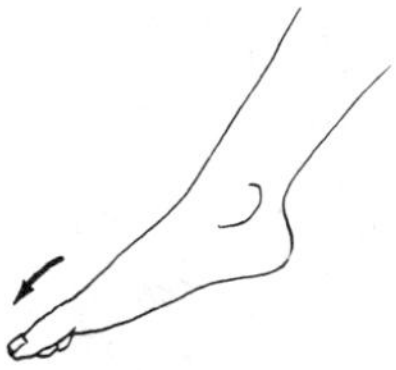

Retraction

HYPEREXTENSION: Movement that bends the part beyond the position taken in extension.

Hyperextension

PLANTAR FLEXION: Movement that flexes the foot toward the sole.

DORSIFLEXION: Plantar extension with upward movement of the foot.

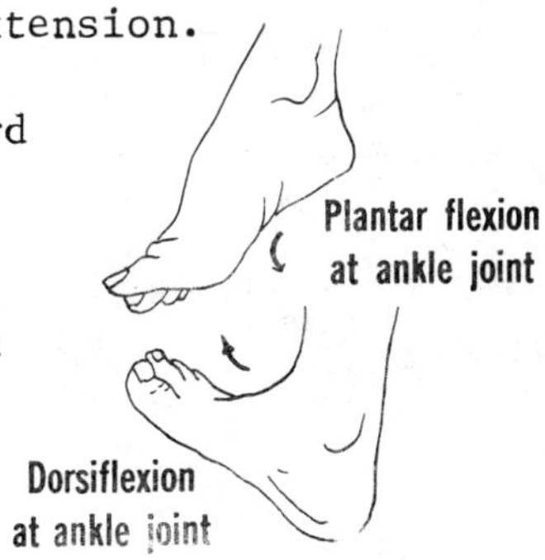

Plantar flexion at ankle joint

Dorsiflexion at ankle joint

FRACTURES

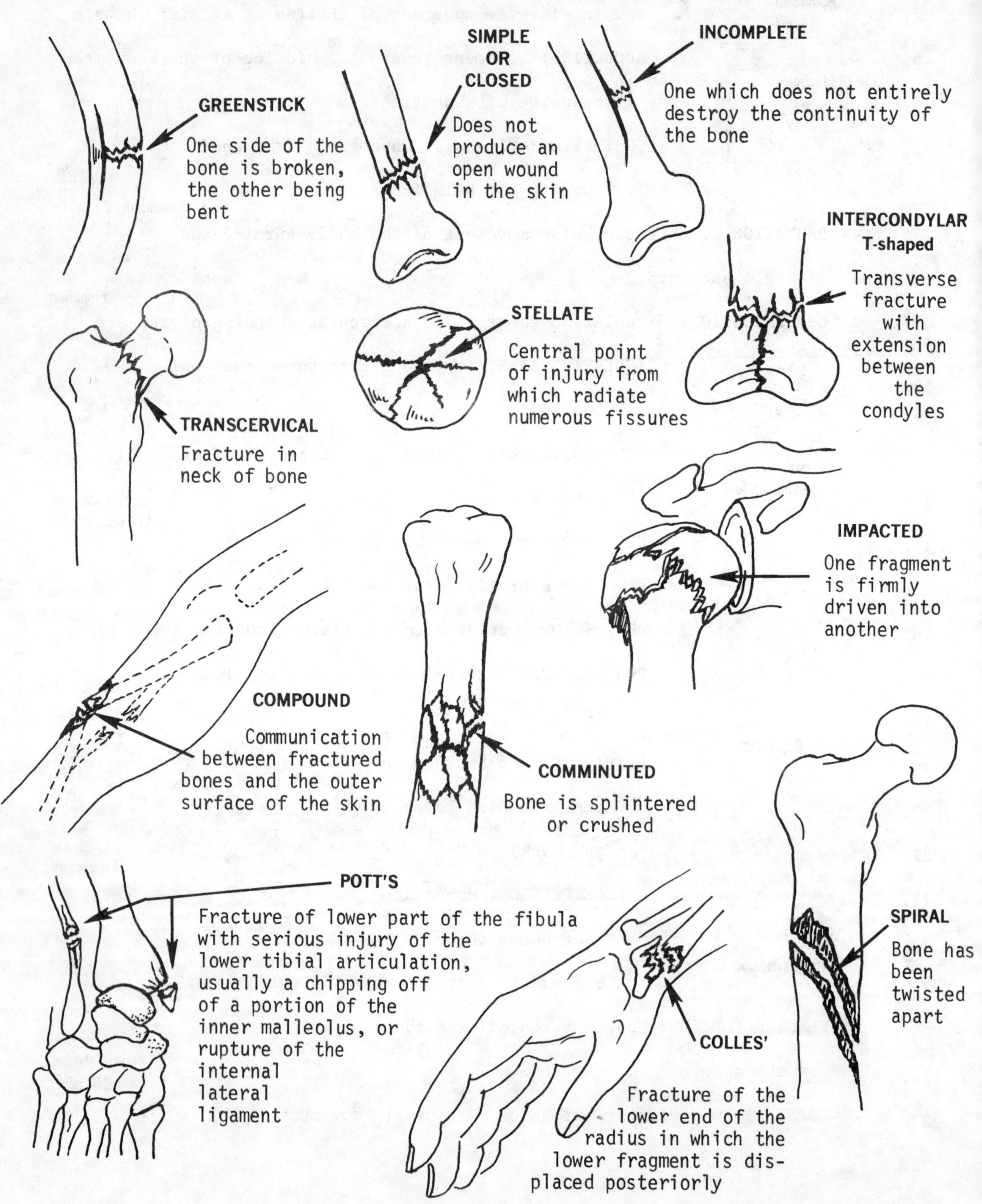
GREENSTICK
One side of the bone is broken, the other being bent
SIMPLE OR CLOSED
Does not produce an open wound in the skin
INCOMPLETE
One which does not entirely destroy the continuity of the bone
INTERCONDYLAR T-shaped
Transverse fracture with extension between the condyles
STELLATE
Central point of injury from which radiate numerous fissures
TRANSCERVICAL
Fracture in neck of bone
IMPACTED
One fragment is firmly driven into another
COMPOUND
Communication between fractured bones and the outer surface of the skin
COMMINUTED
Bone is splintered or crushed
POTT'S
Fracture of lower part of the fibula with serious injury of the lower tibial articulation, usually a chipping off of a portion of the inner malleolus, or rupture of the internal lateral ligament
SPIRAL
Bone has been twisted apart
COLLES'
Fracture of the lower end of the radius in which the lower fragment is displaced posteriorly

FRACTURES

A fracture is a break in the continuity of a bone. As applied to the long bones of the body it usually implies displacement, although there can be a fracture without displacement. Fractures are grouped as simple, compound, com/minuted (KOM-i-nū-ted) and greenstick fractures.
with small

Simple fractures are those which do not have communication between the fractured bones and the outer surface of the skin.

Compound fractures are those which have a tract communicating between the fractured fragments and the outside of the skin.

Comminuted fractures are those in which the bone is broken into more than two fragments. A comminuted fracture may be either simple or compound. It usually occurs in fractures caused by direct violence such as automobile accidents.

Greenstick fractures are those in which the bone is not broken completely through, part of the shaft being broken and the remainder bent. This type of fracture is usually seen in children.

SPRAINS AND DISLOCATIONS

Sprains: If a joint is stretched to such a degree that a ligament or the joint capsule tears at some point it is called a sprain. A sprain is generally a harmless occurrence. After a short period of rest a sprained joint is once more fit for use.

Dislocations: A dislocation is caused when the ligaments, on being put under tension, not only are stretched excessively, but are actually torn to such a degree that the bone escapes from the joint and becomes impacted among the neighboring ligaments and muscles. This type of injury is much more serious than a simple sprain. Under favorable conditions the bone may immediately be replaced in its socket and the dislocation reduced. It generally takes several weeks before torn ligaments and joint capsule heal and the joint is again fit for use.

Sub/luxation *below dislocation* (sub-luks-Ā-shun) and pseudo/luxation *false* (sū"do-luks-Ā-shun) are terms which indicate incomplete or partial dislocation.

DISEASES AND ANOMALIES OF BONES

A/sept/ic *without decay* (ā-SEP-tik) necr/osis *death* (nē-KRŌ-sis) is necrosis or death of the bone without the presence of infection. Interference with the blood supply is the most common cause of aseptic necrosis.

Osteo/chondr/itis *bone cartilage* (os-tē-ō-kon-DRĪ-tis) is inflammation of bone and cartilage.

Epi/phys/itis *on, upon to grow* (ep-i-fis-Ī-tis) is inflammation of the cartilage which joins the infantile epi/physis (ē-PIF-i-sis) to a shaft.

Coxa *hip* (KOK-sah) plana *plane* (PLĀ-nah) or Legg-Perthes'[1] (leg-per-THĒZ) disease is a disease of the upper femor/al *femur* (FEM-or-al) epiphysis wherein the epiphysis is flattened in a typical manner under the influence of weight-bearing and muscle pull.

Deformities of the epiphysis may remain permanently. Other examples of this affection of the epiphyses are calcaneo-apo/phys/itis *heel from to grow* (kal-KĀ-nē-ō-ah-pof"i-SĪ-tis), Freiberg's[2] (FRĪ-bergs) or Kohler's[3] (KŌ-lers) disease of the second metatarsal head, primary and secondary epiphysitis of the patella and vertebral bodies, and epiphysitis of the head of the humerus, crest of the ilium, symphysis pubis, tuberosity of the ischium and proximal tibial epiphysis, and Osgood-Schlatter's[4] (OS-good-SCHLĀ-ters) disease of the tibial tubercle.

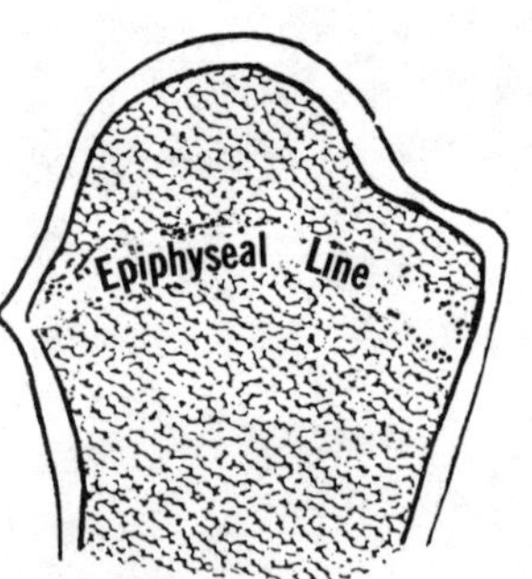

(upper end of humerus)

Osteo/myel/itis *bone marrow* (os"tē-ō-mī-el-Ī-tis) is inflammation of bone-marrow. Acute pyo/gen/ic *pus to produce* (pī-ō-JEN-ik) osteomyelitis in children usually begins in the meta/physis *beyond to grow* (met-AF-i-sis). In adults, the origin is in the peri/osteum (per-ē-OS-tē-am) and the peri/oste/al *around bone* (per-ē-OS-tē-al) vessels that invade the bone.

Osteochondritis dis/secans *apart to cut* (DIS-i-kans) is a joint affection characterized

1. Arthur T. Legg, Boston surgeon, 1874-1939, Georg Clemens Perthes, German surgeon, 1869-1927
2. Albert Henry Freiberg, American surgeon, 1868-1940
3. Alban Kohler, German radiologist, 1874-1947
4. Robert Bayley Osgood, Boston orthopedic surgeon, born 1873. Carl Schlatter, Zurich surgeon, 1864-1934.

by the partial detachment of a fragment of cartilage and underlying bone from the articular surface. It is most common in the knee.

Oste/itis (os-tē-Ī-tis) fibrosa (fiber) (FĪ-BRŌ-zah) cystica (cyst) (SIS-tik-ah) is also known as von Recklinghausen's[1] (von REK-ling-how-senz) disease of the bones. It may be diffuse or local. In generalized osteitis fibrosa cystica, the bone cysts (sists) are the result of an aden/oma (gland) (ad-en-Ō-mah) and hyperactivity of the para/thyr/oid (beside shield) (par-ah-THĪ-royd) gland, and a consequent calcium (limestone) (KAL-sē-um) imbalance which causes the calcium to be withdrawn from the bones. Localized osteitis fibrosa cystica is of a different origin.

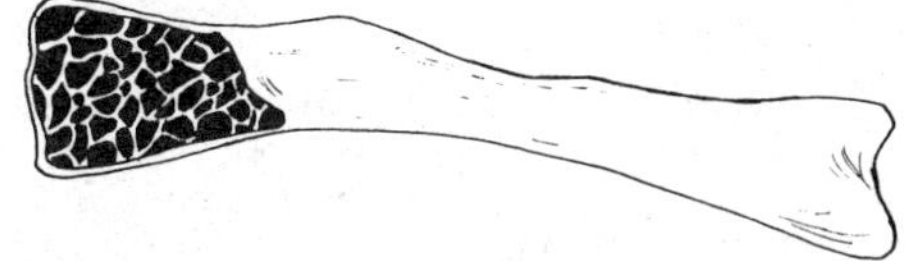

Bone changes due to osteitis fibrosa cystica. Cystic cavities formed inside head of tibia and deformity of the shaft.

Rickets is a disease of childhood in which the bones become crooked and deformed and their earthy salts are diminished. Since the discovery of vitamin D deficiency as the causative agent of rickets, operative treatment has been required in a much smaller number of cases and is undertaken only for the correction of residual deformity after the process has subsided. The deformities which commonly require surgical correction are genu (knee) (JĒ-nū) varum (bow leg) (VAR-um) or bowlegs and genu valgum (knock knee) (VAL-gum) or knock knees.

Talipes (clubfoot)[2] (TĀ-li-pēz) is a congenital deformity in which the foot is twisted out of shape or position. Some of the more common types are talipes equinus (horse) (ē-KWĪN-us), t. calcaneus, t. varus, t. valgus and t. cavus (cave) (KĀ-vus). In talipes equinus the individual walks on the toes of one or both feet. This results from contraction of the Achilles tendon which raises the heel. T. cavus is an exaggeration of the normal arch of

Talipes Equinus

Talipes Cavus

Talipes Calcaneus

1. Friedrich Daniel von Recklinghausen, German pathologist, 1833-1910.
2. "talipes" comes from the Latin "talus" meaning "heel, ankle" and "pes" meaning "foot."

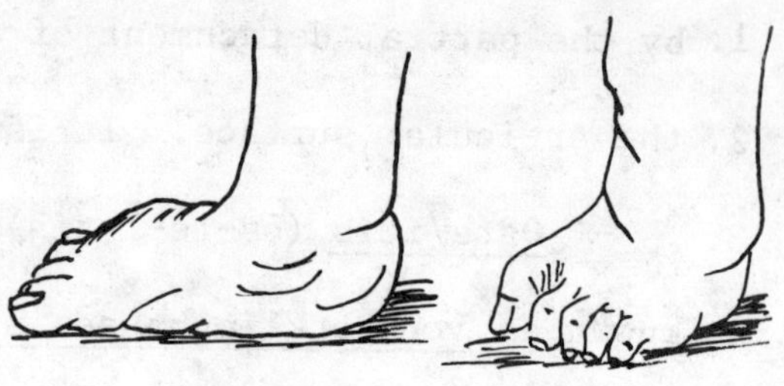
Talipes Valgus Talipes Varus

the foot. T. calcaneus is permanent dorsal flexion of the foot. The weight of the body rests on the heel only. T. valgus is permanent eversion of the foot and the individual walks on the inner border of the foot, the sole being turned outward. It is usually combined with a breaking down of the plantar arch. T. varus is inversion of the foot. The individual walks on the outer border of the foot, the sole being turned inward.

Endo/crine [within to separate] (EN-dō-krin)[1] disturbances: Affections of bones induced by endocrine disturbances are pituit/ary [phelgm] (pi-TŪ-i-tār-ē) dwarfism (DWOR-fiz-em) or giantism (jī"ent-IZ-em), acro/megaly [extremity large] (ak-rō-MEG-ah-lē), hypo/thyr/oid [below] (hī-pō-THĪ-royd) dwarfism (cretin/ism [KRĒ-tin-izm]), and hyper/para/thyr/oid/ism [above] (hī"per-par-ah-THĪ-roy-dizm) (diffuse osteitis fibrosa cystica).

Paget's[2] (PAJ-ets) disease is also known as osteitis deformans (dē-FŌR-menz) and it is characterized by an enlargement, softening and distortion of the bones. The disease, at present, is incurable and the treatment is only palliative [cloaked] (PAL-ē-ah-tiv).

Scoli/osis [crooked] (skō-lē-Ō-sis) is an abnormal curvature of the vertebral column in which the spinal column curves to one side. Among the many causes are improper posture, scarring (cicatrici/al [scar] [sik-ah-TRISH-al] contraction) following necrosis, from disease of a hip resulting in a tilting of the pelvis, paralysis, rickets and weakness of spinal muscles.

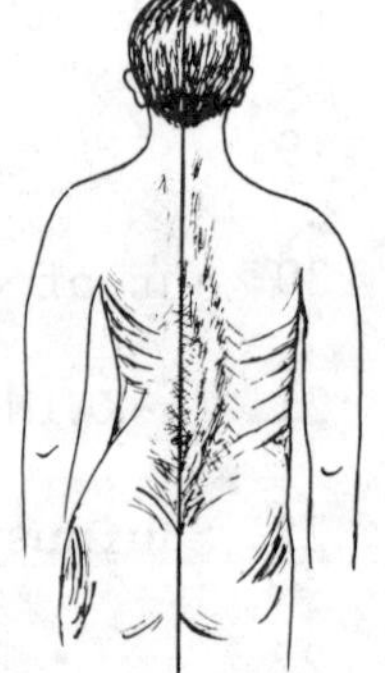
Scoliosis

Kyph/osis [humpback] (kī-FŌ-sis) is an abnormal curvature of the spine with convexity backward due to decay of bone (caries [dry rot] [KĀ-ri-ēz) and destruction of the bodies of the affected vertebrae. Kyphosis may also be called osteo/chondr/osis [bone cartilage] (os"tē-ō-kon-DRŌ-sis) of the vertebrae.

Spondylo/listh/esis [vertebra to slip] (spon"di-lō-lis-THĒ-sis) is an anomaly[3] [irregular] (ah-NOM-ah-lē)

1. Optional pronunciation EN-dō-krīn
2. Sir James Paget, English surgeon, 1814-1899
3. "anomaly" comes from the Greek "an" meaning "not" and "homos" meaning "same."

in which there is a forward displacement of one vertebra over another, usually of the fifth lumbar vertebra over the body of the sacrum, or of the fourth lumbar over the fifth lumbar vertebra.

Tumors of the bones may be primary or meta/stat/ic [beyond a setting] (met"ah-STAT-ik). Primary bone tumors are either osteo/gen/ic [produce] (os-tē-ō-JEN-ik) or non/osteo/gen/ic [not] (non"os-tē-ō-JEN-ik). The more common bone tumors may be classified as follows:

Osteogenic tumors, benign: oste/oma (os-tē-Ō-mah) or ex/ost/osis [out bone] (eks-os-TŌ-sis), osteo/chondr/oma (os-tē-ō-kon-DRŌ-mah), osteo/chondr/omat/osis [tumor] (os-tē-ō-kon-drō-mah-TŌ-sis) (joint mice), chondr/oma (kon-DRŌ-mah) or chondro/myx/oma [mucus] (kon-drō-miks-Ō-mah), giant cell tumors (osteo/clast/oma [to break] [os-tē-ō-klas-TŌ-mah]) and xanth/oma [yellow] (zan-THŌ-mah). The differenti/ation [to distinguish between] (dif"i-ren-she-Ā-shun) between benign and malignant [evil] (me-LIG-nent) giant cell tumors, osteo/lyt/ic [to loosen] (os-tē-ō-LIT-ik) osteogenic sarc/oma [flesh] (sar-KŌ-mah) or media/stat/ic [middle a setting] (mē-dē-ah-STA-tik) carcin/oma [cancer] (kar-sin-Ō-mah) may be difficult.

Osteogenic tumors, malignant: chondro/myxo/sarc/oma (kon-drō-miks-ō"sar-KŌ-mah) (primary and secondary), chondro/sarc/oma (kon-drō-sar-KŌ-mah), and osteolytic osteogenic sarcoma.

Nonosteogenic tumors, benign: angi/oma [vessel] (an-jē-Ō-mah).

Nonosteogenic tumors, malignant: endo/theli/al [within nipple] (en-dō-THĒ-lē-al) myel/oma [marrow] (mī-el-Ō-mah) (Ewing's [Ū-ings] tumor), myeloma, periosteal fibro/sarc/oma [fiber] (fī"brō-sar-KŌ-mah).

Metastatic tumors: carcinoma, lymph/aden/oma [water gland] (limf"ad-i-NŌ-mah), hyper/nephr/oma [above kidney] (hī"per-nē-FRŌ-mah).

Common benign soft tissue tumors are fibr/oma (fī-BRŌ-mah), neuro/fibroma (nū"rō-fī-BRŌ-mah), lip/oma [fat] (lī-PŌ-mah)[1]; osteochondroma, giant cell tumor, xanthoma, hem/angi/oma [blood vessel] (hē-man-jē-Ō-mah), and lymph/angi/oma (limf-an-jē-Ō-mah). The common malignant tumors are fibrosarcoma and epi/theli/oma (ep-i-thēl-ē-Ō-mah). Both benign and malignant types may arise in skin, sub/cutane/ous [below skin] (sub"kyōō-TĀ-nē-us)

1. Optional pronunciation lip-Ō-mah

tissues, tendons, tendon sheaths, fasciae *band* (FASH-ē-ē), vessels or nerves.

Neuro/fibr/omat/osis *tumor* (nū"ō-fī-brō-mah-TŌ-sis) is an affection of the nervous system characterized chiefly by multiple soft tissue tumors distributed along the course of the peri/pher/al *around to bear* (pe-RIF-er-al) nerves, and pigment/ations *deposit of pigment* (pig"men-TĀ-shuns) of the skin, and frequently by elephant/iasis *elephant's disease* (el-i-fan-TĪ-ah-sis), changes in the structure of the bones, and skeletal deformities. The disease is con/genit/al *with to produce "born together"* (kon-JEN-i-tal). Other congenital and developmental anomalies *irregular* (ah-NOM-ah-lēz), glaucoma *opacity of lens* (glaw-KŌ-mah), deafness, spina *spine* (SPĪ-nah) bifida *two parts* (BIF-i-dah), meningo/cele *membrane hernia* (men-IN-gō-sēl), and mental deficiency may be associated.

Congenital deficiences of bone include:

Osteogenesis im/perfecta *not perfect* (im-per-FEK-tah), also known as fragilitas *fragile* (frah-JIL-i-tis) osseum *bone* (OS-sē-um), is a famili/al *family* (fah-MIL-ē-al) disease of the long bones characterized by abnormal brittleness and associated with blue sclerae[1] *hard* (SKLER-ē).

Osteo/scler/osis *bone hard* (os-tē-ō-skler-Ō-sis) is an abnormal hardness of bone which is also known as marble bones.

Chondro/dys/plasia *cartilage bad* (kon"drō-dis-PLĀ-zē-ah) is an abnormality of cartilage growth, with formation of cartilagin/ous *gristle* (kar-til-AJ-in-us) growths in the bones.

Dys/chondro/plasia (dis"kon-drō-PLĀ-zē-ah) is a disease whose etio/logy *cause study of* (ē"tē-OL-i-jē) is unknown and which attacks the long bones and the metacarpal and phalange/al *phalanx* (fah-LAN-jē-al) skeleton of the hand.

A/chondro/plasia *lack* (ā"kon-drō-PLĀ-zē-ah) is a condition of abnormal osteogenesis resulting in the congenital dwarf.

DISEASES OF THE JOINTS

The term arthr/itis *joint* (ar-THRĪ-tis), which actually signifies inflammation of a joint, applies to nearly all diseases of the joints; thus, arthritis is said to be in/fectious *in to do, make* (in-FEK-shus) (true inflammation), ~~degenerative~~, metabolic *a change*

1. The sclera is the white of the eye

(met-ah-BOL-ik), traumat/ic *wound* (traw-MAT-ik), or allerg/ic *allergy* (ah-LER-jik). Arthritis may be acute or chronic.

Acute arthritis is usually infectious, traumatic, or allergic. It is a principal manifestation of rheumat/ic *subject to flux* (rū-MAT-ik) fever and of serum *whey* (SĒ-rum) sickness, and occurs as a complication of many infectious diseases, such as lob/ar *lobe* (LŌ-bar) pneumon/ia *lung* (nū-MŌ-nē-ah), cerebro/spin/al *brain spine* (ser"i-brō-SPĪ-nal) fever, gono/rrhea *seed* (gon-ō-RĒ-ah), typh/oid *stupor, fog* (TĪ-foyd) fever, bacill/ary *bacillum* (BAS-il-ā-rē) dys/entery *bad intestine* (DIS-en-ter-ē), and septic/emia *putrefaction blood* (sep"ti-SĒ-mē-ah). It may follow trauma *wound* (TRAW-mah) if a wound has entered the joint, or organisms may enter from osteomyelitis in an adjacent bone, or by way of the blood stream. If the organisms are pus-producers (strepto/coccus *curved berry* [strep-tō-KOK-us], staphylo/coccus *bunch of grapes* [staf"il-ō-KOK-kus]) pus forms in the joint.

Chronic arthritis may be due to syphilis[1] (SIF-i-lis), tubercul/osis *tubercle* (tū-ber-kyōō-LŌ-sis), or to other specific infections, but its most common varieties are two diseases whose causes are not definitely known. They are known by several names: (1) rheumat/oid (RŪ-mah-toyd) arthritis, arthritis deformans or chronic infectious arthritis; (2) hyper/troph/ic *above to nourish* (hī"per-TRŌ-fik) arthritis, degenerative arthritis or osteo/arthr/itis *bone joint* (os"tē-ō-ar-THRĪ-tis). Rheumatoid arthritis is a chronic inflammatory disease of the joints and the tissues about them. Hypertrophic arthritis is a chronic, noninflammatory disease of the joints which occurs for the most part in elderly people.

Tumors of joints: Tumors may arise primarily from the structures within the joints or may invade the joint from extra-articul/ar *outside of joint* (eks"trah-ar-TIK-ū-lar) tissues. Benign or malignant neo/plasms *new formation* (NĒ-ō-plazms) of joints, although uncommon, are observed most often in the knee. Synovi/oma *synovia* (si-nō-vē-Ō-mah), which arises primarily from the synovial lining, is the most common of the malignant tumors of joints. The benign tumors are lipoma, hemangioma, fibroma, xanthoma and endo/theli/oma *within nipple* (en"dō-thēl-ē-Ō-mah).

1. Named after a shepherd who was infected with the disease. It originally was the title of a poem written in 1530 in which the shepherd was the principal character.

SURGERY OF BONES AND JOINTS

Osteo/tomy [bone] (os-tē-OT-ō-mē) is the manual or surgical breaking of bone and is performed for ankylosis, malunion of fractures, deformities either congenital or uncorrected from injury, nonunion of fractures, irreducible fractures, congenital dislocation, tuberculosis of joints, osteo/dys/trophy [bad] (os-tē-ō-DIS-trof-ē), in rotation deformities, infantile paralysis, epiphyse/al [epiphysis] (ep-i-FIZ-ē-al) growth disturbances.

Osteo/synthesis [a putting together] (os-tē-ō-SIN-the-sis) is the operative fastening of the ends of a fractured bone by sutures, rings, plates or other mechanical means. It is performed for nonunion of bones and pseudoarthrosis (a false joint, as that sometimes seen following a fracture).

Methods of osteosynthesis:

1. Metallic
   - a. metal bands
   - b. nails
   - c. pins
2. Non-metallic
   - a. fiber, cow horn, etc.
   - b. bone graft methods:
     - (1) hetero/gen/ous [other, produce] (het-er-OJ-i-nus), boiled bone, etc.
     - (2) auto/gen/ous [self] (aw-TOJ-i-nus) graft
       - (a) inlay graft (most commonly used)
       - (b) onlay graft (good for bones of the forearm)
       - (c) osteo/peri/oste/al (os"tē-ō-per-ē-OS-tē-al) graft (does not require special equipment)
       - (d) intra/medull/ary [inside, marrow] (in-trah-MED-ū-lār-ē) and spongiosa [sponge]

Smith-Peterson nail with side plate for intertrochanteric fracture of femur

Insertion of Smith-Peterson nail for fracture of neck of femur

(spun-jē-Ō-sah) graft (use of spongi/ous (SPUN-jē-us) bone masses)

3. Bone drilling
4. External appliances.

Bone grafts are used for

1. ununited fractures
2. to repair traumatic bone injuries and defects
3. to supply congenitally absent bone, as in the tibia
4. to replace bone destroyed by infection, as in osteomyelitis
5. to replace bone removed for cyst or tumor
6. to immobilize and stimulate osteogenesis in tuberculous joints
7. to stabilize a relaxed and flail joint, as in infantile paralysis

Equalization operations:

1. Bone shortening is done for shortening of the opposite leg in infantile paralysis, traumatism, infection, congenital deformities, injuries to growth plates, etc.
2. Bone lengthening is done for a leg shortened by tuberculosis of the hips, knee, osteomyelitis, congenital shortening, congenital dislocation of hip, ectro/mel/ia (ek-trō-MĒ-lē-ah) (congenital
miscarriage limb
absence of a limb or limbs), spastic paralysis, fracture of the femur; the majority of cases are shortening from infantile paralysis.
3. Epiphyseal arrest is done to retard the growth of the epiphysis and equalize length of lower extremities.

Indications for amputation surgery:

1. complete severance of the main nerve and blood supply or of the blood supply alone, with or without compound fracture
2. extensive destruction or laceration of the limb likely to lead

to total loss of function

3. infection. Uncontrollable infection endangering the life, or severe tuberculosis

4. malignancies

5. gangrene (GANG-rēn) secondary to arterio/sclerosis (ar-tē"rē-ō-
artery hardening
skle-RŌ-sis) or thrombo-angi/itis (throm-bō-an-jē-Ī-tis)
clot vessel

6. severe deformity if artificial limb promises better function

Guillotine (GIL-o-tēn) amputation is a life-saving procedure and is indicated in septicemia, in gangren/ous (GANG-rin-us) or badly infected feet, and in extensive infectious lymph/ang/itis (limf-an-JĪ-tis).
water

Osteo/clasis (os"tē-ō-KLĀ-sis) is the surgical refracture of a bone in
to break
cases of malunion of fractured parts.

Osteo/plasty (OS-tē-ō-plas-tē) is the reconstruction or repair of a bone.

Ost/ectomy (os-TEK-tō-mē) is the excision of a bone.

Sequestr/ectomy (sē-kwes-TREK-tō-mē) is the surgical removal of a piece of
something laid aside
dead bone that has become separated during the process of necrosis from the sound bone.

Fracture procedures used:

Closed reduction is manipulation and application of casts, splints or traction apparatus.

Open reduction is open surgery with repair of tissues, alignment of bone ends thus reducing the fracture, and, if necessary, osteosynthesis.

Procedures and indications for spinal surgery:

1. Spinal fusion (arthro/desis [ar-thrō-DĒ-sis])[1] is the internal fix-
binding
ation of the spine by fusion where external fixation by appliances is inopportune or inadequate; in scoliosis, in spondylolisthesis.

2. Lamin/ectomy (lam-i-NEK-tō-mē) and hemi/laminectomy (hem"ē-lam-i-NEK-
thin plate half
tō-mē) (stripping the muscles away from one side only) are performed

1. Optional pronunciation ar-THROD-i-sis

for decompression of the spinal cord, to relieve pressure upon the spinal cord or peripheral spinal nerves caused by intraspinal tumors, herniated disk, certain types of spinal fractures, pressure by inflammatory products, from kyphot/ic [humpback] (kī-FOT-ik) or scoliot/ic [crooked] (skō-lē-OT-ik) deformities of the spine.

3. Lamino/tomy (lam-i-NOT-ō-mē) is taking out bits of bone from the lamell/ar (LAM-i-lar) arch to widen the space. It is done for ruptured disk to make more room for the emerging nerve.

4. Costo/trans/vers/ectomy [rib, across, to turn] (kos"tō-trans"ver-SEK-tō-mē) is the removal of the transverse process with adjacent portions of the ribs, head and neck, either unilateral or bilateral for access to the dorsal spine for drainage.

5. Trans/peri/tone/al [around, to stretch] (tranz"per-i-ton-Ē-al) drainage is performed for abscesses in the retro/peri/tone/al [backward] (re"trō-per-i-ton-Ē-al) space in front of the lumbar spine.

6. Trans/sacr/al [sacrum] (tranz-SĀ-kral) drainage is performed for cases of sacral abscess.

7. Trans/vers/ectomy (tranz-ver-SEK-tō-mē) is the excision of the 5th lumbar transverse process for low back pain with its radiations and referred symptoms caused by anatomical variations of the 5th lumbar vertebra.

8. Coccyg/ectomy [coccyx] (kok"si-JEK-tō-mē) (removal of the coccyx) is performed when there is coccygo/dynia [pain] (kok"si-gō-DIN-ē-ah) usually following trauma by blow or a fall upon the end of the spine.

Operations on joints are performed for three reasons:

1. drainage and evacuation done by
   a. puncture and aspiration
   b. arthro/tomy (ar-THROT-ō-mē) for removal of loose bodies

(joint mice), loose cartilage or removal of synovial membrane.

2. The obliteration of the joint by arthrodesis or resection.

   a. Joint resections are performed for traumatic dislocation not reducible by open operation, tuberculosis of the shoulder with mixed infection and suppuration.

   b. Arthrodesis in which only the articular cartilage is removed. It is a fusion of the joint eliminating mobility (free motion).

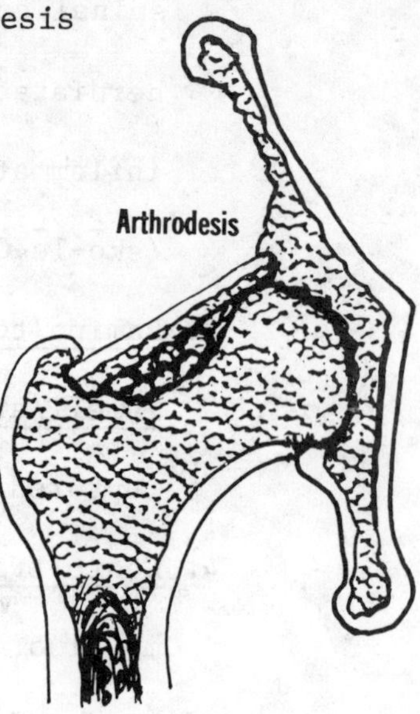

Arthrodesis

Femoral head and acetabulum chiseled to expose cancellous bone, neck roughened, flap of bone from ilium turned down

3. The reconstruction of the joint.

   a. Arthro/plasty (AR-thrō-plas-tē) is a reconstruction operation upon ankylosed or stiffened joints re-establishing the range of motion. The principle of the operation is the formation of a new joint.

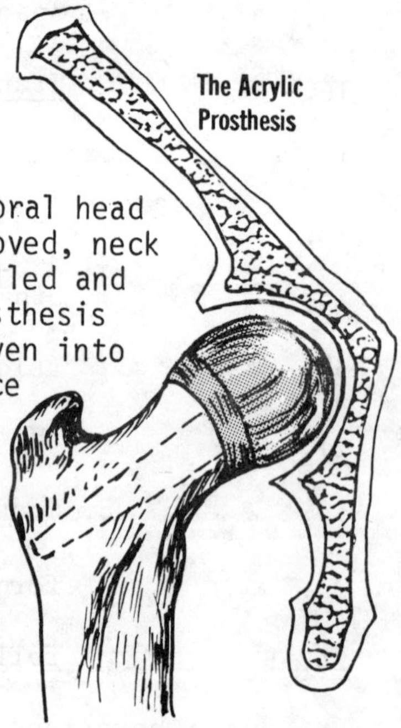

The Acrylic Prosthesis

Femoral head removed, neck drilled and prosthesis driven into place

Surgery of the Joint Capsule:

1. Capsulo/tomy (capsule) (kap-sū-LOT-ō-mē) is performed for contractions.
2. Capsular plasty is performed for deviation of the great toe.
3. Capsular fenestr/ation (window) (fen-es-TRĀ-shun) is performed to relieve joint pressure and congestion.

REVIEW OF THE SKELETAL SYSTEM

Bones of the Cranium		Bones of the Face	
occipital	1	nasal	2
parietal	2	vomer	1
frontal	1	nasal concha	2
temporal	2	lacrimal	2
sphenoid	1	zygomatic (malar)	2
ethmoid	1	palatine	2
Total	8	maxilla	2
		mandible	1
		Total	14

TOTAL BONES OF SKULL - 22

Bones of the Ear		Bones of the Trunk	
malleus	2	cervical vertebra	7
incus	2	thoracic vertebra	12
stapes	2	lumbar vertebra	5
TOTAL BONES OF EAR -	6	sacral vertebra	1
		coccygeal vertebra	1
hyoid bone in the neck	1	TOTAL VERTEBRAE IN THE ADULT	26
		ribs	24
		sternum	1
		TOTAL BONES IN THE TRUNK -	51

Bones of the Upper Extremities		Bones of the Lower Extremities	
clavicle	2	hip bone (os coxae)	2
scapula	2	femur	2
humerus	2	patella	2
ulna	2	tibia	2
radius	2	fibula	2
carpus		tarsus	
navicular (scaphoid)	2	calcaneus (calcaneum)	2
lunate (semilunar)	2	talus	2
triangular (cuneiform)	2	cuboid	2
pisiform	2	navicular (scaphoid)	2
greater multangular (trapezium)	2	third cuneiform	2
lesser multangular (trapezoid)	2	second cuneiform	2
capitate (os magnum)	2	first cuneiform	2
hamate (unciform)	2		
metacarpus	10	metatarsus	10
phalanges	28	phalanges	28
TOTAL BONES OF UPPER EXTREMITIES -	64	TOTAL BONES OF LOWER EXTREMITIES -	62

TOTAL NUMBER OF BONES IN THE SKELETON - 206

INDEX
CHAPTER II

PAGE	LINE	
35	19	trapezium
35	20	trapezoid
49	9	trauma
49	1	traumatic
36	21	trochanters
34	13	trochlea
33	23	tubercles
49	13	tuberculosis
33	14	tuberosity
29	13	turbinated
27	21	tympanic
49	7	typhoid
34	14	ulna
35	22	unciform
45	18	valgum
45	17	varum
32	2	vertebra
31	16	vertebrae
32	1	vertebral
38	28	viscid
29	16	vomer
45	4	von Recklinghausen's
47	11	xanthoma
32	17	xiphoid
29	18	zygomatic

CHAPTER III
THE MUSCULAR SYSTEM

The movements of the body are produced by the action of the muscles. This is made possible because muscles have a special development of function known as contractility which occurs when the muscles are stimulated. Muscle cells are long fibers which are arranged in compact bundles. Therefore, in addition to being contractile, muscular tissue is also noted for irritability or excitability, extensibility and elasticity.

Forty to fifty percent of body weight is composed of muscular tissue.

Muscles are classified by structure and location. There are three types of muscle fibers: striated [striped] (STRĪ-āt-ed) or cross-striped, nonstriated or smooth, and indistinctly striated.

The striated muscles are skeletal and are known as voluntary muscles. These are the muscles which are concerned with voluntary action such as raising an arm, walking, writing and speaking. In other words, the individual's will can make these muscles operate. The function of the skeletal muscles is to operate the bones of the body for the purpose of producing motion.

NUCLEUS

STRIATED (VOLUNTARY) MUSCLE

Muscles over which we have no control are known as involuntary muscles. They occur in the stomach, intestines, blood vessels and are called nonstriated or smooth muscles because there is no cross-striping in their cyto/plasm [cell shape] (SĪ-tō-plazm). The function of these smooth muscle cells is to produce any changes in shape and size which occurs in these organs. Peri/stalsis [around contraction] (per-i-STAL-sis) of the alimentary canal is an example of this function.

NUCLEUS

SMOOTH (INVOLUNTARY) MUSCLE

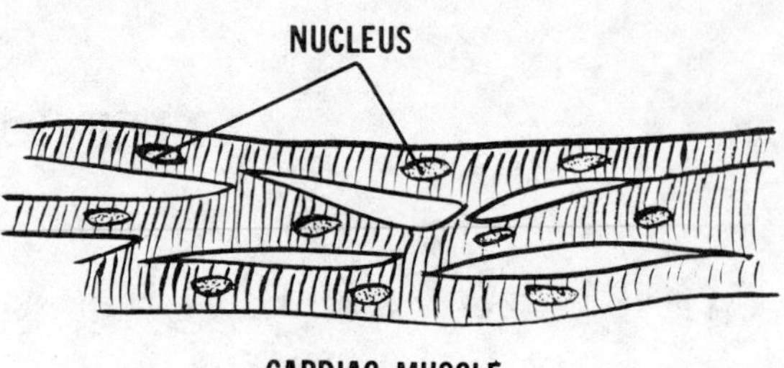

CARDIAC MUSCLE

The heart is formed of cardiac muscle tissue which is indistinctly striated.

Striated or skeletal muscles in most instances pass over joints. Some of these joints are movable, some are immovable. If the joint is movable, the origin and insertion of the muscle are mentioned. The attachment nearer the center of the body is usually described as the origin and the attachment which is more peripheral (farther out in the body) is termed the insertion. The origin of the muscle is the end attached to the less movable bone while the insertion is the attachment of the muscle to a bone which moves in the ordinary activity of the body. When a muscle contracts lengthwise it increases in diameter and pulls the attachments at each end nearer to each other. For example, bend the arm, bringing the hand toward the shoulder. Notice how the biceps muscle in the upper arm becomes larger.

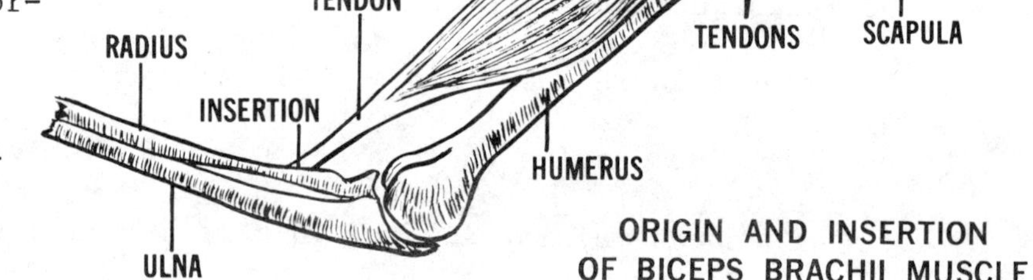

ORIGIN AND INSERTION OF BICEPS BRACHII MUSCLE

The fleshy portion of a muscle is occasionally attached directly to bone, but attachment is usually achieved by means of a fibrous tissue, tendon or <u>apo/neurosis</u> (apo = from, neurosis = sinew, tendon) (ap"on-ū-RŌ-sis)[1]. A tendon is a dense white cord and the <u>apo/neuroses</u> (ap"on-ū-RŌ-sēz)[1] are broad flat sheets or, what might be called, flattened tendons. Tendons are exceedingly strong, inextensible but at the same time flexible. It could be said they resemble cables.

Tone is the property of muscle tissue whereby a steady, partial contraction varying in degree is maintained. It is by means of this tonic contraction

1. Optional pronunciation ap"ō-nū-RŌ-sis, ap"ō-nū-RŌ-sez

in skeletal muscle that posture is maintained for long periods of time with little or no evidence of fatigue.

Most skeletal muscles occur in pairs. There are a few single muscles situated in the midline which represent the fusion of two muscles. The skeletal muscles are usually arranged so they oppose each other. The opposing muscles to the flexors would be the extensors. In the arm the flexors cause the arm to bend and the extensors extend or straighten the arm.

The following listing covers those muscles most frequently encountered in various medical specialties.

Name of Muscle	Action
Muscles of the Skull and Face[1]	
epi/crani/al (ep-i-KRĀ-nē-al) or on skull occipito/front/alis (ok-sip"i-tō-fron-TAL-is)[2] back of head forehead	occipit/al (ok-SIP-i-tal) portion draws scalp backward; frontal portion elevates eyebrows, pulls scalp forward
superior rectus (REK-tus) straight	rolls eyeball upward
inferior rectus	rolls eyeball downward
medial rectus	rolls eyeball inward
lateral rectus	rolls eyeball outward
superior oblique (ob-LĪK) slanting	rotates eyeball directing the cornea (KOR-nē-ah) downwards and outwards
inferior oblique	rotates eyeball directing the cornea upwards and outwards
levator (lē-VĀ-tor) palpebrae (PAL-pe-brē) lifter eyelid superioris (su-PĒ-rē-or-is) above	raises the upper lid and opens the eye
orbicularis (or"bik-ū-LAR-is) oculi (OK-ū-lī) a small disk eye	closes lids, wrinkles forehead, compresses lacrimal sac

1. Most of the muscles of the skull and face are known as "expression" muscles. Those who study for an acting career find it a great aid to learn the function of these muscles.

2. Muscles ending in "alis" have an optional pronunciation as ok-sip"i-to-fron-TAH-lis.

Muscles of the Head

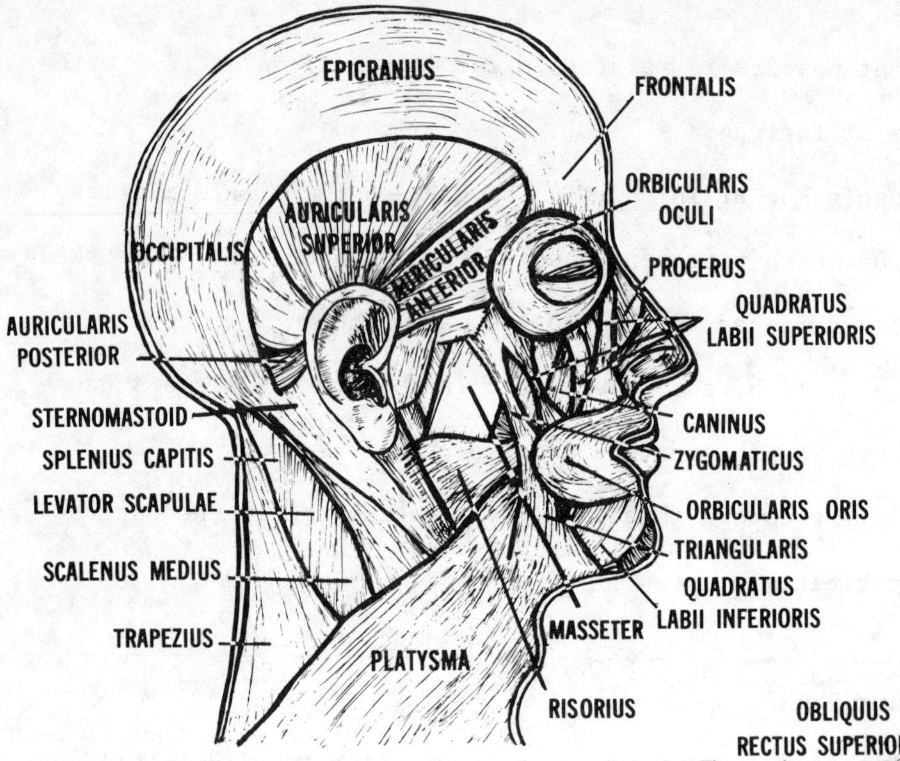

EPICRANIUS
FRONTALIS
ORBICULARIS OCULI
AURICULARIS SUPERIOR
AURICULARIS ANTERIOR
OCCIPITALIS
PROCERUS
QUADRATUS LABII SUPERIORIS
AURICULARIS POSTERIOR
STERNOMASTOID
CANINUS
SPLENIUS CAPITIS
ZYGOMATICUS
LEVATOR SCAPULAE
ORBICULARIS ORIS
TRIANGULARIS
SCALENUS MEDIUS
QUADRATUS LABII INFERIORIS
MASSETER
TRAPEZIUS
PLATYSMA
RISORIUS

Muscles of the Eye

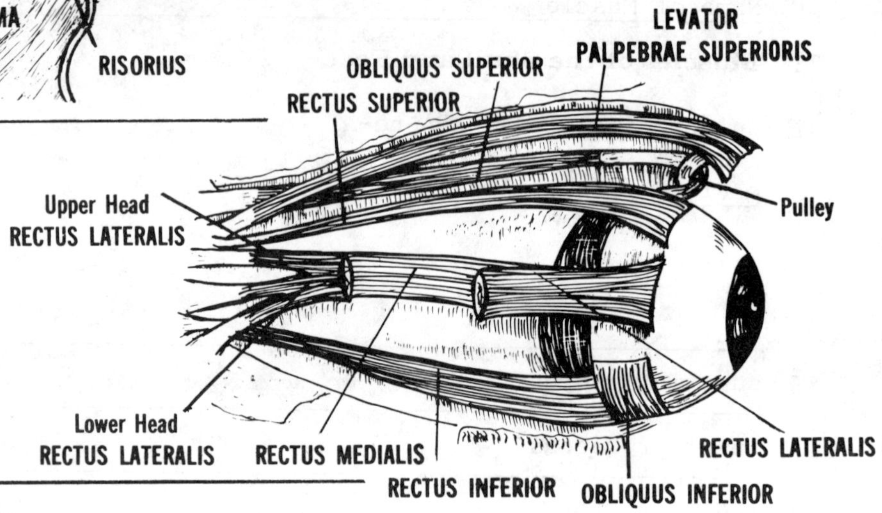

LEVATOR PALPEBRAE SUPERIORIS
OBLIQUUS SUPERIOR
RECTUS SUPERIOR
Upper Head RECTUS LATERALIS
Pulley
Lower Head RECTUS LATERALIS
RECTUS MEDIALIS
RECTUS INFERIOR
OBLIQUUS INFERIOR
RECTUS LATERALIS

Muscles of the Neck

STYLOHYOID
MASTOID PROCESS
MANDIBLE (Lower Jaw Bone)
STERNOCLEIDOMASTOID
DIGASTRIC
SPLENIUS
MYLOHYOID
HYOID BONE
GREATER CORNUA
LEVATOR SCAPULAE
THYROHYOID
OMOHYOID
SCALENUS POSTERIOR
STERNOHYOID
TRAPEZIUS
Sternal origin STERNOCLEIDOMASTOID
CLAVICLE

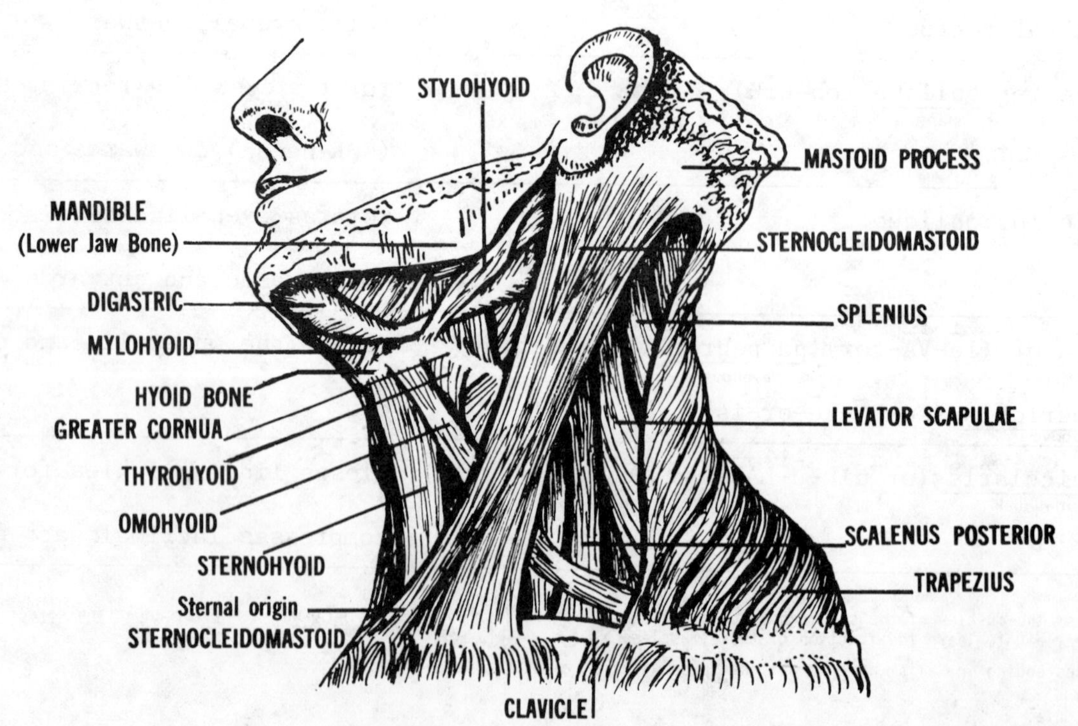

Muscle	Action
procerus (long) (prō-SER-us)	draws down medial angle of eyebrows; causes wrinkles over bridge of nose
nasalis (nose) (NĀ-zal-is)	depresses cartilagin/ous (gristle) (kar-ti-LAJ-i-nus) part of nose and draws ala (wing) (Ā-lah) toward septum (wall off) (SEP-tum)
depressor septi (SEP-tī)	draws ala of nose downward, constricting aperture (opening) (AP-er-chūr) of naris (nose) (NAR-is)
dilator naris anterior	enlarges aperture of naris
dilator naris posterior	enlarges aperture of naris
masseter (masticator) (MAS-i-ter)[1]	raises the mandible (a jaw) (MAN-di-bl) and closes the mouth
tempor/alis (time, temple) (tem-pō-RAL-is)	raises the mandible, closes the mouth; draws the mandible backward
internal pteryg/oid (wing) (TER-i-goyd)	raises mandible and closes mouth; assists in protruding the mandible
external pterygoid	assists in opening mouth; protrudes mandible
orbicularis oris (mouth) (OR-is)	protrudes lips and pushes them forward; closes the lips, the sphincter (a band) (SFINK-tur) of the mouth
buccinator (trumpeter) (BUK-si-nā-tur)	compresses the cheeks and retracts the angles of the mouth
quadratus (square) (kwod-RĀ-tus) labii (lip) (LĀ-bē-ī) superioris	Has 3 heads: angular head raises upper lip and dilates nostril; infra/orbit/al (below circle) (in"frah-OR-bi-tal) head gives expression of sadness; zygomat/ic (yoke together) (zī-gō-MAT-ik) head draws upper lip upward and outward

1. Optional pronunciation mas-Ē-ter

Muscle	Action
quadratus labii inferioris	depresses lower lip as in the expression of irony
caninus (kā-NĪ-nus) caninus: dog	raises angle of mouth; produces the naso/labi/al (nā-zō-LĀ-bē-al) furrow (FUR-ō) naso: nose; labi: lip; furrow: groove
ment/alis (men-TAL-is) ment: chin	raises and protrudes lower lip and wrinkles skin of chin; produces expression of doubt and disdain
zygomatic	draws angle of mouth backward and upward as in laughing
triangularis (trī-ang-gū-LAR-is) triangularis: triangle	pulls down corners of the mouth
risorius (rī-SAW-rē-us) risorius: to laugh	draws angle of mouth causing an expression of grinning
Muscles of the Tongue	
genio/glossus[1] (jē"nē-ō-GLOS-us) genio: chin; glossus: tongue	retracts, depresses and protrudes the tongue; raises the hyoid bone
stylo/glossus (stī"lō-GLOS-us) stylo: pillar, pole	raises and retracts the tongue
Muscles of the Neck	
platysma (plah-TIZ-mah) platysma: flat plate	wrinkles skin of neck; depresses lower jaw and lower lip
sterno/cleido/mast/oid[2] (stur"nō-klī"dō-MAS-toyd) sterno: sternum; cleido: clavicle; mast: breast	depresses and rotates head; flexes head on chest or neck
scalenus (skah-LĒ-nus) anterior scalenus: uneven scalenus medius scalenus minimus scalenus posterior	help raise 1st and 2nd ribs and bend vertebral column

1. "geni(o)" is Greek for "chin;" "mentum" is Latin for "chin."
2. This term is often shortened to "sternomastoid."

MUSCLES OF THE BODY

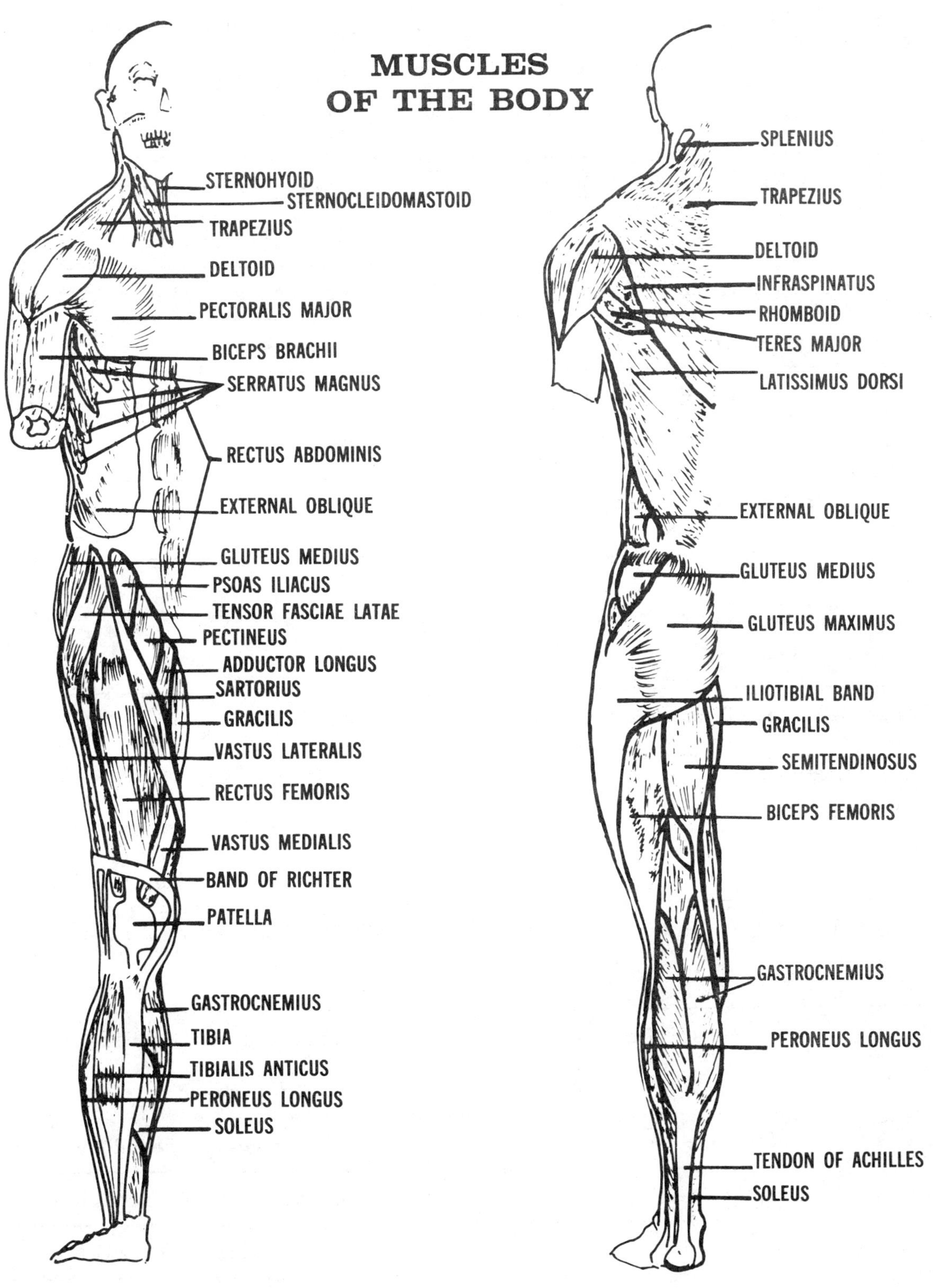
STERNOHYOID
STERNOCLEIDOMASTOID
TRAPEZIUS
DELTOID
PECTORALIS MAJOR
BICEPS BRACHII
SERRATUS MAGNUS
RECTUS ABDOMINIS
EXTERNAL OBLIQUE
GLUTEUS MEDIUS
PSOAS ILIACUS
TENSOR FASCIAE LATAE
PECTINEUS
ADDUCTOR LONGUS
SARTORIUS
GRACILIS
VASTUS LATERALIS
RECTUS FEMORIS
VASTUS MEDIALIS
BAND OF RICHTER
PATELLA
GASTROCNEMIUS
TIBIA
TIBIALIS ANTICUS
PERONEUS LONGUS
SOLEUS
SPLENIUS
TRAPEZIUS
DELTOID
INFRASPINATUS
RHOMBOID
TERES MAJOR
LATISSIMUS DORSI
EXTERNAL OBLIQUE
GLUTEUS MEDIUS
GLUTEUS MAXIMUS
ILIOTIBIAL BAND
GRACILIS
SEMITENDINOSUS
BICEPS FEMORIS
GASTROCNEMIUS
PERONEUS LONGUS
TENDON OF ACHILLES
SOLEUS

Muscle	Action
Muscles of the Back	
trapezius *(table or counter)* (trah-PĒ-zē-us)	draws head backward or sidewise, retracts scapula, elevates point of shoulder, depresses scapula and rotates it
latissimus *(broad)* (lat-IS-i-mus) dorsi *(back)* (DOR-sī)	draws humerus downward and backward, rotates it inward
rhomboideus[1] *(a lozenge shaped figure)* (rom-BOYD-ē-us) major	retracts and elevates the scapula
rhomboideus minor	retracts and elevates the scapula
levator scapulae *(shoulder blade)* (SKAP-ū-lē)	raises upper angle of scapula; aids in rotating head
sacro/spin/alis *(sacrum, spine)* (sā"krō-spi-NAL-is) ilio/cost/alis *(ilium, rib)* (il"ē-ō-kos-TAL-is) longissimus *(long)* (lon-JIS-i-mus) spinalis	serve to maintain the vertebral column in the erect posture
Muscles of the Chest (Thorax)	
pector/alis *(breast bone)* (pek-tō-RAL-is) major	depresses arm to side, adducts and draws it forward, rotates it; helps to raise ribs in forced inspiration
pectoralis minor	draws down scapula; helps in raising ribs
serratus *(a saw)* (ser-Ā-tus) anterior	raises ribs in inspiration; carries scapula forward
sub/clavius[2] *(beneath, clavicle)* (sub-KLĀ-vē-us)	depresses shoulder down and forward
external inter/costals *(between, ribs)* (in-ter-KOS-tals)	contract during inspiration
internal intercostals	contract during expiration
levatores *(lifter)* (lē-vah-TŌ-res) costarum *(rib)* (kō-STAH-rum)	rotate vertebral column and flex it laterally

1. Also called "rhomboid"
2. Clavicle comes from Latin diminutive "claviculum" which in turn comes from the Latin "clavis" meaning "key." "cleid(o)" and "clid(o)" are Greek for "clavicle."

diaphragm *a partition* (DĪ-ah-fram)	principal muscle of inspiration; modifies size of chest and abdominal cavity; aids in expulsion of substances from body

Muscles of the Abdominal Wall - Anterior and Posterior

external or descending oblique (obliquus [ō-BLĪ-kus] externus abdominis [ab-DOM-i-nis])	compresses abdominal viscera, flexes thorax, aids in expulsive acts
internal or ascending oblique (obliquus internus abdominis)	compresses abdomen, flexes thorax and aids in expiration
trans/versus *across / to turn* (trans-VER-sus) or trans/vers/alis (trans-ver-SAL-is) abdominis	compresses the viscera and flexes the thorax
rectus abdominis	compresses abdomen and flexes vertebral column
pyramid/alis *pyramid* (pi-ram-i-DAL-is)	tenses linea *line* (LIN-ē-ah) alba *white* (AL-bah); aids in inspiration
psoas *muscles of the loin* (SŌ-as) major	flexes and rotates thigh outward; flexes thigh on pelvis; abducts and flexes lumbar spine
psoas minor	tensor of the ili/ac *ilium* (IL-ē-ac) fascia
iliacus *ilium* (il-Ē-ak-us)	aids psoas major to flex thigh upon pelvis and tilt pelvis forward
quadratus lumborum *loin* (lum-BOR-um)	flexes chest laterally and forward; draws down last rib and aids in inspiration

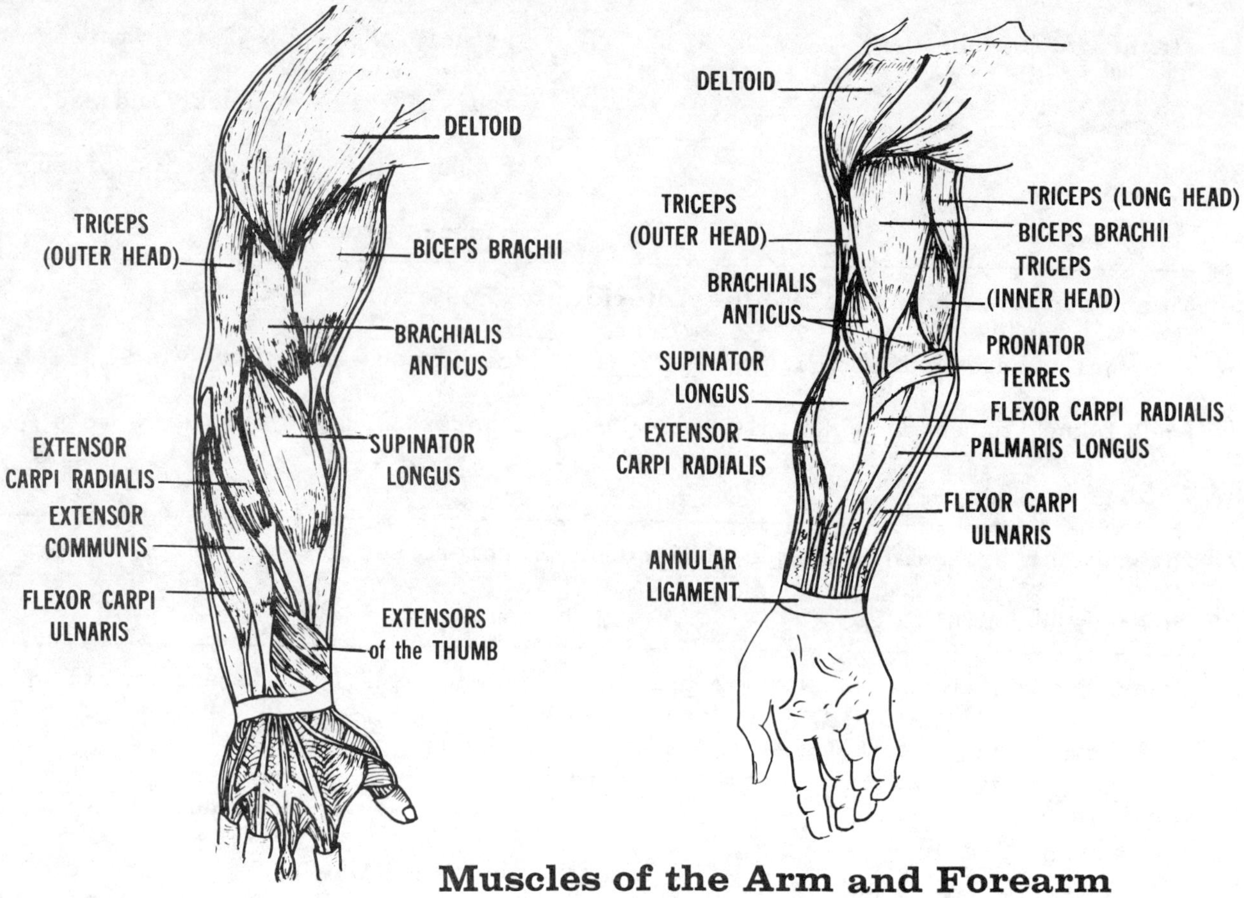

DELTOID
TRICEPS
(OUTER HEAD)
BICEPS BRACHII
BRACHIALIS
ANTICUS
EXTENSOR
CARPI RADIALIS
SUPINATOR
LONGUS
EXTENSOR
COMMUNIS
FLEXOR CARPI
ULNARIS
EXTENSORS
of the THUMB
DELTOID
TRICEPS (LONG HEAD)
TRICEPS
(OUTER HEAD)
BICEPS BRACHII
TRICEPS
(INNER HEAD)
BRACHIALIS
ANTICUS
PRONATOR
TERRES
SUPINATOR
LONGUS
FLEXOR CARPI RADIALIS
EXTENSOR
CARPI RADIALIS
PALMARIS LONGUS
FLEXOR CARPI
ULNARIS
ANNULAR
LIGAMENT

Muscles of the Arm and Forearm

Muscles of the Hand - Palmar View

TRANSVERSE
CARPAL LIGAMENT
FLEXOR DIGITI QUINTI
ABDUCTOR DIGITI QUINTI
Common sheath of FLEXORES
DIGITORUM SUBLIMIS and
PROFUNDUS
FLEXOR POLLICIS
BREVIS (cut)
Tendon Sheath
Terminal Phalanx
ABDUCTOR
POLLICIS BREVIS
Sheath of FLEXOR
POLLICIS LONGUS
Insertion of FLEXOR
DIGITORUM SUBLIMIS
FLEXOR POLLICIS
BREVIS (cut)
Insertion of FLEXOR
DIGITORUM PROFUNDUS
ADDUCTOR POLLICIS

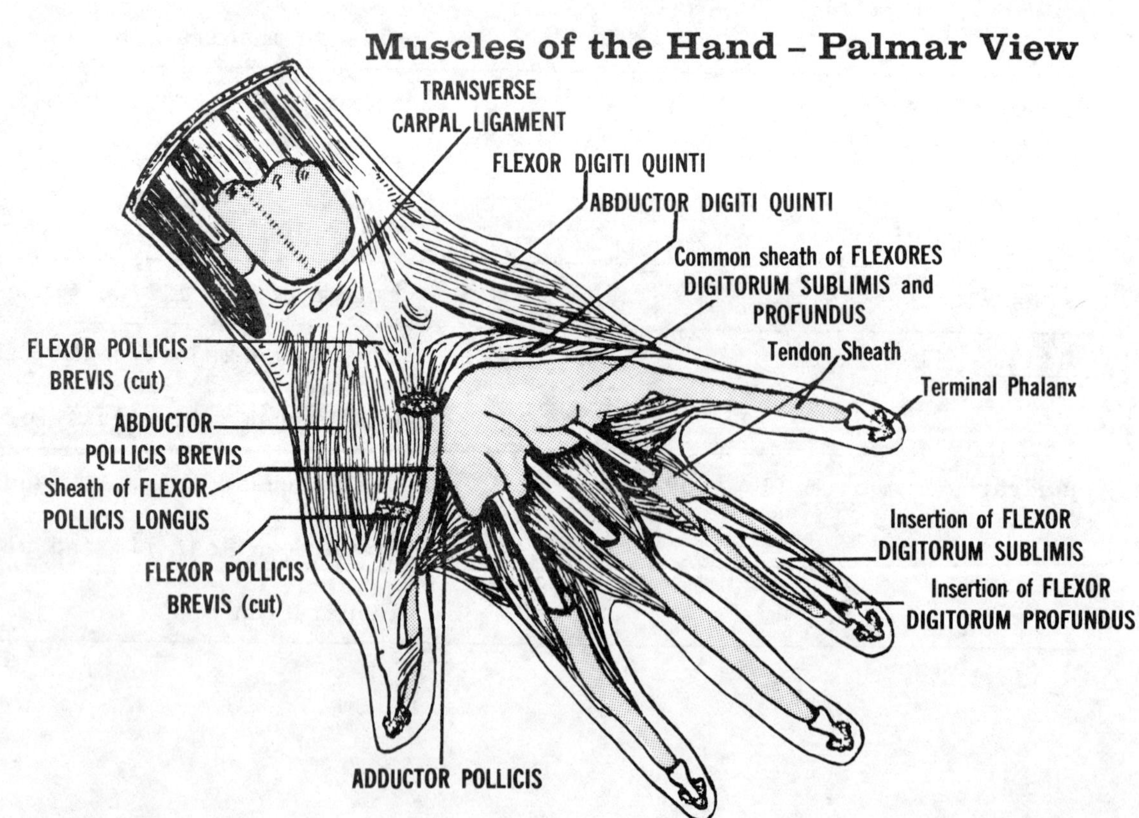

Muscles of Shoulder, Arm, Forearm

Muscle	Action
delt/oid[1] (DEL-toyd) or deltoideus (del-TOY-dē-us) triangle	abducts, flexes, extends and rotates the arm
sub/scapularis (sub"skap-ū-LAR-is) below scapula	inward rotation of arm
supra/spinatus (sū"prah-spi-NĀ-tus)[2] above spine	abducts the arm
infra/spinatus (in"frah-spi-NĀ-tus) below	outward rotation of arm
teres (TER-ēz)[3] minor long and round	outward rotation of arm
teres major	draws raised arm down and backward; rotates it inward
bi/ceps (BĪ-seps) brachii (BRĀ-kē-ī) two head arm	flexes elbow and shoulder and supinates forearm
tri/ceps (TRĪ-seps) brachii three	great extensor of forearm
coraco/brachi/alis (kor"ah-kō-brā-kē-AL-is) like a crow's beak arm	flexes the arm at the shoulder
brachialis	flexes the elbow
pronator (prō-NĀ-ter) teres to bend forward	rotates radius upon ulna, renders the hand prone
flexor carpi (KAR-pī) radi/alis (rā-dē-AL-is) wrist radius	flexes and abducts the wrist
palmaris (pal-MAR-is) longus palm of hand	flexes the wrist joint, assists in flexing the elbow
flexor carpi ulnaris (ul-NAR-is) elbow, arm	flexes and abducts wrist; assists in bending elbow
flexor digitorum (dij-i-TOR-um) sublimis (SUB-li-mis) finger or toe high, superficial	flexes middle and proximal phalanges (fah-LAN-jēz), assists in flexing the wrist and elbow a line of soldiers
flexor digitorum profundus (prō-FUN-dus) deep	flexes distal phalanges
flexor pollicis (POL-li-sis) longus thumb	flexes thumb
pronator quadratus	pronates and rotates hand

1. "delt" in "deltoid" comes from the Greek letter "delta" Δ
2. Optional pronunciation sū"prah-spi-NAH-tus
3. Optional pronunciation TĒ-rēz

brachio/radi/alis (brā″kē-ō-rā-dē-AL-is) arm radius	flexes forearm and assists in supination
extensor carpi radialis longus	extends wrist and abducts hand
extensor carpi radialis brevis (BREV-is) short	extends wrist and abducts hand
extensor digitorum communis (KOM-ū-nis) common	extends fingers; helps extend forearm
extensor digiti (DIJ-i-tī) quinti (KWIN-tī) proprius (PRŌ-prē-us) digiti: finger or toe; quinti: five; proprius: one's own	extends little finger
extensor carpi ulnaris	extends and abducts wrist
anconeus (an-KON-ē-us) elbow	assists triceps in extending forearm
supinator (sū-pi-NĀ-ter) to bend backward	supinates hand
ab/ductor (ab-DUK-ter) pollicis brevis away from; to draw	carries thumb laterally from palm of hand
extensor pollicis brevis	extends and abducts proximal phalanx (FĀ-lanks) of thumb phalanx: line or array of soldiers
extensor pollicis longus	extends terminal phalanx of thumb; helps extend and abduct wrist
extensor indicis (IN-di-sis) proprius one that points out	extends index finger

Muscles of the Pelvis

obturator (OB-tū-rā-tur) internus to stop up	rotates and abducts femur
obturator externus	rotates femur outward
levator ani (Ā-nī) anal orifice	helps to form pelvic floor; constricts the lower end of the rectum and vagina
coccygeus (kok-si-JĒ-us) the coccyx	supports and raises coccyx (KOK-siks) and closes pelvic outlet coccyx: a cuckoo

Muscles of the Lower Extremities

Muscle	Action
gluteus (glu-TĒ-us) maximus (MAK-si-mus) gluteus: buttock; maximus: greatest	extends, abducts and rotates thigh outward
gluteus medius	rotates, abducts and extends thigh
gluteus minimus	rotates, abducts and extends thigh
tensor (TEN-ser) fasciae (FASH-ē-ē) latae (LAH-tē) tensor: to stretch; fasciae: band; latae: broad	tightening of the fascia lata
piri/formis (pir-i-FOR-mis) piri: pear; formis: shape	rotates thigh outward
quadratus femoris (FEM-o-ris) femoris: femur	rotates thigh outward
gemelli (jeh-MEL-ī)[1] gemelli: twin gemellus (jeh-MEL-lus) inferior gemellus superior	rotates extended thigh; abducts it when flexed
sartorius[2] (sar-TŌ-rē-us) sartorius: tailor	flexes leg on thigh and thigh on pelvis; abducts and rotates thigh outward
quadri/ceps (KWOD-ri-seps) femoris quadri: four; ceps: head arises by four heads: 1. rectus femoris 2. vastus (VAS-tus) later/alis (lat-er-AL-is) vastus: huge; lateralis: side 3. vastus medialis 4. vastus intermedius	rotates thigh outward
gracilis (GRAH-sil-is) gracilis: slender or delicate	flexes and adducts knee and adducts thigh
ad/ductor (ad-DUK-tor) longus ad: toward; ductor: to draw	rotates outward, adducts and flexes thigh
adductor brevis	adducts, rotates outward and flexes thigh upon pelvis

1. Optional pronunciation ge-MEL-lī
2. The muscle used in crossing the legs in the tailor's position.

1.	adductor magnus	adducts thigh and everts it
2.	pectineus [comb] (pek-tin-Ē-us)	flexes hip, adducts and rotates
3.		thigh outward
4.	biceps femoris	flexes knee, extends thigh and
5.		rotates leg outward
6.	semi/tendinosus [half / tendon] (sem"ē-ten-di-NŌ-sus)	rotates leg inward
7.	extensor hallucis [great toe] (HAL-lu-sis)	extends phalanges of great toe
8.	extensor digitorum longus	extends phalanges of toes; flexes
9.		foot and turns it out
10.	gastro/cnemius [belly / leg] (gas-trok-NĒ-mē-us)	extends foot at ankle; flexes
11.		femur upon tibia
12.	soleus [sole of foot] (sō-LĒ-us)	helps extend foot on ankle, raising
13.		the heel; steadies leg upon foot
14.	plantaris [sole of foot] (plan-TĀR-is)	extends ankle; bends the knee
15.	popliteus [back of knee] (pop-li-TĒ-us)[1]	flexes leg; rotates flexed leg
16.		inward
17.	flexor hallucis longus	flexes great toe and extends foot
18.	flexor digitorum longus	flexes toes and extends foot
19.	tibi/alis [tibia] (tib-ē-AL-is) anterior or	flexes foot at ankle and elevates
20.	anticus [anterior] (AN-ti-kus)	inner border of foot
21.	tibialis posterior or posticus [posterior] (POS-ti-kus)	extends foot at ankle and turns in
22.		the foot
23.	peroneus [brooch, fibula] (per-ō-NĒ-us) longus	extends, abducts and everts foot
24.	peroneus brevis	extends and abducts foot
25.	extensor digitorum brevis	extends proximal phalanges of toes
26.	flexor digitorum brevis	flexes toes
27.	abductor hallucis	abducts and flexes proximal phalanx
28.		of great toe

1. Optional pronunciation pop-LIT-ē-us

Muscle	Action
abductor digiti quinti	abducts little toe, flexes its proximal phalanx
quadratus plantae (PLAN-tē) plantae: sole of foot	assists flexor digitorum longus in flexing the toes
lumbricales (lum-bri-KĀ-lēz) lumbricales: an earthworm	extends last phalanges of toes and flexes the first phalanges
flexor hallucis brevis	flexes great toe
adductor hallucis	adducts and flexes proximal phalanx of great toe
flexor digiti quinti brevis	flexes little toe
inter/ossei (in-ter-OS-ē-ī) dorsales (dor-SAL-is) inter: between; ossei: bones; dorsales: back	flex proximal and extend middle and distal phalanges; abduct 2nd, 3rd and 4th toes
interossei plantares (plan-TAR-ēz) plantares: sole of foot	adduct proximal phalanges of three outer toes; flex proximal and extend middle and distal phalanges

Muscles of the Leg

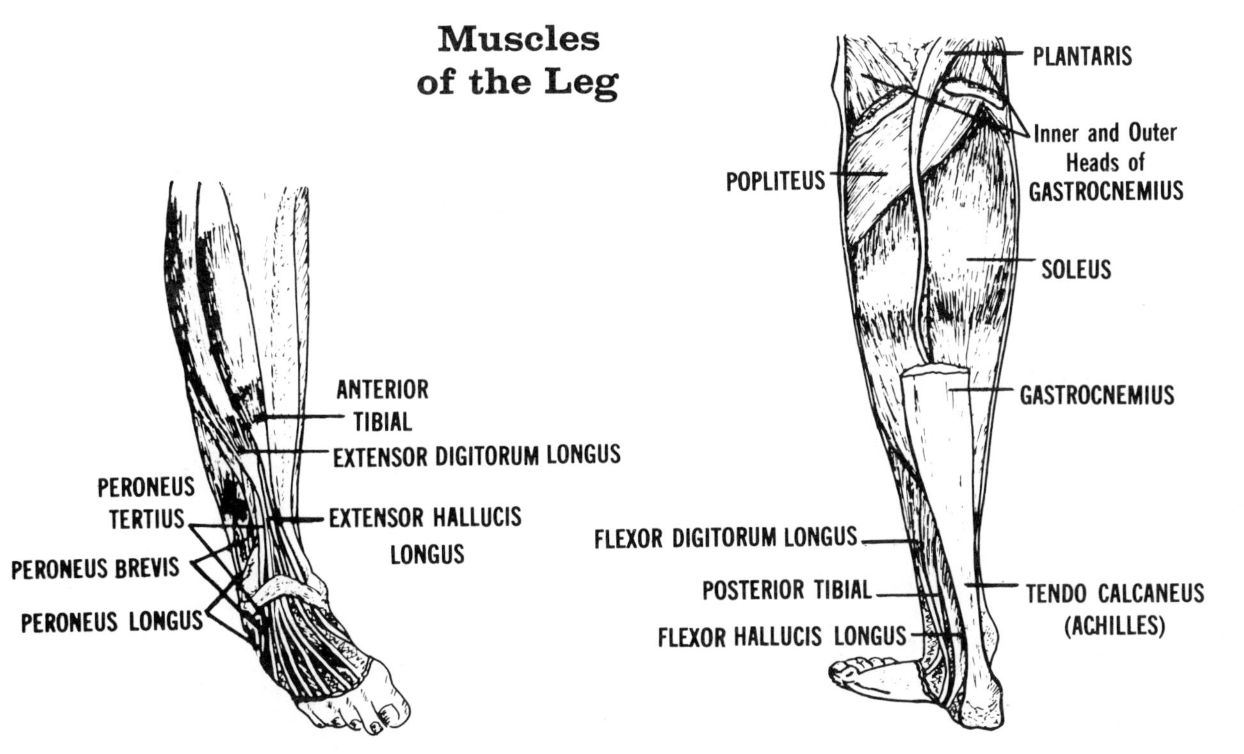

DISEASES AND ANOMALIES

Burs/itis [a purse] (bur-SĪ-tis): bursae (BUR-sē) are sacs lined by endo/theli/al [within nipple] (en-dō-THĒ-lē-al) membrane, usually located around joints or at some point where skin, tendon or muscle moves over a bony prominence. Various types of inflammation of the bursae and their locations are as follows: bursitis of the knee or pre/patell/ar [before a small plate] (prē-pah-TEL-ar) bursitis, infra/patell/ar [below] (in-frah-pah-TEL-ar) bursitis, semi/membranosus [half membrane] (sem"ē-mem-brah-NŌ-sus) bursitis, medial gastrocnemius bursitis, trochanter/ic [the runner] (trō-kan-TER-ik) bursitis or bursitis of the hip, ilio/pectine/al [ilium comb] (il"ē-ō-pek-TIN-ē-al) bursitis (also in the hip), ischio/glute/al [hip buttock] (is"kē-ō-GLŪ-tē-al) bursitis also known as weaver's bottom. Bursitis of the spine, of the shoulder or sub/delt/oid [below triangle] (sub-DEL-toyd) or sub/acromi/al [tip of shoulder] sub-ah-KRŌ-mē-al) bursitis, olecranon [head or point of elbow] (ō-LEK-ra-non) or bursitis of the elbow are other areas where infection may occur.

Torti/collis [twist neck] (tor-te-KŌ-lis)[1] or wry neck is usually caused by contracture of the sternocleidomastoid muscle, associated, as a rule, with contracture of the cervic/al [neck] (SER-ve-kal) fascia and platysma muscle. Scoli/osis [curved, crooked] (skō-lē-Ō-sis) of the cervical spine may also accompany torticollis.

Inflammation of the skeletal muscles include sup/purative [under pus] (SUP-ū-ra-tive) myos/itis [muscle] (mī-ō-SĪ-tis) characterized by pus formation; nonsuppurative myositis characterized by inflammation without pus formation. There are five types of nonsuppurative myositis: dermato/myos/itis [skin muscle] (der"mah-tō-mī-ō-SĪ-tis), myositis fibrosa [fiber] (fī-BRŌ-sah), intra/muscul/ar [within muscle] (in-trah-MUS-kū-lar) fibros/itis [fiber] (fī-brō-SĪ-tis), myositis ossi/ficans [bone to make] (os-IF-i-kanz), and trichin/ous [hair (larval worm)] (TRIK-in-us) myositis.

The term muscular dys/trophies [difficult nourishment] (DIS-tro-fēz) is applied to a group of diseases usually heredit/ary [heir] (he-RED-i-ter-ē) and famili/al [family] (fah-MIL-ē-al), in which marked weakness of the muscles occurs. The best known type is called pseudo/hyper/troph/ic [false excessive nourishment] (sū"dō-hī-per-TRŌ-fik)[2] muscular dystrophy.

1. Optional pronunciation tor-te-KOL-lis

2. Optional pronunciation sū"dō-hī-per-TROF-ik

Other muscular affections are congenital myo/ton/ia *muscle tone* (mī-ō-TŌ-nē-ah) (Thomsen's disease) and my/asthenia *weakness* (mī-as-THĒ-nē-ah) gravis *heavy* (GRAV-is).

SURGERY OF MUSCLES, BURSAE, TENDONS

Operative measures on muscles, tendons or tendon sheaths are carried out for the following conditions: acute pyo/gen/ic *pus produce* (pī-ō-JEN-ik) infections of muscles, isch/em/ic *keep back blood* (is-KEM-ik)[1] myositis (Volkmann's paralysis), local myositis ossificans, inter/stiti/al *between spaces* (in-ter-STISH-al) ossi/fication *bone to make* (os"i-fi-KĀ-shun) and ossi/fying *bone to make* (OS-i-fī-ing) hemat/oma *blood* (hē-mah-TŌ-mah)[2] or rupture of muscles and tendons, sten/osis *narrow* (ste-NŌ-sis) of tendon sheaths, muscle hernia, tennis elbow, ganglion *a subcutaneous tumor, a knot* (GANG-glē-on) and trigger finger.

Procedures and indications for surgery of the bursae:

1. aspiration in simple ser/ous *whey* (SĒ-rus) effusions combined with pressure bandages
2. incision and drainage (I & D) in chronic inflammation with thick inflammatory deposits (calcium); in pyogenic infections
3. excision in chronic bursitis with thickened walls, adhesions, recurrent effusions; in bursae communicating with a joint, in tuberc/ul/ous *node small* (tū-BER-kū-lus) bursae, in large serous bursae causing functional disturbances.

Tendon surgery is performed for contractures, torn tendons or muscles, separation of tendons from bone, ruptured tendons, paralyzed tendons, joint dislocations, adhesions and thickening of tendon sheaths.

Types of procedures performed and their indications:

1. teno/tomy *tendon* (ten-OT-ō-mē) and tendon lengthening done for release of contracture
2. teno/rrhaphy (ten-OR-af-ē) is tendon suture and repair for torn muscles, separation of tendons from bone, ruptured tendons

1. Optional pronunciation is-KĒ-mik
2. Optional pronunciation hem-ah-TŌ-mah

Tendon Lengthening and Repair

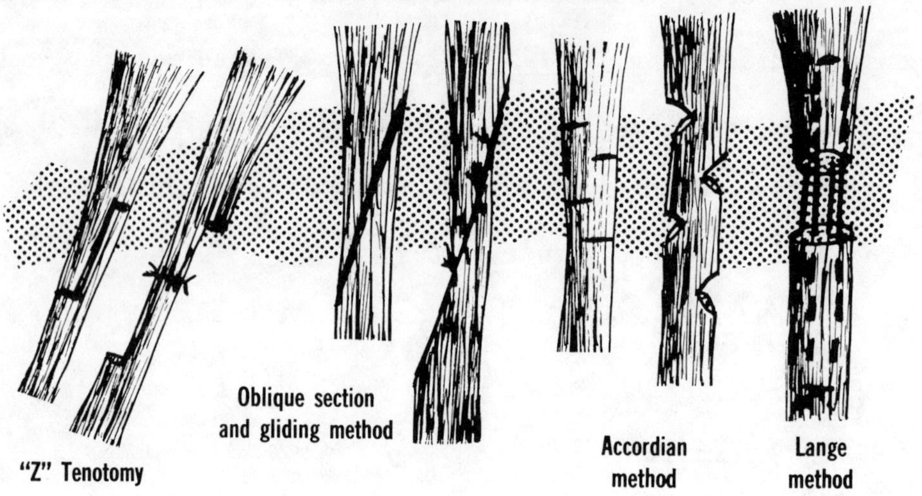

"Z" Tenotomy

Oblique section and gliding method

Accordian method

Lange method

3. tendon or muscle stripping is done for reduction of soft tissue contracture
4. <u>teno/plasty</u> (TEN-ō-plas-tē) is tendon sheath plasty for trigger finger
5. tendon graft is performed by bridging of tendon with other tendons used as grafts
6. <u>teno/lysis</u> (ten-OL-i-sis)[1] or tendon ensheathing is performed for <u>stenosing</u> (ste-NŌ-zing) <u>teno/synov/itis</u> [synovia] (ten"ō-si-nō-VĪ-tis)[2] (constriction of tendons due to <u>proli/ferative</u> [offspring / to bear] [prō-LIF-er-ah-tiv] thickening of their sheaths) and is done to allow free movement of the tendon
7. tendon transplantations are substitution for paralyzed tendons. They are done for <u>thenar</u> [palm of hand] (THĒ-nar) <u>palsy</u> [paralysis] (PAWL-zē).
8. tendon suspension is performed for dislocations
9. <u>teno/desis</u> (ten-ō-DĒ-sis)[3] is the suturing of the end of a tendon to the skeletal attachment. It is done for cases of weakness of extensor tendons.
10. <u>teno/synov/ectomy</u> (ten"ō-si-nō-VEK-tō-mē) is the removal of a tendon and its sheath.

1. Optional pronunciation tē-nō-LĪ-sis
2. Optional pronunciation tē"nō-si-nō-VĪ-tis
3. Optional pronunciation ten-OD-i-sis

Methods of Tendon Shortening

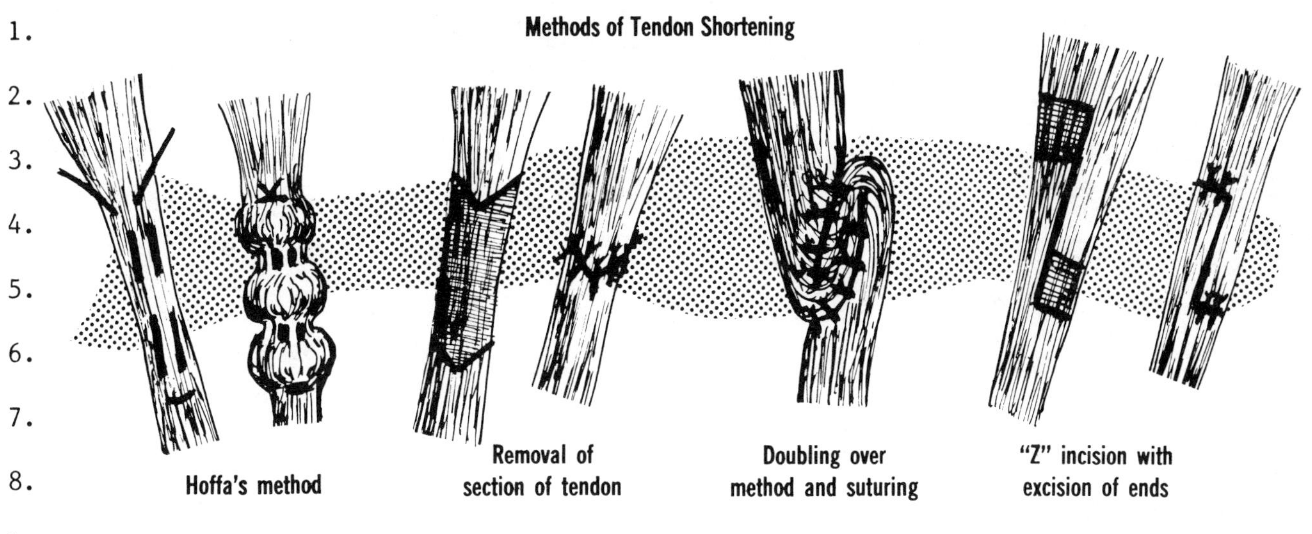

Ligament reconstruction: fascia [band] (FASH-ē-ah) lata [broad] (LAH-tah) is used as a fasci/al (FASH-ē-al) suture for reconstruction in dislocations. It is also used for reinforcement of paralyzed muscles.

Myo/plasty [muscle] (MĪ-ō-plas-tē) is the surgical repair of a muscle by free muscle graft or pedicle graft.

Myo/rrhaphy (mī-OR-ah-fē) is the suturing of a muscle.

Myo/tasis [stretching] (mī-OT-ah-sis) is the stretching of a muscle.

INDEX
CHAPTER III

PAGE	LINE	
74	12	soleus
65	20	sphincter
77	9	stenosis
78	17	stenosing
66	21	sternocleidomastoid
61	9	striated
66	17	styloglossus
76	11	subacromial
68	24	subclavius
76	11	subdeltoid
71	4	subscapularis
71	23	sublimis
63	25	superioris
72	12	supinator
76	18	suppurative
71	5	supraspinatus
65	13	temporalis
78	24	tenodesis
78	16	tenolysis
78	12	tenoplasty
77	26	tenorrhaphy
78	27	tenosynovectomy
78	17	tenosynovitis
77	24	tenotomy
73	6	tensor fasciae latae
71	7	teres
78	22	thenar palsy
74	19	tibialis
76	14	torticollis
69	11	transversalis
69	11	transversus
68	2	trapezius
66	11	triangularis
71	12	triceps
76	23	trichinous
76	8	trochanteric

PAGE	LINE	
77	18	tuberculous
71	21	ulnaris
73	19	vastus
65	28	zygomatic

CHAPTER IV
THE NERVOUS SYSTEM

The central nervous system (CNS) consists of the en/cephalon [in head] (en-SEF-ah-lon) or brain contained within the cranium [skull] (KRĀ-nē-um) and the medulla [marrow] (me-DUL-ah) spin/alis [spine] (spi-NAL-is) or spinal cord lodged in the spinal canal.

The peri/pher/al [around to bear] (peh-RIF-er-al) nervous system consists of a series of nerves by which the central nervous system is connected with the various tissues of the body. These nerves may be arranged in two groups: cerebro/ [brain] spin/al [spine] (ser"i-brō-SPĪ-nal) and sym/pathet/ic [together suffer] (sim-pah-THET-ik). The cerebrospinal nerves are 43 in number on either side: 12 cranial, attached to the brain, and 31 spinal, attached to the medulla spinalis. They are associated with the functions of the special and general senses and the volunt/ary [will] (VOL-un-tār-ē) movements of the body.

The auto/nom/ic [self law] (aw-tō-NOM-ik) nervous system transmits the impulses which regulate the movements of the viscera [organs] (VIS-er-ah), determine the caliber of the blood vessels, and control the phenomena [thing seen] (fe-NOM-i-nah) of secretion. In relation with them are two rows of central ganglia [knot (plural)] (GANG-glē-ah), situated one on either side of the middle line in front of the vertebral column. The sympathetic nerves emerging from the ganglia form three great pre/vertebr/al [before vertebra] (prē-VER-te-bral) plexuses [network] (PLEK-se-sez) which supply the thorac/ic [chest] (thō-RAS-ik), abdominal and pelvic viscera.

THE CENTRAL NERVOUS SYSTEM

The medulla spinalis or spinal cord forms the elongated, nearly cylindrical, part of the central nervous system which occupies the upper two-thirds of the vertebral canal. Above, it is continuous with the brain; below it ends in a conical extremity, the conus [cone] (KŌ-nus) medullaris [marrow] (med-ū-LAR-is), from the apex of which a delicate filament, the filum [thread] (FĪ-lum) terminale [end] (ter-min-AH-lē),

NERVE CELLS

Neuron

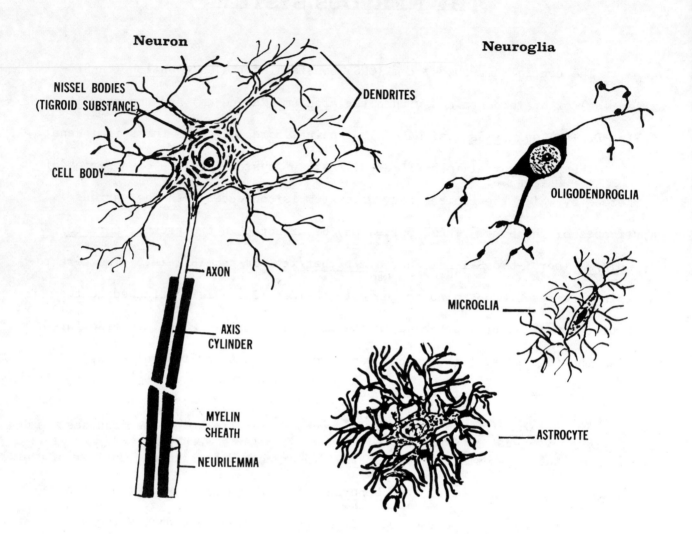

NISSEL BODIES
(TIGROID SUBSTANCE)
DENDRITES
CELL BODY
AXON
AXIS CYLINDER
MYELIN SHEATH
NEURILEMMA

Neuroglia

OLIGODENDROGLIA
MICROGLIA
ASTROCYTE

Bipolar Neurons

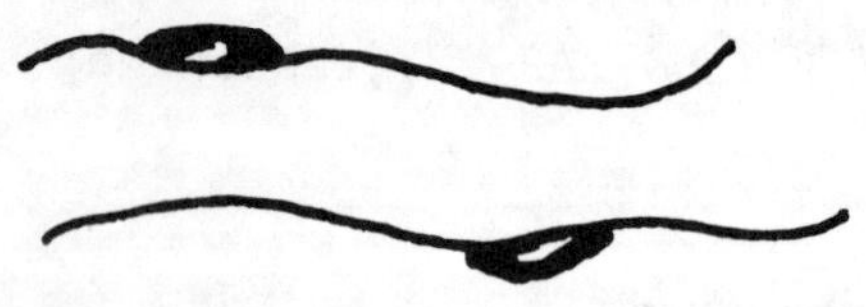

Unipolar Neuron

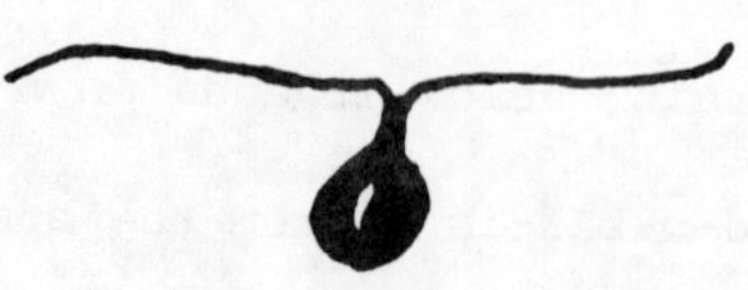

Motor "End Plate" on Skeletal Muscle Fiber

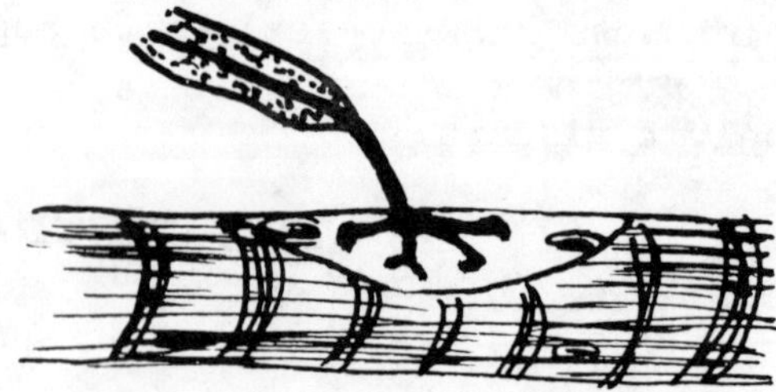

Motor Termination Upon Smooth Muscle Fiber

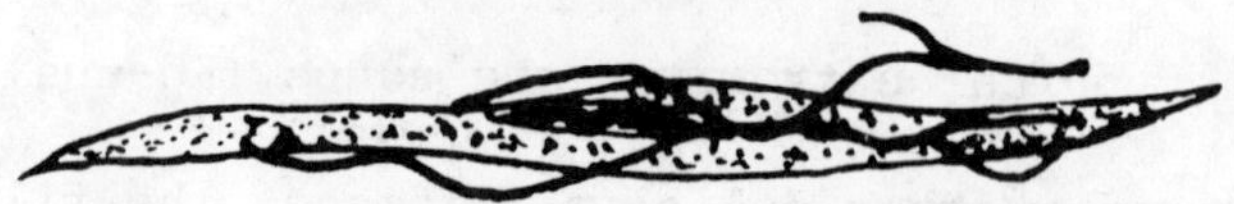

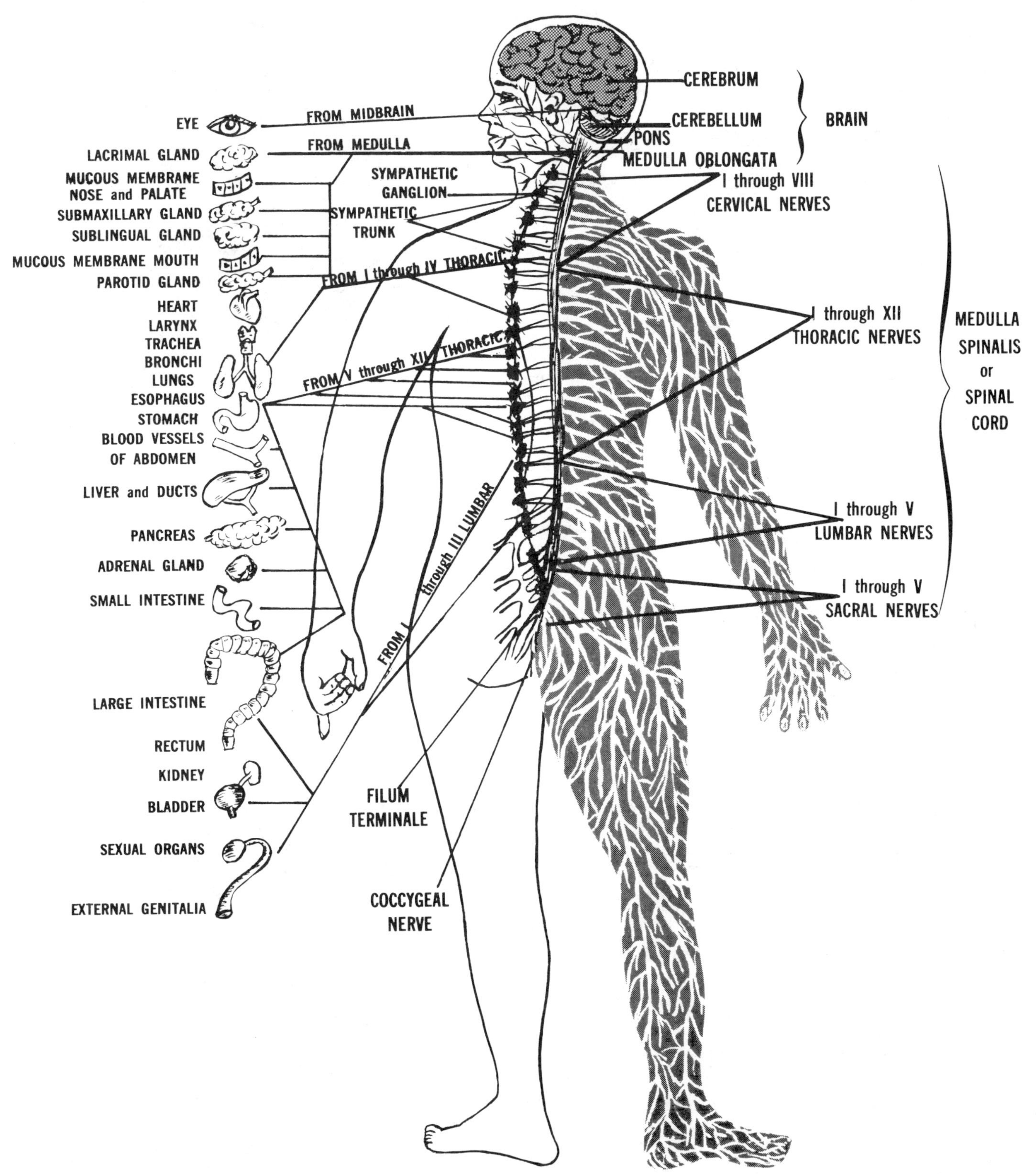
AUTONOMIC
NERVOUS SYSTEM
CENTRAL
NERVOUS SYSTEM
EYE
FROM MIDBRAIN
LACRIMAL GLAND
FROM MEDULLA
MUCOUS MEMBRANE
NOSE and PALATE
SUBMAXILLARY GLAND
SUBLINGUAL GLAND
MUCOUS MEMBRANE MOUTH
PAROTID GLAND
HEART
LARYNX
TRACHEA
BRONCHI
LUNGS
ESOPHAGUS
STOMACH
BLOOD VESSELS
OF ABDOMEN
LIVER and DUCTS
PANCREAS
ADRENAL GLAND
SMALL INTESTINE
LARGE INTESTINE
RECTUM
KIDNEY
BLADDER
SEXUAL ORGANS
EXTERNAL GENITALIA
SYMPATHETIC
GANGLION
SYMPATHETIC
TRUNK
FROM I through IV THORACIC
FROM V through XII THORACIC
FROM I through III LUMBAR
FILUM
TERMINALE
COCCYGEAL
NERVE
CEREBRUM
CEREBELLUM
PONS
MEDULLA OBLONGATA
BRAIN
I through VIII
CERVICAL NERVES
I through XII
THORACIC NERVES
MEDULLA
SPINALIS
or
SPINAL
CORD
I through V
LUMBAR NERVES
I through V
SACRAL NERVES

descends as far as the first segment of the coccyx [a cuckoo] (KOK-siks).

The medulla spinalis is en/ [in] sheathed [a case] (en-SHĒTH-d) by three protective membranes, the meninges [membrane] (me-NIN-jēz) named from without inward, the dura mater [hard mother] (DŪ-rah MĀ-ter), the arachn/oid [spider] (ah-RAK-noyd), and the pia mater [tender] (PĪ-ah MĀ-ter).

Thirty-one pairs of spinal nerves spring from the medulla spinalis. They are grouped as follows: 8 cervical, 12 thoracic, 5 lumbar, 5 sacral, 1 coccyge/al [coccyx] (kok-SIJ-ē-al).

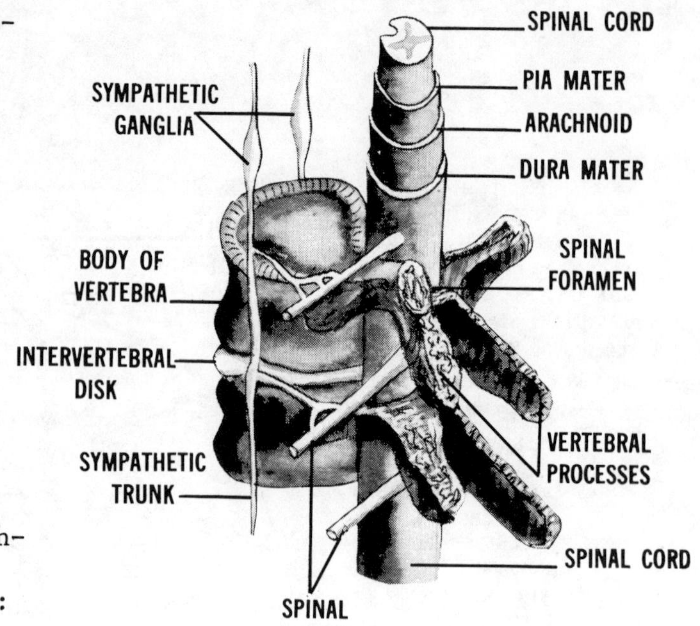

SPINAL CORD AND MENINGES

The brain is composed of the cerebrum [brain] (SER-i-brum), the cerebellum [small brain] (ser-i-BEL-um), the medulla oblongata [rather long] (ob-long-GAH-tah), and the pons [bridge] (ponz) (pons varolii[1] [var-Ō-lē-ī]).

The cerebrum is the most conspicuous portion of the brain and in man reflects the extent of his development toward intelligence. The outermost part of the cerebrum is called the cortex. It consists of gray matter folded many times, making numerous con/volutions [together to twist] (kon"ve-LŌŌ-shens) or gyri [ring or circle] (JĪ-rī), with intervening grooves, called fissures [to split] (FISH-ūrs) or sulci [trench] (SUL-sī).

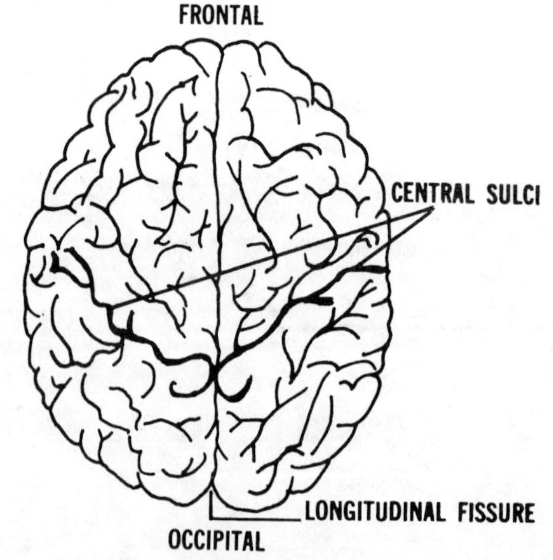

THE CEREBRUM

There are three important fissures: the lateral or sylvian (SIL-vē-an) fissure, the central or fissure of Rolando [Italian anatomist] (rō-LAN-dō) and the longitudinal

1. Named for an Italian anatomist, Constanzio Varolio, 1543-1575.

fissure. The cerebrum presents two hemispheres, separated from each other by the great longitudinal fissure. At the bottom of this cleft is white matter composed of fibers crossing between the two hemispheres. This crossing is called the corpus [body] (KOR-pus) callosum [hard] (kal-LŌ-sum).

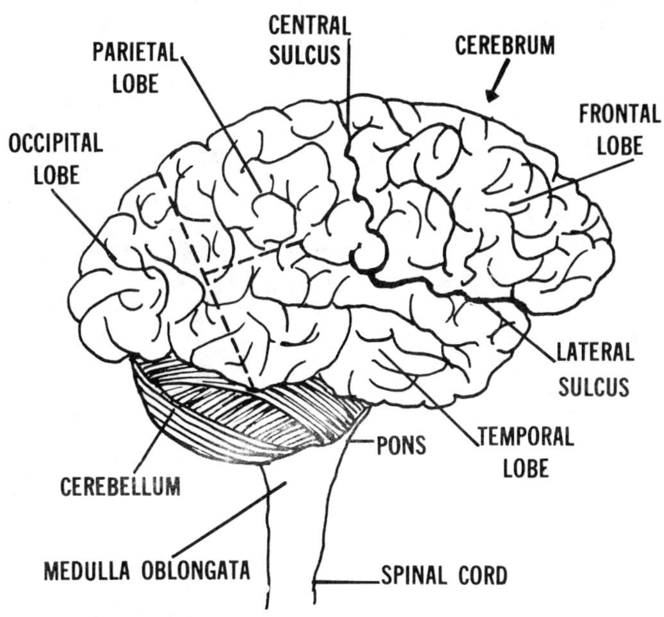

LOBES OF THE BRAIN

The cerebrum being bilateral there are a total of ten lobes. These are the frontal, pariet/al [wall] (pah-RĪ-i-tal), occipit/al [back of head] (ok-SIP-i-tal), temporal and the insula [island] (IN-se-lah).

There are four ventricles in the brain. The first and second ventricles form the lateral ventricle. The fourth ventricle is also called the aque/ [water] duct [canal] (AK-we-duct) of Sylvius[1] or aquae/ductus (ak"we-DUK-tes) cerebri (SER-i-brī).

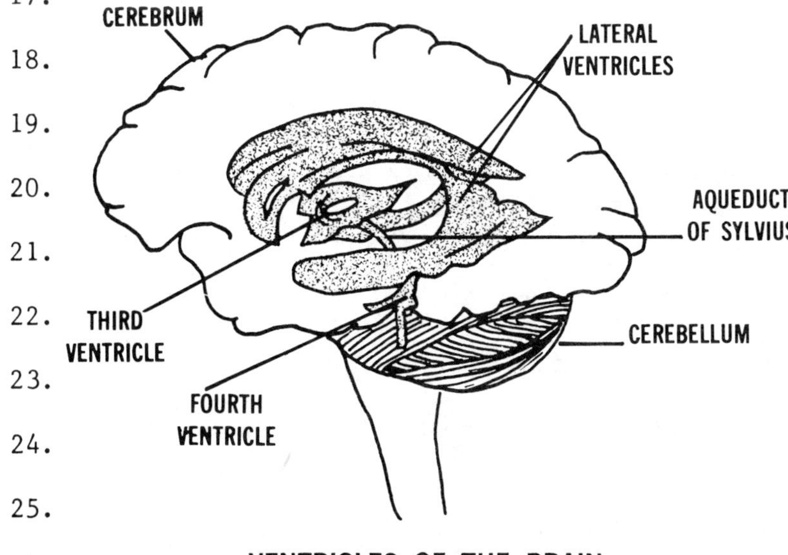

VENTRICLES OF THE BRAIN

The lateral ventricle is connected to the third ventricle by the foramina[2] [opening] (fo-RĀ-mi-nah) of Monro[3] (foramina inter/ventric/ulares [between belly small] [in"ter-ven-trik-u-LAR-is]).

The cerebellum lies below the cerebrum in the posterior region of the skull cavity. It consists, like the cerebrum, of two halves, known as hemispheres, and a central portion, the vermis [worm] (VER-mis).

The cerebellum is connected to the brain stem by three paired bands of white

1. Named for Francois de la Boe Sylvius, French anatomist, 1614-1672.
2. Optional pronunciation fo-RAM-i-nah
3. Alexander Monro an English surgeon, 1737-1817

fibers called ped/uncles [foot small] (pe-DUNG-kls) or brachia [arm (plural)] (BRĀ-kē-ah): the brachium (BRĀ-kē-um) con/junctivum [with joining, yoke] (kon"junk-TĪ-vum), the brachium pontis [bridge] (PON-tes) and the resti/form [rope] (RES-te-form) body. The substance of the cerebellum consists of both gray and white matter.

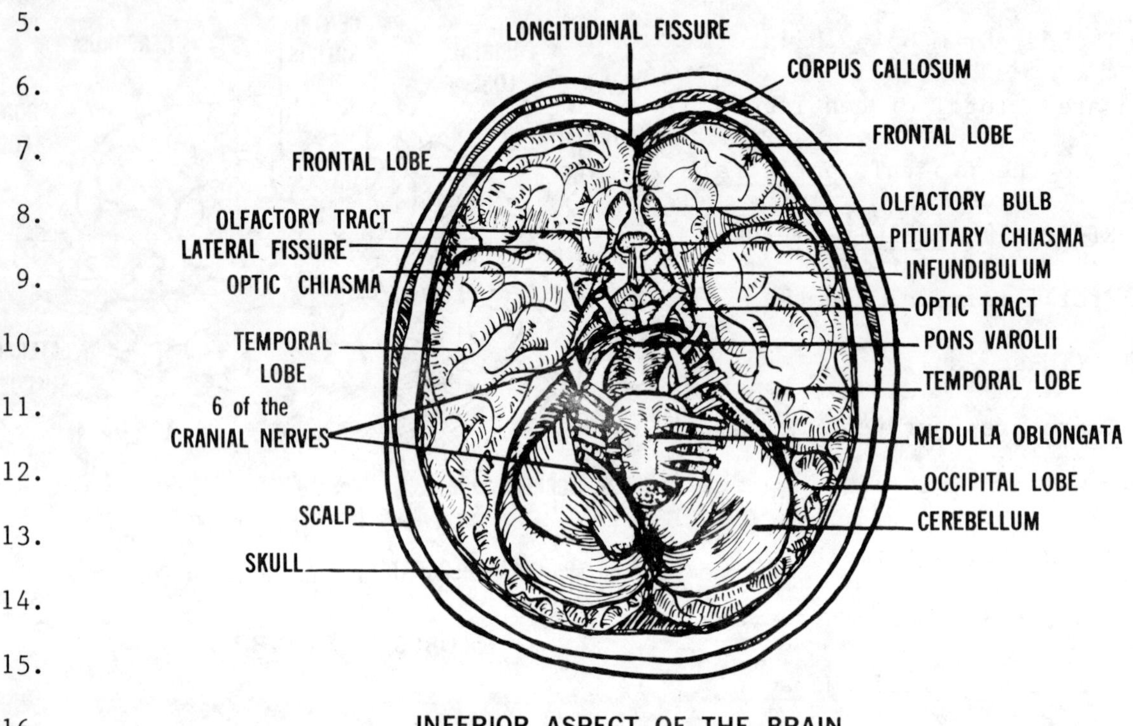

INFERIOR ASPECT OF THE BRAIN

The medulla oblongata is a mass of white and gray matter which connects the pons above with the spinal cord below. It is about an inch in length, and is broader above, where it is continuous with the pons.

The functions of the cerebrum and the cerebellum are not of vital importance, so that death does not instantly follow the removal or destruction of these portions of the brain. But the functions of the medulla oblongata are so necessary that instant death is the result of its destruction. It governs those involuntary movements which constitute the acts of breathing and heart beat.

The pons is composed mostly of fibers passing between the other three parts of the brain. The pons lies in front of the cerebellum.

Through the entire length of the cord extends a narrow central canal which is continued anteriorly into the brain where in four locations it widens out to form the ventricles of the brain. The central canal and ventricles, as well as the space between the arachnoid and the pia mater, are filled with a fluid known as the cerebrospinal fluid. It serves as a support and a cushion for the soft structures of the central nervous system.

THE AUTONOMIC NERVOUS SYSTEM

While separate and distinct in its anatomy and physio/logy (nature) (fiz-ē-OL-ō-jē), the autonomic system is an integral part of the nervous mechanism of the body and closely related with the cerebrospinal system. It comprises a chain of ganglia running from the brain to the coccyx, with connecting fibers to the cord and neurons (nerve cells) (NŪ-rons) that reach out to various outlying parts. The ganglia are the prominent portions, and particularly the ones situated on each side of the vertebral column. The autonomic nervous system has two divisions: the sympathetic and the para/sym/pathet/ic (beyond with suffer) (par"ah-sim-pah-THET-ik). The functions of these two divisions are opposite and antagonistic in effect. For example, the parasympathetic (the cranial part) slows the heart, the sympathetic accelerates its action.

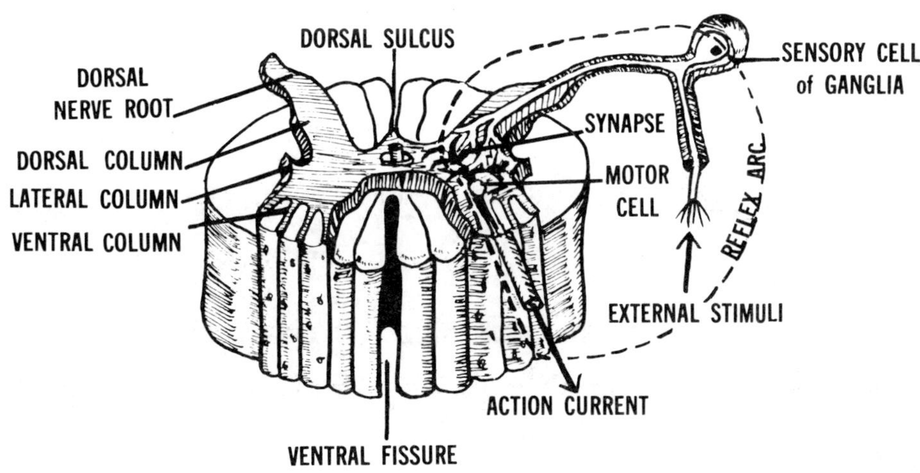

SPINAL CORD (cross section)

THE CRANIAL NERVES

NUMBER	NAME	FUNCTION
I	olfact/ory (ol-FAK-tō-rē) *to smell*	sense of smell
II	opt/ic (OP-tik) *eye*	sense of sight
III	oculo/motor (ok"ū-lō-MŌ-ter) *eye mover*	motor to eye muscles
IV	trochle/ar (TRŌ-klē-ar)[1] *pulley*	motor to eye muscles
V	tri/gemin/al (trī-JEM-i-nal) *three twin*	chief sensory nerve of face and head
VI	ab/ducent (ab-DŪ-sent) *away from to draw*	motor to eye muscle
VII	facial	mixed nerve; motor to face muscles; sensory to tongue
VIII	acoust/ic (ah-KOOS-tik) or audit/ory (AW-de-tō-rē) *hearing* / *hearing*	sense of hearing and equilibrium
IX	glosso/pharynge/al (glos"ō-fah-RIN-jē-al) *tongue pharynx*	sensory to mucous membrane of mouth and tongue, motor to pharyngeal muscles
X	vagus (VĀ-gus) or pneumo/gastr/ic (nū-mō-GAS-trik) *wandering* / *lungs stomach*	sensory and motor to vocal organs and lungs, motor to pharynx, esophagus, stomach and heart. Inhibits action of heart.
XI	spinal accessory	motor to palate (PAL-at), neck muscles and trapezius (trah-PĒ-zē-us) *palate: roof of mouth; trapezius: table or counter*
XII	hypo/gloss/al (hī-pō-GLOS-al) *below tongue*	motor to muscles of tongue and hy/oid (HĪ-oyd) bone *hy/oid: letter 'U'*

DISEASES AND ANOMALIES

The symptoms and signs of disease of the nervous system fall into three groups:

1. Irritative, due to excessive stimulation of the functions of various parts of the nervous system. Among irritative symptoms are convulsions, muscular twitchings, spasms, tremors, exaggerated sensibility (hyper/esthesia (hī"per-es-THĒ-zē-ah), and mental excitement.
   hyper: excessive; esthesia: feeling

1. Optional pronunciation TROK-lē-ar

2. Para/lyt/ic *beyond to loosen* (par-ah-LIT-ik), caused by cessation of functions of various parts of the nervous system. Paralytic symptoms include paralysis of various portions of the body, stupor and coma, mental deterioration, lack of coordination, certain types of blindness and deafness, loss of the sense of touch and of the sensations of pain and temperature, a/trophy *lack* (AT-rof-ē) of muscles, etc.

3. Increased pressure within the cranial cavity. This increased pressure causes headache, projectile vomiting, swelling of the head of the optic nerve as seen with the ophthalmo/scope *eye* (of-THAL-mō-skōp), and in some cases, irritative or paralytic symptoms.

A reflex is the involuntary response of an individual to a given type of stimulation applied to a specific area. Generally speaking, two types of reflexes are tested during a physical examination:

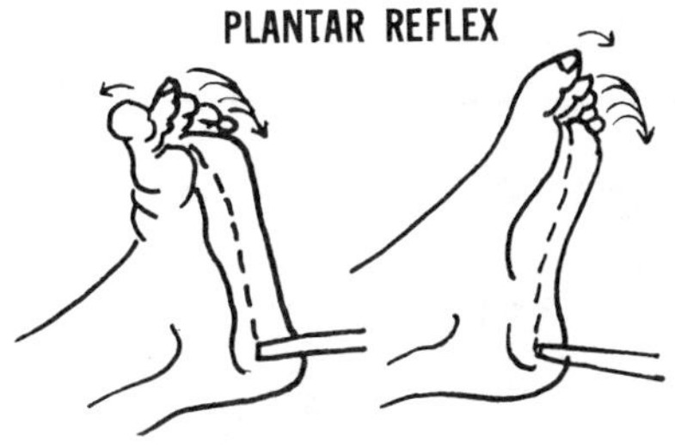

PLANTAR REFLEX

BABINSKI REFLEX

NORMAL REFLEX

1. Deep reflexes, which consist of contraction of a group of muscles in response to a light blow over a muscle or tendon. The most frequently tested deep reflexes are: patell/ar *kneepan* (pah-TEL-ar) reflex or knee jerk; Achilles (ah-KIL-ēz) reflex or ankle jerk; the biceps and triceps reflexes; and the jaw or masseter *masticator* (MAS-i-ter) reflex.

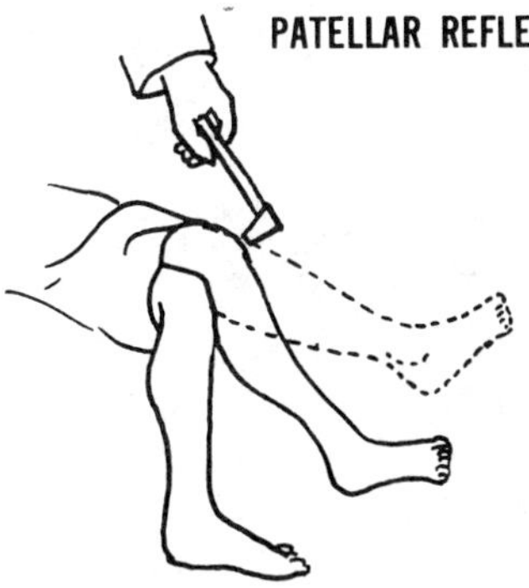

PATELLAR REFLEX

2. Superficial reflexes consist of certain responses to touching, stroking, or pinching the surface of the body in various areas. The most frequently tested superficial reflexes are: the plant/ar *sole of foot* (PLAN-tar) reflex, the cremaster/ic *to suspend* (krē-mas-TER-ik) reflex, the abdominal reflex, and the corne/al *horny* (KOR-nē-al) reflex.

Besides these and similar tests, which are part of the physical examination, other important tests are examination of the cerebrospinal fluid and the use of x-ray. The ventricles of the brain may be visualized indirectly by replacing some of the cerebrospinal fluid with air (ventric/ulo/graphy *belly small* [ven-trik-ū-LOG-rah-fē] or encephalo/graphy *brain* [en-sef-ah-LOG-rah-fē]) and the position of a block in the spinal cord may be determined by the injection of a radio-opaque *ray shady* (rā-dē"ō-ō-PĀK) oil (pant/opaque *all shady* [pant-ō-PĀK]) into the spinal canal (myelo/gram *marrow* [MĪ-el-ō-gram]). The electro/encephalo/graph *amber, electricity* (ē-lek"trō-en-SEF-ah-lō-graf) is used to record brain waves to determine the site of lesions and in the study and diagnosis of epi/lepsy *on* (EP-i-lep-sē). An electro/myo/gram *muscle* (ē-lek"trō-MĪ-ō-gram) is a tracing which records the electric response in a contracting muscle. It may be used to denote nerve injury from the spinal cord.

The cerebr/al *brain* (SER-i-bral) cortex *rind* (KOR-teks) is concerned with thought, reason, memory, emotion, the conscious perception of all types of sensation and with the initiation of voluntary actions. Disease of this area of the brain results in disturbance of these functions, either of an irritative or paralytic nature. The principal factors which cause disease are trauma *wound* (TRAW-mah), arterio/sclerosis *artery hardening* (ar-tē"rē-ō-skle-RŌ-sis), syphilis (SIF-i-lis) and tumors.

The portion of the interbrain (the optic thalamus *chamber, bedroom* [THAL-ah-mus] which is concerned with sensation is seldom diseased but other portions of the interbrain are frequently affected by arteriosclerosis or the epidemic type of encephal/itis *brain* (en-sef"ah-LĪ-tis). Such a condition is known as parkinson/ism[1] (PAR-kin-sun-izm) and, when it is caused by arteriosclerosis, as Parkinson's[2] (PAR-kin-sunz) disease or paralysis agitans *restless* (AJ-i-tans). Irritable phenomena due to disease of the interbrain occur in chorea *dance* (kō-RĒ-ah) and consist of purposeless movements of the facial muscles, arms and hands, and sometimes of the feet and legs.

The portion of the white matter that is most frequently attacked by disease

1. A group of nervous conditions resembling and including Parkinson's disease.
2. Named after the English physician, James Parkinson, 1755-1824.

is the internal capsule whose fibers in the anterior portion have to do with the performance of voluntary movement. The fibers in the posterior portion of the internal capsule have to do with the conscious perception of sensation. Thus, a lesion in the anterior portion of the capsule on one side will cause a paralysis of the entire opposite side of the body -- face, arm and leg -- a condition known as hemi/plegia [half] (hem-ē-PLĒ-jē-ah). A lesion in the posterior portion of the capsule, which occurs less commonly, will cause loss of sensation in the opposite side of the body, a condition called hemi/an/esthesia [lack feeling] (hem"ē-an-es-THĒ-zē-ah). The most common cause of disease in this region of the brain is hemo/rrhage [blood] (HEM-or-ij) into the anterior portion of the capsule due to rupture of the lentic/ulo/striate [lens small striped] (len-tik"ū-lō-STRĪ-āt) branch of the middle cerebral artery, in patients with high blood pressure. This condition, known as "stroke" or apo/plexy [from] (AP-ō-plek-sē), occurs with dramatic suddenness. A lesion with similar effects may be due to thromb/osis [clot] (throm-BŌ-sis) of the middle cerebral artery, or one of its branches, with the formation of an infarct [to stuff into] (IN-farkt) in the region of the internal capsule. Lesions of the internal capsule may also result from pressure due to tumors or ab/scesses [away to go] (AB-ses-sez).

The cerebellum is concerned principally with the maintenance of equilibrium and with the coordination of muscular acts. If cerebell/ar [small brain] (ser-i-BEL-ar) disease occurs only on one side, the incoordination is limited to the side of the lesion. The common causes of cerebellar disease are tumors, abscesses, arteriosclerosis, and certain heredit/ary [heir] (he-RED-i-ter-ē) and famili/al [family] (fah-MIL-ē-al) diseases.

In the brain stem, comprising the midbrain, pons, and medulla oblongata, small lesions are apt to cause serious and widespread manifestations. In addition, in the medulla oblongata is situated the vital re/spirat/ory [again to breathe][1] (re-SPĪ-rah-tō-rē) center, a lesion of which will cause cessation of breathing and sudden death. Large lesions in the midbrain or pons may cause paralysis of both arms and legs (quadri/plegia [four] [kwod-re-PLĒ-jē-ah]). Lesions of the brain stem are most

1. Optional pronunciation RES-pi-rah-tō-rē

commonly due to pressure by tumors and to epidemic encephalitis, but may also be due to rupture or thrombosis of vessels or to trauma.

The important diseases of the meninges are inflammatory ones. Inflammation of the meninges is called mening/itis [membrane] (men-in-JĪ-tis). The important organisms which cause meningitis are the meningo/coccus [berry] (me-ning"gō-KOK-us), pneumo/coccus [lung] (nū-mō-KOK-us), strepto/coccus [twist] (strep-tō-KOK-us), staphylo/coccus [bunch of grapes] (staf"il-ō-KOK-kus), hemo/philus[1] [blood, to love] (hē-MOF-i-lus) influenzae [influence] (in-flū-EN-zē), tuber/cle [node, small] (TŪ-ber-kl) bacillus [rod, staff] (bah-SIL-us), the virus [poison] (VĪ-rus) of lympho/cyt/ic [water, cell] (limf-o-SIT-ik) meningitis, and the spiro/cheta [coil, hair] (spī-rō-KĒ-tah) pallida [pale] (PAL-i-dah) of syphilis.

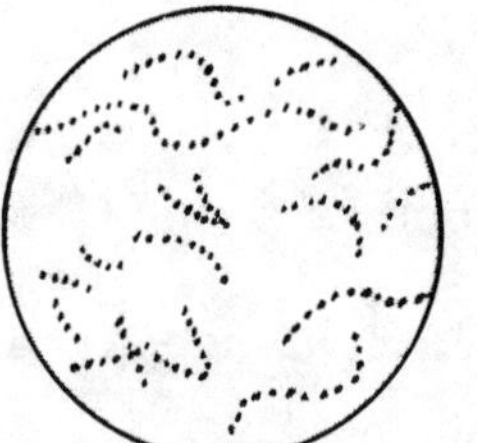

STREPTOCOCCI

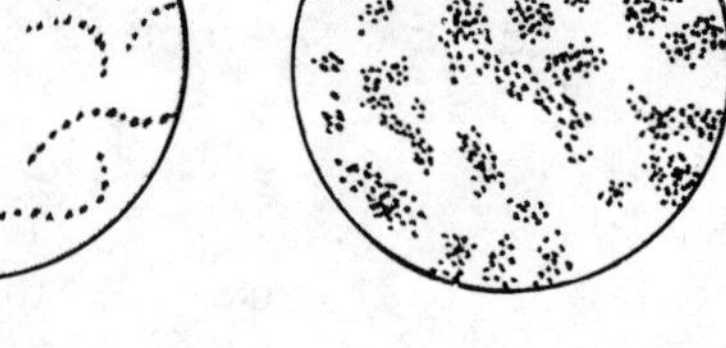

STAPHYLOCCI

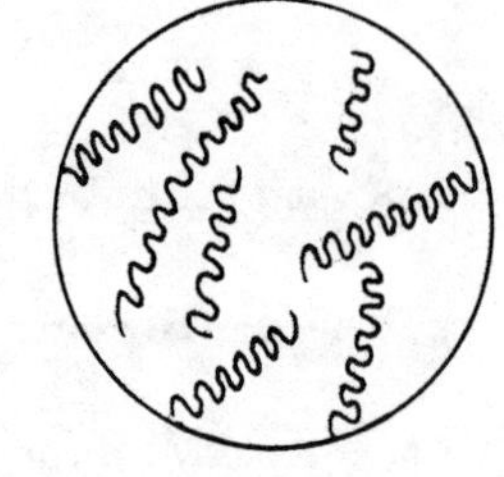

TRIPONEMA PALLIDUM OF SYPHILIS (SPIROCHETES)

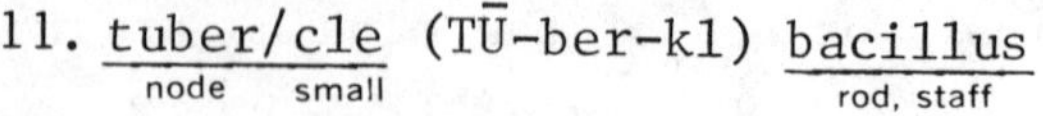

Abscess of the brain is caused by the organisms which cause abscesses in other parts of the body, most commonly the staphylococcus.

Tumors within the skull may be primary or meta/static [beyond, to stand] (met-ah-STAT-ik).

Epilepsy is a chronic disease characterized by attacks of brief or prolonged loss of consciousness, frequently accompanied by convulsions. Two types of attacks are recognized: major attacks or grand [great] mal [evil] (grahn mahl), and minor attacks or petit [small] mal (pe-TĒ mahl).

The common causes of disease of the spinal cord are trauma, tumors, infections of the substance of the cord itself or of neighboring structures and nutritional deficiency. The spinal cord may be involved in certain specific infectious diseases such as polio/myel/itis [gray, marrow] (pō"lē-ō-mī-el-Ī-tis) and syphilis, and degenerative lesions may occur in pernici/ous [destructive] (per-NISH-us) an/emia [lack, blood] (ah-NĒ-mē-ah) and in a number of familial diseases and conditions of obscure cause.

Tumors within the spinal canal may arise within the substance of the cord itself, from the meninges, or from the bone or peri/osteum [around, bone] (per-ē-OS-tē-um) of

1. Optional pronunciation hē-mō-FIL-us

the vertebrae. Tumors give rise to symptoms by destroying or compressing the spinal cord or the roots of the spinal nerves in the region of the tumor.

The most common causes of disease of the 12 cranial nerves are "pinching" by ex/udate [out sweat] (EKS-ū-dāt) due to meningitis about the brain stem and pressure upon them by brain tumors.

The most common cause of disease of individual peripheral nerves is trauma; they may be severed or torn by various types of violence, such as gunshot and stab wounds, injuries sustained in automobile accidents, etc. Individual nerves, especially the uln/ar [elbow] (UL-nar) nerve in the arm may be attacked by leprosy [scaly] (LEP-ro-sē).

Poly/neur/itis [many nerve] (pol"ē-nū-RĪ-tis), otherwise known as multiple neuritis or peripheral neuritis, is a disease characterized patho/log/ically [disease study of] (path-ō-LOJ-i-kal-ē) by widespread degenerative changes of peripheral nerves throughout the body, and clinically by muscular weakness, sym/metr/ical [with measure] (si-MET-re-kal) flacc/id [weak] (FLAK-sid) paralysis, and tenderness of muscles. The most frequent cause of poly-neuritis is nutritional deficiency. There are other causes, however. It may be due to chemical agents or to the toxin [poison] (TOK-sin) of diphtheria [leather, membrane] (dif-THĒ-rē-ah), or perhaps to specific involvement of the nerves or nerve roots by one or more filtr/able [to strain] (FIL-tra-bl) viruses.

The term neur/algia [nerve] (nū-RAL-jē-ah) refers to the presence of pain over the course of a nerve or over its cutane/ous [skin] (kyo͞o-TĀ-nē-us) distribution. The most common cause is pressure upon the nerve or its roots by such conditions as aneurisms[1] [a widening] (AN-ū-rizms), syphilit/ic (sif-i-LIT-ik) meningitis and hyper/troph/ic [excessive] (hī-per-TRŌ-fik)[2] arthr/itis [joint] (ar-THRĪ-tis); sometimes focal infection is apparently responsible. In many instances, no cause can be found. The most common types are trigeminal neuralgia, inter/cost/al [between rib] (in-ter-KOS-tal) neuralgia, and sciat/ic [hip joint] (sī-AT-ik) neuralgia. Trigeminal neuralgia is also known as tic [spasm] (tik) douloureux [painful] (do͞o-lo͞o-RŌ).

1. The older spelling but still correct is "aneurysm."

2. Optional pronunciation hī-per-TROF-ik

Localized portions of the autonomic nervous system may be affected by organic disease with characteristic symptoms resulting. Thus, a tumor in the neck may compress the superior cervical ganglion (sympathetic) and cause constriction of the pupil, drooping of the eyelid, and flushing of one side of the face (Horner's syn/drome [together a running] [SIN-drōm]); exudate around the communicating branches to the sympathetic ganglia, such as occurs in tabes [a wasting away] (TĀ-bēz) dors/alis [back] (dor-SAL-is), may irritate these fibers and cause violent painful spasms of the stomach and intestines.

SURGERY OF THE CRANIUM AND BRAIN

The covering of the skull consists of five distinct layers:

1. skin
2. superficial fascia
3. galea [helmet] (GĀ-lē-ah) apo/neurotica [from / sinew, tendon] (ap"o-nū-ROT-ik-ah), the tendin/ous [to stretch] (TEN-di-nus) expansion of the occipito/front/alis [back of head / forehead] (ok-sip"i-tō-fron-TAL-is) muscle
4. loose areol/ar [space] (ah-RĒ-ō-lar) tissue
5. peri/cranium [around / skull] (per-ē-KRĀ-nē-um) or peri/oste/al [bone] (per-ē-OS-tē-al) layer

SUBCUTANEOUS TISSUE
GALEA APONEUROTICA
PERICRANIUM
CRANIAL BONE
DURA MATER
ARACHNOID
PIA MATER
SUPERIOR SAGITTAL SINUS
BRAIN

DIAGRAMMATIC SECTION OF SCALP

Fractures of the skull: Linear fractures or more extensive fractures of the skull with displacement of fragments, present a surgical problem only when they are complicated with intra/crani/al [inside / skull] (in-trah-KRĀ-nē-al) hemorrhage, when foreign material may be driven into the fragment lines or when the fractures are compound.

Depressed fractures: the majority of these fractures require operative repair by piecemeal or bloc removal of bone and suture of the dura [hard] (DŪ-rah) if it has been lacerated. The surgery is known as decompression, suture of dura mater.

Methods used for control of brain hemorrhage:

1. Silver clip of Cushing used and left in place.
2. Electro/coagul/ation [electricity, to curdle] (ē-lek"trō-kō-ag-ū-LĀ-shun)
3. Small muscle stamps placed on venous bleeders.
4. Use of spongy, porous foam such as gel/foam [congeal] (JEL-fōm) or oxidized [to combine with oxygen] cellul/ose [little cell] (SEL-ū-lōs).

Types of grafts used to cover dural defects:

1. temporal fascia
2. fascia lata from the thigh
3. amniot/ic [lamb] (am-nē-OT-ik) membrane
4. tantalum foil
5. fibrin film

If bone fragments cannot be replaced to overcome a skull defect a non-reactive metal plate such as tantalum or acryl/ic[1] (ah-KRIL-ik) plastic can be used to repair the defect.

For middle meninge/al [membrane] (me-NIN-jē-al) hemorrhage which results from tearing of the meningeal artery a sub/tempor/al [below, temple] (sub-TEM-por-al) decompression is performed.

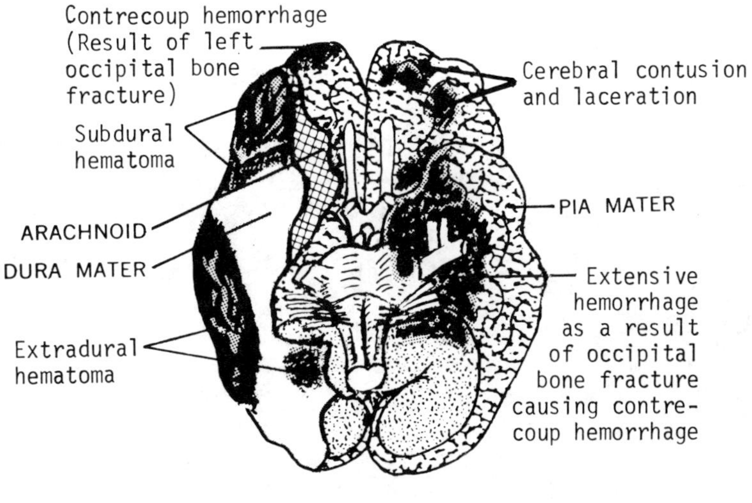

BRAIN INJURIES

For sub/dur/al [hard] (sub-DŪ-ral) hemat/omas [blood] (hē-mah-TŌ-mahs) drainage of the subdural space is performed with cranio/tomy [skull]

1. Often used incorrectly as a noun.

(krā-nē-OT-ō-mē) and evacuation of the hematoma.

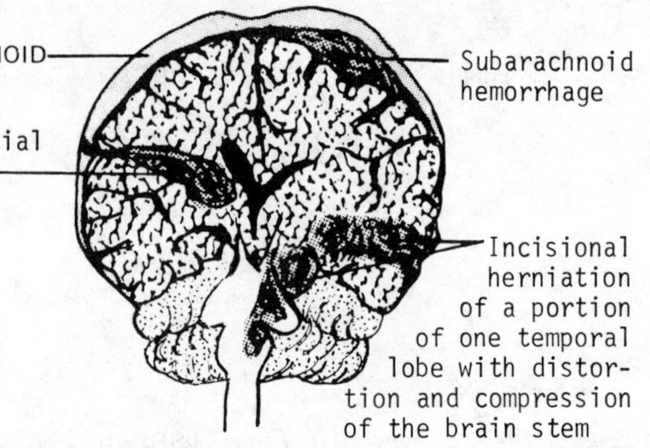

Ligation of the carotid (to put to sleep) (kah-ROT-id) artery and intracranial clipping or ligation of aneurism is performed for sub/arachn/oid (spider) (sub-ah-RAK-noyd) hemorrhage from ruptured aneurism of an intracranial artery.

Intracranial hemorrhages (bleeding which occurs in the brain substance itself) may require craniotomy and evacuation of the clot.

Infection:

1. Superficial infections require only simple drainage to evacuate infected material and allow cleansing.
2. Osteo/myel/itis (bone marrow) (os"tē-ō-mī-el-Ī-tis) of the skull requires radical removal of all infected bone.
3. Brain abscesses are treated by
    a. the closed method (drainage of abscess)
    b. the open method (excision of lesion and drainage)
    c. complete ex/tirp/ation (out root) (eks-tur-PĀ-shun) which is a more dangerous procedure because of the danger of rupture of the abscess with the complication of a spread of infection.

Tumors of the skull:

1. Benign tumors:
    a. oste/omas (bone) (os-tē-Ō-mahs)--bloc removal of the bone and repair of the skull defect with tantalum or acrylic plastic plate.
    b. hem/angi/omas (blood vessel) (hē-man-jē-Ō-mahs) may be single or multiple. Bloc removal of bone in single lesions.

c. epi/derm/oid [on skin] (ep-i-DER-moyd) tumors are of congenital character. Bloc removal or e/nucle/ation [out kernel] (ē-nū-klē-Ā-shun) of the contents of the cavity.

d. meningi/omas [membrane] (men-in-jē-Ō-mahs)--craniotomy with excision of meningioma and intracranial extension of the tumor.

2. Malignant tumors: Metastatic tumors may involve the skull. Operation is seldom indicated in such lesions.

Brain tumors:

Methods of radio/graph/ic [ray to record] (rā"dē-ō-GRAF-ik) diagnosis:

1. Cerebral angio/graphy [vessel] (an-jē-OG-rah-fē) is the injection of a contrast medium into the common carotid or vertebral artery which demonstrates the cerebral blood vessels in the x-rays and may detect brain tumors with specific vascular patterns.

2. Encephalography and pneumo/encephalo/graphy [air brain] (nū"mō-en-sef-ah-LOG-rah-fē) are the introduction of air or oxygen into the spaces normally occupied by the cerebrospinal fluid through a needle in the lumbar subarachnoid space. Immediately following this x-rays are taken in various planes to demonstrate the location of the lesion.

3. Pneumo/ventric/ulo/graphy [air belly small] (nū"mō-ven-trik-ū-LOG-rah-fē) is done when there is an appreciable increase in intracranial pressure or where a posterior fossa tumor is suspected. In this procedure air is introduced directly into the ventricles through burr holes in the skull.

4. Radio/encephalo/gram (rā"dē-ō-en-SEF-ah-lō-gram), radio/iso/tope [equal place] (rā"dē-ō-Ī-sō-tōp) uptake study is the injection of radio/iodine (rā"dē-ō-Ī-ō-dīn) tagged human serum albumin [white] (al-BŪ-min) to detect brain tumors or determine their localization. After 24 hours a systemic scanning of the skull is done with a radiation detector.

The surgery performed for removal of brain tumors is craniotomy with resection of tumor (opening into skull, osteo/plast/ic *(to form)* [os"tē-ō-PLAS-tik] flap for operative exposure above the tentorium *(tent)* [ten-TŌ-rē-um], and removal of tumor).

Types of scalp incisions for intracranial operations: temporal, parietal, occipital, frontal, occipital-posterior fossa. Tumors which lie below the tentorium are approached through a sub/occipit/al (sub-ok-SIP-i-tal) crani/ectomy (krā-nē-EK-tō-mē).

For internal hydro/cephalus *(water, head)* (hī-drō-SEF-ah-lus), obstructive, noncommunicating, a ventric/ulo/cisterno/stomy *(belly, small, cistern)* (ven-trik"ū-lō-sis"ter-NOS-tō-mē) is performed which consists of shunting cerebrospinal fluid from the lateral ventricle to the cisterna *(cistern)* (sis-TER-nah) magna *(great)* (MAG-nah) by means of a plastic catheter; or a ventric/ulo/-uretero/stomy *(ureter)* (ven"trik-ū-lō-ū-rē"ter-OS-tō-mē) may be performed which is a shunting of the cerebrospinal fluid from the lateral ventricle of the brain into the upper end of the ureter after a nephr/ectomy *(kidney)* (nef-REK-tō-mē) has been performed.

Pallido/tomy *(globus pallidus)* (pal-i-DOT-ō-mē) or thalamo/tomy *(a bed, bedroom)* (thal-ah-MOT-o-me) by injection of alcohol into the globus *(a sphere)* (GLŌ-bus) pallidus *(pale)* (PAL-i-dus) or ventro/later/al *(side)* (ven-trō-LAT-er-al) nucleus *(kernel, nut)* (NU-klē-us) of the thalamus is done in Parkinson's disease.

Pre/front/al *(before, forehead)* (prē-FRON-tal) lobo/tomy *(lobe)* ((lō-BOT-ō-mē) or leuco/tomy *(white)* (lū-KOT-ō-mē) is a unilateral or bilateral transection of the white matter of the frontal bones in the plane of the coron/al *(crown)* (kō-RŌ-nal) suture and is performed for a psych/osis *(mind)* (sī-KŌ-sis) of chronic agitated depression.

SURGERY OF THE AUTONOMIC NERVOUS SYSTEM

Peri/arteri/al *(around, artery)* (per-ē-ar-TĒ-rē-al) sym/path/ectomy *(with, suffer)* (sim"pah-THEK-tō-mē) in the cervical portion of the sympathetic chain is performed for de/nerv/ation *(from, nerve)* (dē-ner-VĀ-shun) of the carotid sinus in cases of irritable carotid body resulting in a/sy/stole[1] *(not, with, contraction)* (ah-SIS-tō-lē), a fall in blood pressure or a change in cerebral circulation.

1. Optional pronunciation ā-SIS-tō-lē

When pain is intolerable and cannot be relieved by removal of its cause, it is sometimes necessary to divide the pathways in the nervous system which conduct the pain in order to make life bearable for the patient. Various procedures performed are as follows:

1. Cervico/thorac/ic *neck chest* (ser"ve-kō-thō-RAS-ik) sympathectomy is done for relief of angina *quinsy* (AN-ji-nah) pectoris *breast bone* (PEK-to-ris)[1]. It is also performed for treatment of severe types of hyper/hidr/osis *above sweat* (hī"per-hi-DRŌ-sis) and caus/algia *heat* (kaw-ZAL-jē-ah).

2. Thoracic sympathectomy and vag/ectomy *wandering* (vā-GEK-tō-mē) are done to denervate the upper extremity, the heart and the splanchn/ic *viscera* (SPLANK-nik) bed, for relief of abdominal pain of visceral origin.

3. Supra/diaphragmat/ic *above* (sū"prah-dī-ah-frag-MAT-ik) splanchnic/ectomy (splank-ne-SEK-tō-mē) is performed for relief of hypertension and hypertensive cardio/vascul/ar *heart vessel* (kar"dē-ō-VAS-cū-lar) disease.

4. Lumbar sympathectomy is performed for denervation of vessels in the lower extremities to inhibit vaso/con/striction *vessel together to draw* (vas"ō-kon-STRIK-shun) in the presence or absence of known vascular disease and for relief of hyperhidrosis. It may be indicated in certain motility disorders of the left colon.

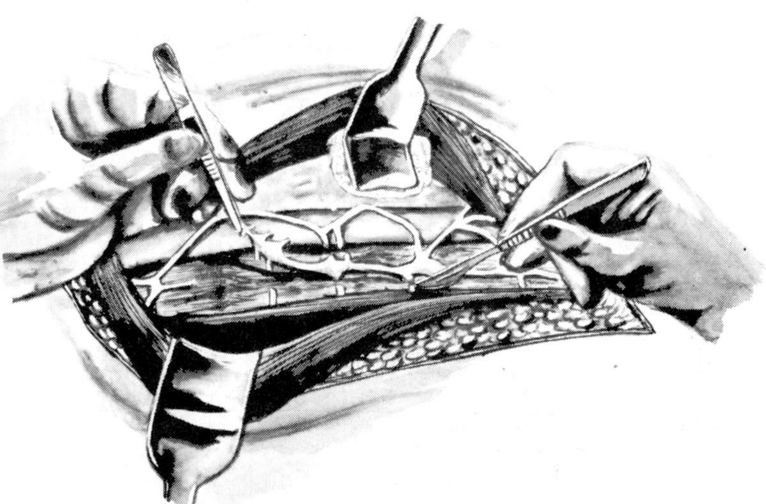

LUMBAR SYMPATHECTOMY

5. Pre/sacr/al *before sacrum* (prē-SĀ-kral) neur/ectomy *nerve* (nū-REK-tō-mē) with exposure by laparo/tomy[2] (lap-ah-ROT-ō-mē) is helpful in the management of severe dys/meno/rrhea *bad month* (dis"men-ō-RĒ-ah).

1. Often pronounced an-JĪ-nah pek-TOR-us although this is no longer considered the correct pronunciation.
2. The modern translation is "abdomen" although "flank" is the correct and original translation.

6. Peripheral sympathectomy is done for management of peripheral vascular disease under certain definite circumstances. It is indicated in patients with obliterative vascular disorders having painful localized gangrene or ulceration. It sometimes allows time for healing while alleviating pain thus preventing the need for amputation.

7. Tracto/tomy [a drawing out] (trak-TOT-ō-mē) is done for intractable pain due to any cause and consists of transection of pain tracts in the spinal cord. Anterolateral tractotomy is section of the anterolateral spino/thalam/ic [spine, thalamus] (spī"nō-thah-LAM-ik) tract.

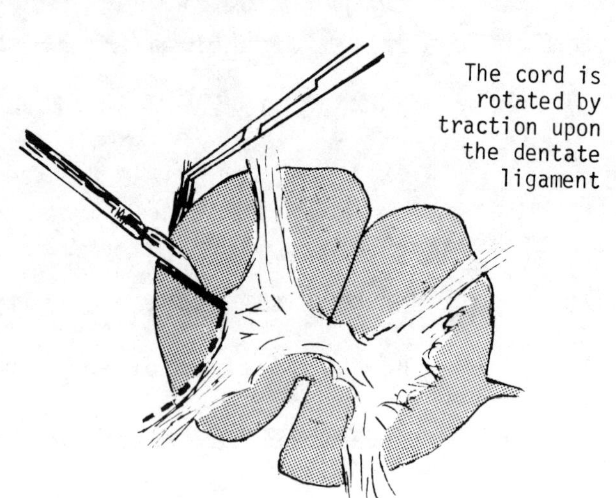

The cord is rotated by traction upon the dentate ligament

ANTEROLATERAL TRACTOTOMY (CHORDOTOMY)

8. Posterior rhizo/tomy [root] (rī-ZOT-ō-mē) is section of the posterior spinal roots.

POSTERIOR RHIZOTOMY

9. Paravertebral sympathetic block: the sympathetic rami [a branch] (RĀ-mī) and ganglia can be blocked paravertebrally with procaine. The effect is temporary but serves as a diagnostic test. For a more lasting effect, ethyl alcohol, 95% or absolute, can be injected in 3 to 5 cc amounts in each needle. It may be used for intractable visceral pain, particularly angina pectoris, in cases in which the risk of surgical excision is deemed too great and for management of minor causalgias and deep thrombo/phleb/itis [clot, vein] (throm"bō-fle-BĪ-tis) involving the femoral and iliac veins with phlegmasia [flame] (fleg-MĀ-zē-ah) alba [white] (AL-bah) dolens [causing pain] (DŌ-lenz) (phlebitis of the femoral vein -- known as "milk leg").

10. Thoracic paravertebral block is done for hypertension and angina pectoris.

11. Lumbar paravertebral block is done to <u>de/sympath/ectom/ize</u> [from / to cut out] (dē-sim" pah-THEK-tō-mīz) the lower extremity.

SURGERY OF THE SPINAL CORD

Acute injuries of the spinal cord are among the most discouraging lesions in surgery since function lost as the result of violent trauma to the spinal cord is rarely recovered.

The most common fractures and fracture dislocations occur in the 5th and 6th cervical vertebrae and the 1st and 5th lumbar vertebrae. Cervical cord injuries result usually from falls on the head and may accompany severe brain injuries.

APPLICATION OF CRUTCHFIELD TONGS

for skeletal traction in cervical injuries

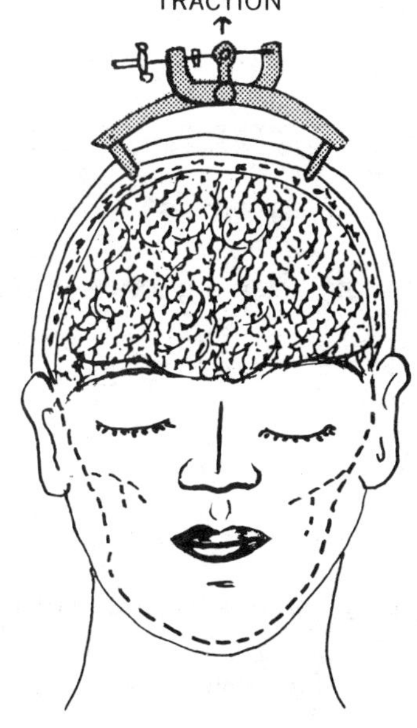

Cervical spine dislocations are reduced by the use of Crutchfield tongs.

Decompression of acute cord injuries is done by simple laminectomy.

Exploratory laminectomy is performed for penetrating wounds of the spinal canal and in transverse <u>myel/itis</u> [marrow] (mī-el-Ī-tis) to rule out tumors.

The <u>inter/vertebr/al</u> [between / vertebra] (in-ter-VER-te-bral) disc syndrome: <u>Myelo/graphy</u> (mī-el-OG-rah-fē) with the use of pantopaque as a radio-opaque medium is performed to verify or ascertain a diagnosis of a herniated intervertebral disc with compression of the emerging root. The majority occur at the 4th and 5th lumbar vertebral spaces. Laminotomy is performed.

Unilateral laminotomy is performed for herniated nucleus <u>pulposus</u> [pulp] (pul-PŌ-sus). In some cases spinal fusion may be done.

For tuberculosis of the spine with compression of the cord an open decompressive laminectomy is performed.

In chronic adhesive and cyst/ic *cyst* (SIS-tik) arachn/oid/itis *spider* (ah-rak"noyd-Ī-tis) the operative procedure consists of loosening of the adhesions (lysis *loosen* [LĪ-sis] of adhesions).

Neo/plasms *new formation* (NĒ-ō-plazms): Tumors which compress the spinal cord may be extra/dur/al *outside dura* (eks-trah-DŪ-ral), intra/dur/al *inside* (in-trah-DŪ-ral) but extra/medull/ary *marrow* (eks"trah-MED-ū-lār-ē), or intramedullary. It is not always possible to distinguish among the three types.

Laminectomy with removal of the tumor to secure adequate decompression of the cord is done for extradural tumors which consist of lip/omas[1] *fat* (lī-PŌ-mahs), chondr/omas *cartilage* (kon-DRŌ-mahs), fibro/sarc/omas *fiber flesh* (fī"brō-sar-KŌ-mahs), epi/derm/oid (ep-i-DER-moyd), metastatic carcinoma (particularly from the prostate, kidney, breast or uterus), myel/oma (mī-el-Ō-mah), benign giant cell tumor, Ewing's[2] (Ū-ingz) sarcomas; for intradural extramedullary tumors which with rare exceptions are meningiomas or neuro/fibr/omas *nerve* (nū"rō-fī-BRŌ-mahs); and for intramedullary tumors (ependym/omas[3] *upper garment* [ep-en-de-MŌ-mahs] or astro/cyt/omas *star cell* [as"trō-sī-TŌ-mahs]).

Syringo/myel/ia *pipe, fistula* (si-ring"gō-mī-Ē-lē-ah) is not a true neoplasm but its symptoms are similar to those produced by tumors. It is an accumulation of fluid which eventually forms a cyst in the central canal of the spinal cord causing compression. The syringo/myel/ic (si-ring"gō-mī-Ē-lik) cysts may be evacuated thus alleviating the symptoms but the condition cannot be cured surgically.

SURGERY OF THE INTRACRANIAL NERVES

Intracranial nerve disorders consist of trigeminal neuralgia (tic douloureux), Ménierè's[4] (mān-YAIRS) syndrome, facial spasm, glossopharyngeal neuralgia, spasmod/ic *draw, pull* (spaz-MOD-ik) torti/collis *twist neck* (tor-te-KŌ-lis).

1. Optional pronunciation lip-Ō-mah
2. A New York pathologist, 1866-1943
3. Ependyma is the lining membrane of the ventricles of the brain and of the central canal of the spinal cord.
4. A French physician, 1799-1862

Trigeminal neuralgia is the most common and its treatment consists of various surgical procedures:

1. alcohol injection of one or the other of the three branches of the trigeminal nerve (supra/orbit/al (above, circle) [sū-prah-OR-bi-tal], maxill/ary (jawbone) [MAK-se-ler-ē] or mandibul/ar (a jaw) [man-DIB-ū-lar]);
2. surgical section of the sensory root of the trigeminal nerve known as posterior root section or retro/gasserian (backward)[1] (re"trō-gas-Ē-rē-an) neuro/tomy (nū-ROT-ō-mē);
3. avulsion of the supraorbital branch of the trigeminal nerve.

The operative procedure for exposure of nerves in the posterior fossa is known as unilateral suboccipital craniectomy.

SURGERY OF THE PERIPHERAL NERVES

Peripheral nerve damage occurs from compound comminuted fractures where there is extensive damage of the surrounding tissue, vessels and nerves and in traumatic wounds such as caused by bullets and knives. There can be complete physiological loss of function without anatomical severance of a nerve. As peripheral nerves will regenerate slowly and incompletely when their ends are joined various surgical procedures may be performed on them. These consist of

1. neuro/rrhaphy (nū-ROR-ah-fē)-- the suture of an injured nerve;
2. neuro/lysis (nū-ROL-i-sis) -- the freeing of a nerve of adhesions;
3. neuro/anastomosis (to furnish with a mouth) (nū"rō-ah-nas-tō-MŌ-sis) -- the joining of nerve ends;
4. neurotomy -- the transection of a nerve;
5. neuro/plasty (NŪ-rō-plas-tē) -- the plastic repair of a nerve;
6. neurectomy -- the excision of a nerve or lesion of a nerve, for example, a solitary neur/oma (nū-RŌ-mah);
7. ganglion/ectomy (a knot) (gang"glē-ō-NEK-tō-mē) -- the excision of a ganglion;
8. the transplantation of a nerve to a new anatomical environment in order that the tension on the suture line may be reduced.

1. A ganglion named for Johann Laurentius Gasser, professor of anatomy, Vienna, in the 18th Century.

REVIEW OF THE NERVOUS SYSTEM

The encephalon or brain consists of

1. the cerebrum, the most conspicuous portion of the brain, which has
   two hemispheres
   the outermost part of the cerebrum is called
   the cortex which consists of gray matter folded many times making
   convolutions or gyri with intervening grooves called
   fissures or sulci. The three most important fissures are
   - the lateral or sylvan
   - the central or fissure of Rolando
   - the longitudinal fissure

   the cerebrum has 5 lobes which occur in pairs
   - frontal
   - parietal
   - occipital
   - temporal
   - insula

   there are 4 ventricles
   - the first and second ventricles form the lateral ventricle
   - the fourth ventricle is also called aqueduct of Sylvius or aquaeductus cerebri
   - the lateral ventricle is connected to the third ventricle by the foramina of Monro (foramina interventriculares)
2. the cerebellum which lies below the cerebrum in the posterior region of the skull cavity. It consists of two halves known as
   hemispheres
   and a central portion called
   the vermis
3. the pons varolii is composed mostly of fibers passing between the other three parts of the brain. It lies in front of the cerebellum.
4. the medulla oblongata is a mass of white and gray matter which connects the pons above with the spinal cord below. It is about an inch in length, and is broader above, where it is continuous with the pons.
5. There are 12 Cranial Nerves

I Olfactory	VII Facial
II Optic	VIII Acoustic
III Oculomotor	IX Glossopharyngeal
IV Trochlear	X Vagus
V Trigeminal	XI Spinal Accessory
VI Abducent	XII Hypoglossal

The medulla spinalis or spinal cord is elongated, nearly cylindrical, extends from the upper border of the atlas to the lower border of the first, or upper border of second, lumbar vertebra. It is continuous with the brain above. Below it ends in a conical extremity, the conus medullaris from the apex of which a delicate filament, the filum terminale, descends as far as the first segment of the coccyx.

the meninges are three membranes which protect the spinal cord. They are

the dura mater, the outside membrane, which is strong and fibrous and forms a wide tubular sheath

the arachnoid, the middle membrane, is a thin, transparent sheath

the pia mater, the inner membrane, closely invests the spinal cord

There are 31 pairs of spinal nerves

cervical - 8

thoracic -12

lumbar - 5

sacral - 5

coccygeal- 1

The autonomic nervous system is divided into

sympathetic which sends nerves to all organs, glands and blood vessels supplied with parasympathetic fibers

parasympathetic which is divided into

the cranial and sacral parts

the cranial portion carries nerve fibers to the iris of the eye, salivary glands, thyroid, and smooth muscles of blood vessels of face and neck region. From the medulla fibers pass in the vagus nerve which are widely distributed to heart, lungs, stomach, upper intestine, liver, pancreas, kidneys, and blood vessels of upper extremities and upper trunk.

the sacral portion supplies nerves to over half the colon, to the bladder and genitalia

the functions of the sympathetic and parasympathetic divisions are opposite and antagonistic in effect. When the parasympathetic (cranial) slows the heart, the sympathetic accelerates its action.

The cerebrospinal fluid runs through the entire length of the spinal cord and the ventricles of the brain. It serves as support and cushion for the soft structures of the central nervous system.

INDEX
CHAPTER IV

THE CIRCULATORY SYSTEM

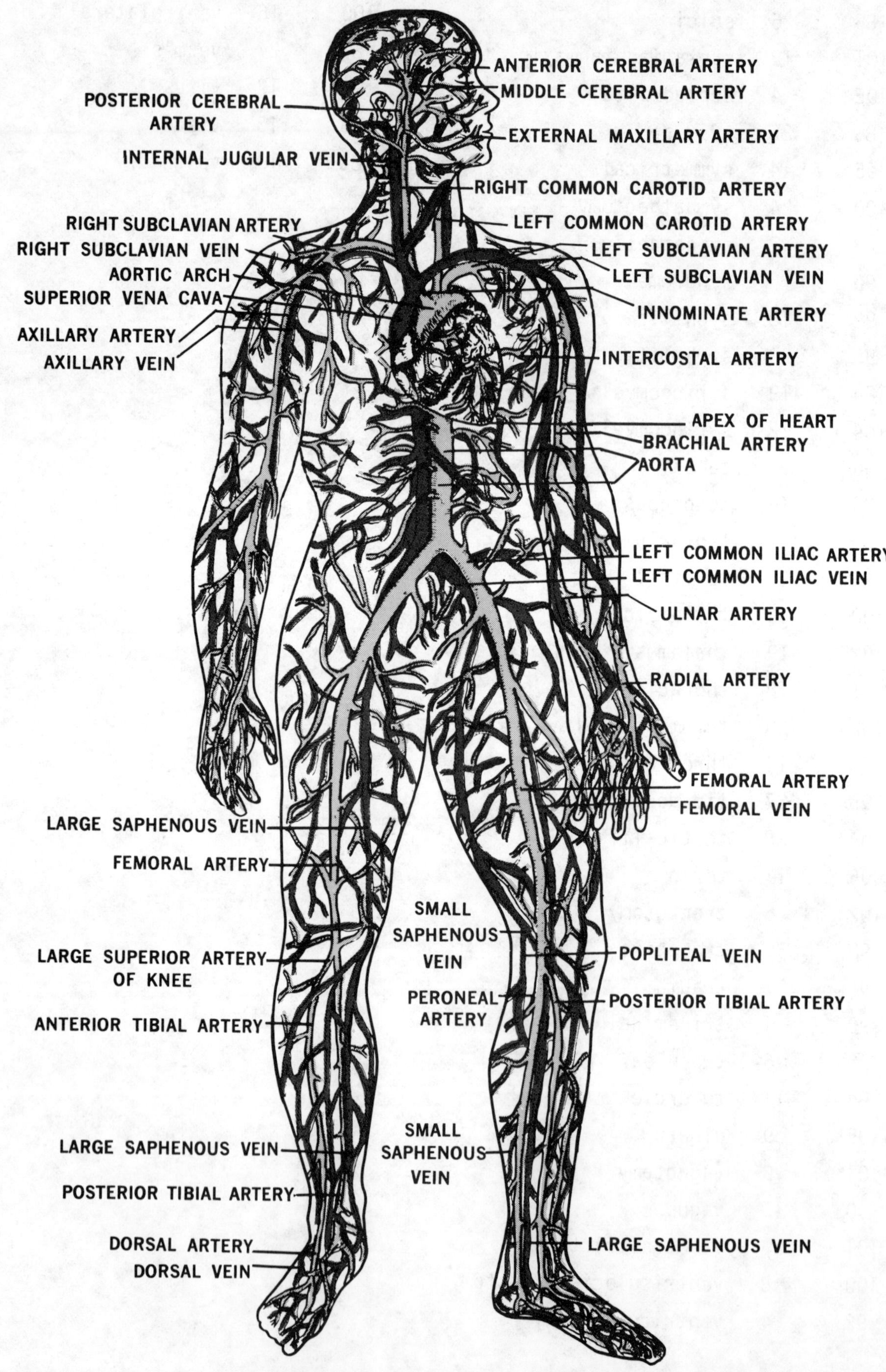
ANTERIOR CEREBRAL ARTERY
MIDDLE CEREBRAL ARTERY
POSTERIOR CEREBRAL ARTERY
EXTERNAL MAXILLARY ARTERY
INTERNAL JUGULAR VEIN
RIGHT COMMON CAROTID ARTERY
RIGHT SUBCLAVIAN ARTERY
LEFT COMMON CAROTID ARTERY
RIGHT SUBCLAVIAN VEIN
LEFT SUBCLAVIAN ARTERY
AORTIC ARCH
LEFT SUBCLAVIAN VEIN
SUPERIOR VENA CAVA
INNOMINATE ARTERY
AXILLARY ARTERY
AXILLARY VEIN
INTERCOSTAL ARTERY
APEX OF HEART
BRACHIAL ARTERY
AORTA
LEFT COMMON ILIAC ARTERY
LEFT COMMON ILIAC VEIN
ULNAR ARTERY
RADIAL ARTERY
FEMORAL ARTERY
FEMORAL VEIN
LARGE SAPHENOUS VEIN
FEMORAL ARTERY
SMALL SAPHENOUS VEIN
LARGE SUPERIOR ARTERY OF KNEE
POPLITEAL VEIN
PERONEAL ARTERY
POSTERIOR TIBIAL ARTERY
ANTERIOR TIBIAL ARTERY
SMALL SAPHENOUS VEIN
LARGE SAPHENOUS VEIN
POSTERIOR TIBIAL ARTERY
DORSAL ARTERY
LARGE SAPHENOUS VEIN
DORSAL VEIN

CHAPTER V
THE CIRCULATORY AND LYMPH VASCULAR SYSTEM

The circulatory system is made up of four functionally different parts: (1) the heart, a muscular pump, (2) the arteries and arteri/oles [artery small] (ar-TĒ-rē-ōls), the conducting and distributing vessels; the capillaries [hair like] (KAP-i-lar-ēz), the functional part; the ven/ules [vein small] (VĒ-nūls) and veins, the collecting vessels; (3) a circulatory fluid, the blood; and (4) an auxiliary system for returning fluids from the tissue spaces, the lymphat/ic [water] (lim-FAT-ik) system (also called the lymph vascular system).

The heart is a hollow muscular organ situated in the thorax between the lungs and above the central depression of the diaphragm. It is about the size of a closed fist. Its walls are composed of three coats: the endo/cardium [within heart] (en-dō-KAR-dē-um), the innermost layer; the myo/cardium [muscle] (mī-ō-KAR-dē-um), the middle layer, which forms the bulk of the muscular wall and which is covered by the epi/cardium [on,upon] (ep-i-KAR-dē-um), a serous [whey] (SĒ-rus) membrane, which is reflected at the upper portion of the heart to form a sac, the peri/cardium [around] (per-ē-KAR-dē-um) in which the heart is lodged.

The heart has four cavities: the right aur/icle [ear small] (AW-re-kl) or atrium [chamber] (Ā-trē-um) into which the superior and inferior venae [vein] cavae [hollow] (VĒ-nē KĀ-vē) empty (it always contains venous blood); the right ventricle or ventr/iculum [belly small] (ven-TRIK-ū-lum) from which the pulmon/ary [lung] (PUL-mo-nār-ē) arteries leave (always contains venous blood which the pulmonary artery takes to the lungs for oxygen and to give up carbon dioxide); the left auricle into which the four pulmonary veins empty the oxy/genated [sour to produce] (OK-se-je-nā-ted) blood from the lungs (it always contains arterial blood); the left ventricle from which the aorta [to lift up] (ā-OR-tah) leaves (it always contains arterial blood which the aorta distributes to the arteries and capillaries throughout the body).

Between the auricles and ventricles are the cardiac valves which open into the ventricles. The valves open when blood passes through the auricle into the ventricle but close during contraction of the ventricle to prevent re/gurgitation [back / to flood] (rē-gur-ji-TĀ-shun) of the blood into the auricle. The tri/cuspid [three / point] (trī-KUS-pid) valve is made up of three flaps or cusps and is on the right side of the heart. The bi/cuspid [two] (bī-KUS-pid) or mitr/al[1] [miter] (MĪ-tral) valve is composed of two flaps or cusps and is on the left side. The chordae [cords] (KŌR-dē) tendinae [tendons] (TEN-din-ē) are many small but very strong cords attached at one end to the border of the valves. At the other end they are attached to fleshy columns, the papill/ary[2] [nipple] (PAP-i-lār-ē) muscles, of the ventr/icul/ar (ven-TRIK-ū-lar) wall. Their function is to keep the valves from bulging into the auricles.

Just above the attached margins of the aort/ic (ā-OR-tik) valve the aorta gives off two

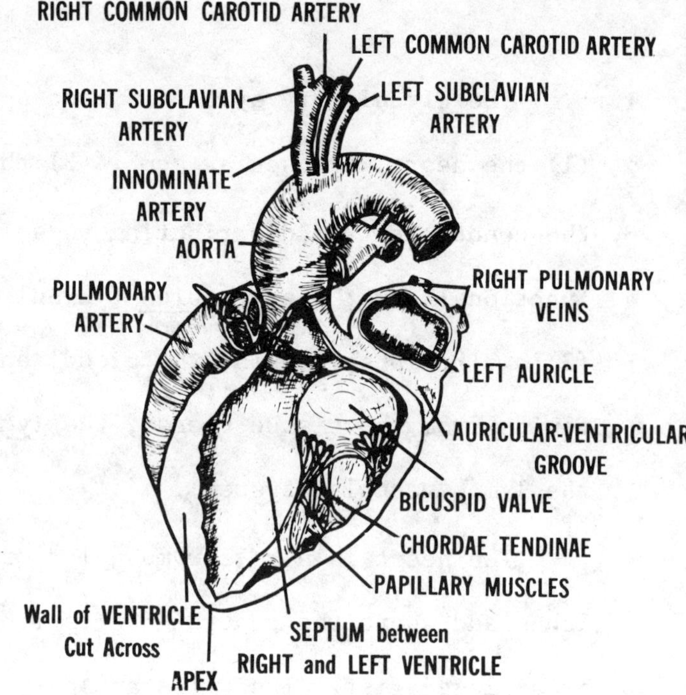

LEFT AURICLE AND LEFT VENTRICLE LAID OPEN

LEFT COMMON CAROTID ARTERY
INNOMINATE ARTERY
LEFT SUBCLAVIAN ARTERY
AORTA
SUPERIOR VENA CAVA
PULMONARY ARTERY
SEMILUNAR VALVE
RIGHT AURICLE
RIGHT VENTRICLE
AURICULAR-VENTRICULAR GROOVE
INFERIOR VENA CAVA
PAPILLARY MUSCLES
CHORDAE TENDINAE
HEPATIC VEINS
TRICUSPID VALVE

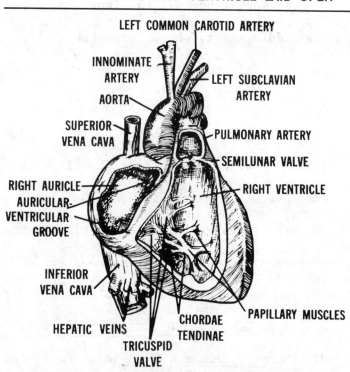

RIGHT AURICLE AND RIGHT VENTRICLE LAID OPEN

1. A tall cap worn by church dignitaries. In outline it resembles a pointed arch.
2. A diminutive of "papilla" meaning "a pimple."

branches called the right and left coron/ary *(crown)* (KOR-ō-nār-ē) arteries. They encircle the heart like a crown and for this reason are called coronary. They supply the substance of the heart with blood as the blood contained within the cavities of the heart only nourishes the endocardium. The blood distributed by the coronary arteries is returned by two sets of veins.

The arteries arise from the ventricles to carry blood away from the heart. The wall of an artery is both extensile and elastic. It is considerably thicker and stronger than that of a corresponding vein because the pressure in an artery is always greater than that in a vein. The walls of larger vessels are nourished by small blood vessels called vasa *(vessel)* (VĀ-sah) vasorum *(vessel)*[1] (vā-SŌ-rum). Arteries do not collapse when empty. Arteries are usually accompanied by a nerve and one or two veins. The arterial walls are made up of three coats: the inner coat, the tunica *(coat)* (TŪ-nē-kah) interna *(inside)* (in-TER-nah) or intima *(innermost)* (IN-ti-mah); the middle coat or tunica media and the outer coat, the tunica externa or ad/ventitia *(to / to come)* (ad-ven-TISH-yah).

The main arteries arising from the heart are the aorta which arises from the left ventricle and the pulmonary artery which arises from the right ventricle. Each is supplied with semilunar valves which open into the arteries only, preventing regurgitation of the blood back into the ventricles.

The arterioles are small arteries formed by the branching out of the arteries.

The capillaries are microscopic vessels formed by the branching out of arterioles and are found in practically every tissue of the body. The blood performs its function of nourishing tissues while it is passing through the capillaries and at no other place. The venules are the larger tubes formed by the reuniting of capillaries. The veins are the merging of

VALVES OF VEINS

EXTERNAL VIEW | INSIDE VIEWS

DILATATION AT SITE OF VALVE | VALVES OPENED | VALVES CLOSED

1. Literally "a vessel upon a vessel."

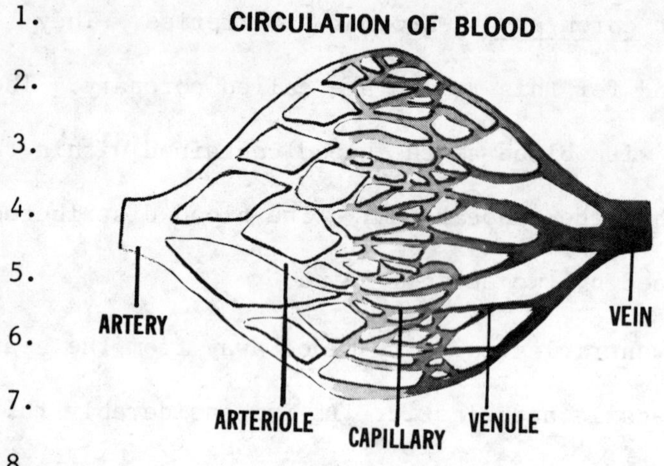

venules to bring blood back to the auricles. They are less elastic than arteries, but are well supplied with valves to prevent regurgitation of blood into the capillaries. The veins like the arteries are supplied with blood vessels.

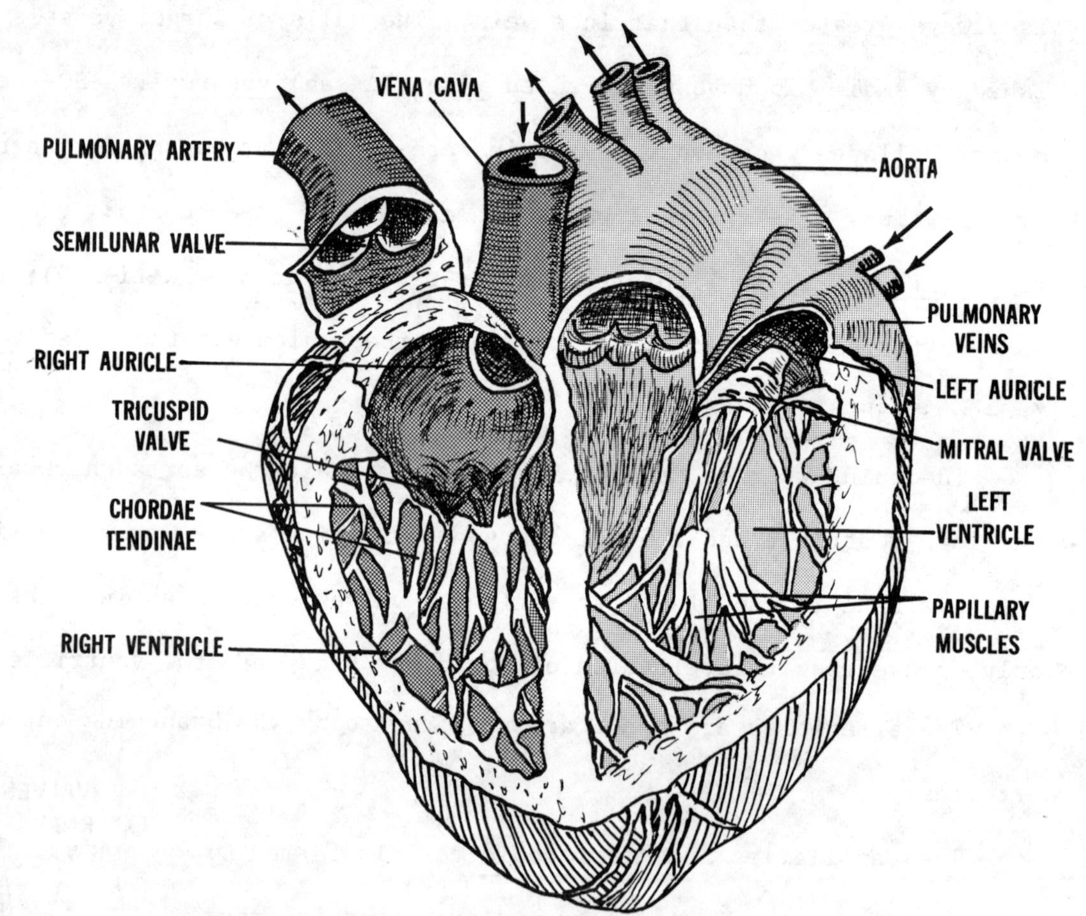

CIRCULATION OF BLOOD THROUGH THE HEART

The blood enters the right auricle from the superior and inferior venae cavae. Contraction of the right auricle expresses blood into the right ventricle from where it is forced by contraction of the ventricle through the semilunar valve into the pulmonary artery. Upon its return from the lungs where it gave up its carbon dioxide the blood is now oxygenated and enters the left auricle by way of the pulmonary veins. It is then forced into the left ventricle and from there into the aorta.

The blood has three important functions: 1. transporting food from the alimentary canal to the cells, carrying oxygen from the lungs to the cells, carrying waste products from the cells to the organs of excretion, distributing heat formed in the more active tissues to all parts of the body thus aiding in the regulation of body temperature, and carrying the hormones made by the ductless glands (thyr/oid (*shield*) [THĪ-royd], ad/renals (*near kidney*)[1] [ad-RĒ-nals], etc.) to all parts of the body; 2. maintaining the proper acid-base balance; and, 3. immuno/logic (*safe*) (i-mū"ni-LOG-ik) reaction.

NORMAL BLOOD CELLS

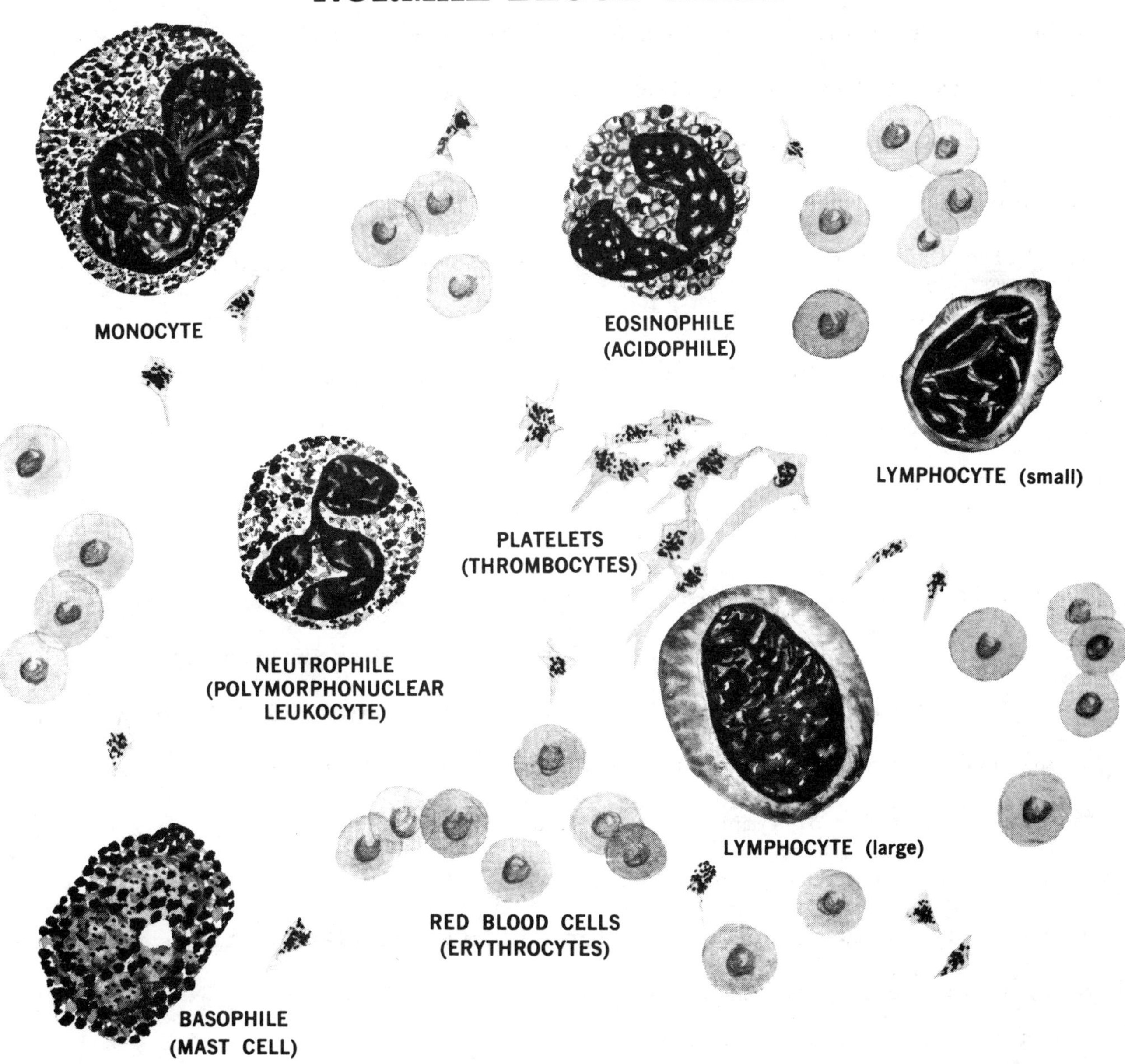

1. This adjective is often used incorrectly as a noun.

The blood is composed of plasma *(to mold)* (PLAZ-mah) and solids. The plasma is a light, yellow liquid of which nine-tenths is water. The solids or formed elements are 40 to 50% of the blood. The solids are composed of red blood cells (erythro/cytes *(red / cells)* [ē-RITH-rō-sīts]), white blood cells (leuko/cytes *(white)* [LŪ-kō-sīts]), and platelets (thrombo/cytes *(clot)* [THROM-bō-sīts]). The erythrocytes contain hemo/globin *(blood / a protein)* (hē-mō-GLŌ-bin) which gives the red color and is the carrier of oxygen and carbon dioxide. The amount of red cells in a cubic millimeter of healthy blood is five million for men and four and one-half million for women. The leukocytes are known as scavengers or immune agents. The amount of white cells in a cubic millimeter of healthy blood is from 5,000 to 7,000 or a proportion of about one white cell to 700 red. The white cells consist of lympho/cytes *(water)* (LIM-fō-sīts) (small and large) and leukocytes of different types: poly/morpho/nucle/ar *(many / shape / nucleus)* (pol"ē-mor-fō-NŪ-klē-ar) or neutro/philes *(neither / to love)*[1] (NŪ-trō-fils), eosino/philes *(dawn)*[1] (ē-ō-SIN-o-fils)[2] or acido/philes *(sour)*[1] (ah-SID-ō-fils), mast cells or baso/philes *(base)*[1] (BĀ-sō-fils) and mono/cytes *(single)* (MON-ō-sīts). The platelets or thrombocytes aid in blood coagulation.

The amount of blood in the human body is generally stated to be from six to eight percent of the body weight.

The lymphatic system begins in the meshes of connective tissues as closed capillaries which anastomose to form rich plexuses or networks. These capillaries unite to form the first collecting trunks or afferent vessels which go to regional lymph nodes. A node is an encapsulated mass of lymphocytes. Because the process of lymph formation is continual, edema *(swelling)* (ē-DĒ-mah) results from the accumulation of lymph if some system of drainage were not provided to return the lymph to the blood. This drainage is accomplished through the lymph vascular system. It is possible for fluid to accumulate in tissue spaces in spite of the drainage this system provides.

1. The suffix ending of these words is also spelled "phil."
2. Optional pronunciation ē-SIN-ō-fils

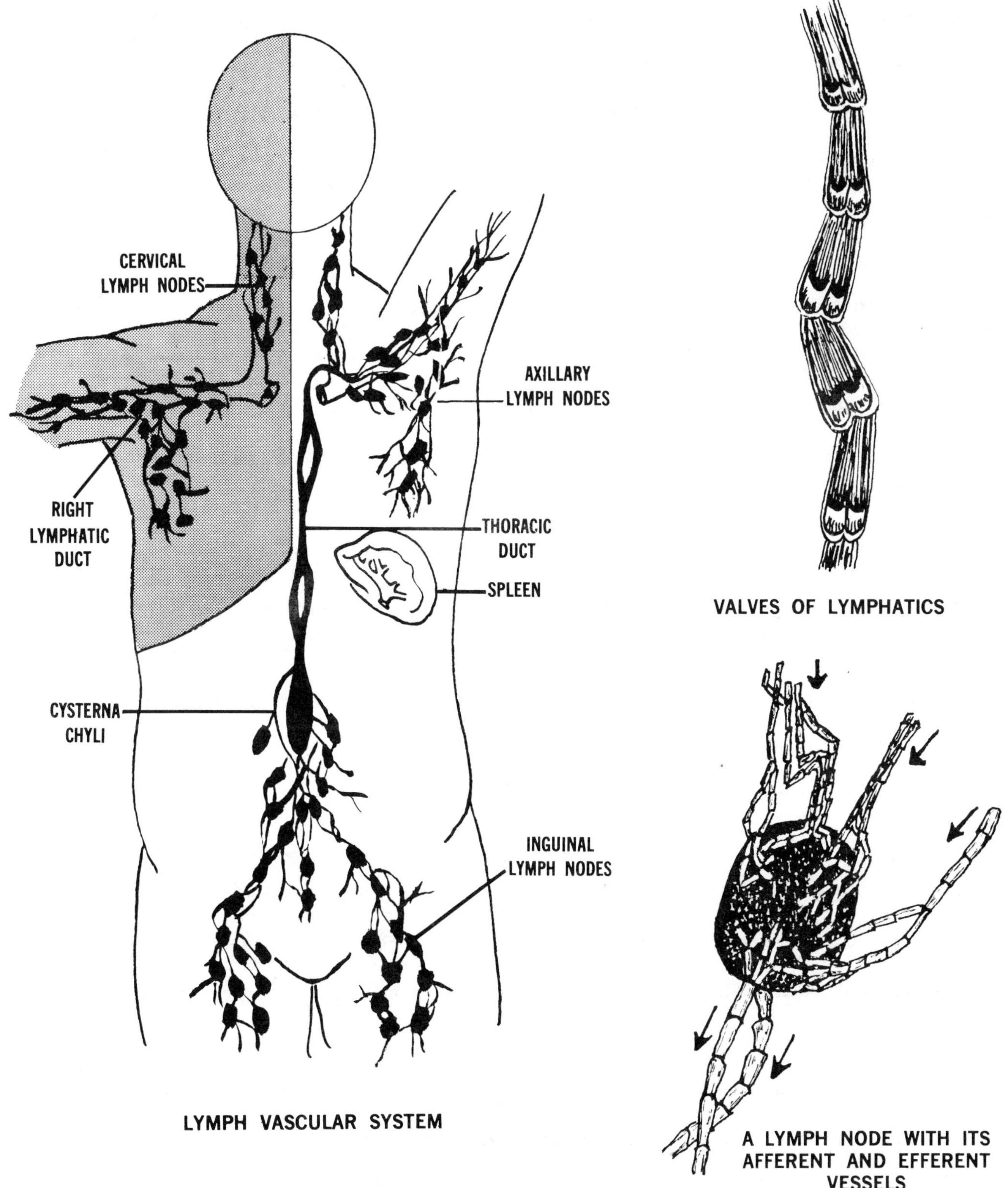

LYMPH VASCULAR SYSTEM

VALVES OF LYMPHATICS

A LYMPH NODE WITH ITS AFFERENT AND EFFERENT VESSELS

The lymph vascular system is made up of three divisions: (1) the lymph vessels which are made up of the lymph capillaries, lymphatics, thoracic duct, right lymphatic duct, lacteals (*milky*) (LAK-tē-als); (2) the expanded lymph spaces made up of the pleur/al (*rib*) (PLŌŌR-al) cavity, the peri/cardi/al (*around*) (per-ē-KAR-dē-al) cavity, the peri/tone/al (*to stretch*) (per-i-tō-NĒ-al) cavity, the meninge/al (*membrane*) (me-NIN-jē-al) spaces, the lymph spaces of the eye and ear, the syn/ovi/al (*together egg*) (si-NŌ-vē-al) bursae (*purse*) (BUR-sē); and, (3) the lymph nodes.

Just as the blood capillaries unite to form veins, the lymph capillaries unite to form larger vessels called lymphatics. The lymphatics continue to unite and form larger and larger vessels until finally they converge into two main channels, the thoracic duct and the right lymphatic duct.

The thoracic duct receives the lymph from the left side of the head, neck, and chest, all of the abdomen and both lower limbs, also the chyle (*juice*) (kīl) (the lymph that fills the lacteals of the intestinal villi (*shaggy hair of beasts*) [VIL-ī]).

The right lymphatic duct pours its contents into the innominate vein at the junction of the right internal jugul/ar (*neck*) (JUG-ū-lar) and sub/clavian (*below clavicle*) (sub-KLĀ-vē-an) veins. The lymphatics from the right side of the head, neck, the right arm, and the upper part of the trunk enter the right lymphatic duct.

The lymphatics resemble the veins in their structure as well as their arrangement.

Lymph vessels have been found in nearly every tissue and organ which contain blood vessels. The cartilage, nails, cut/icle (*skin small*) (KYŌŌ-ti-kl), and hair are without them. The lymph, like the blood in the veins, is returned from the limbs and viscera by a superficial and deep set of vessels.

The function of the lymphatics is to carry from the tissues to the veins all the materials which the tissues do not need.

The lymph nodes are small, oval or bean-shaped bodies varying in size from a pinhead to an almond and placed in the course of the lymphatics. They generally present a slight depression called the hilus [a depression] (HĪ-lus) on one side. The blood vessels enter and leave through the hilus.

There is a superficial and a deep set of nodes just as there is a superficial and a deep set of lymphatics and veins. Occasionally a node exists alone, but they are usually in groups or chains at the sides of the great blood vessels. Lymph nodes are found on the back of the head draining the scalp, around the sterno/cleido/mast/oid [sternum clavicle breast] (ster"nō-klī-dō-MAS-toyd) muscle draining the back of the tongue; the pharynx, nasal cavities, roof of the mouth, and face; and under the rami of the mandible draining the floor of the mouth. All of these nodes are subject to infection particularly from tonsils and teeth. Such infection causes an inflammatory condition called aden/itis [gland] ad-eh-NĪ-tis). The nodes around the sternocleidomastoid muscle are very often infected with tuber/cle [node small] (TŪ-ber-kl) bacilli [staff or rod] (bah-SIL-ī).

In the upper extremities there are three groups, a small one at the bend of the elbow, which drains the hand and forearm, a larger group in the axill/ary [armpit] (AK-si-lār-ē) space into which the first group drains, and a still larger group under the pector/al [breast] (PEK-tō-ral) muscles. The last named drains the mamm/ary [breast] (MAM-mah-rē) gland, skin, and muscles of the chest.

In the lower extremities there is usually a small node at the upper part of the anterior tibi/al [tibia] (TIB-ē-al) vessels, and in the poplite/al [back of knee] (pop-LIT-ē-al) space back of the knee there are several, but the greater number are massed in the groin. These nodes drain the lower extremities and the lower part of the abdominal wall.

The lymph nodes have two important functions: 1. In its passage through the node the lymph takes up fresh lymphocytes, which are continually multiplying by cell division in the substance of the node (considered to be the birthplace of these cells). 2. They are placed in the course of the lymph vessels and the lymph has to take a tortuous course among the cells of the nodes. For this reason it is believed they serve as filters and are a defense against the spread of infection.

The lymph in the various tissues of the body varies in amount from time to time, but under normal circumstances remains fairly constant. Under abnormal conditions, the amount of lymph may be exceeded and the result is known as edema or dropsy [water] (DROP-sē). Excessive accumulations of lymph may also occur in the larger lymph spaces, the serous cavities.

The functions of the spleen are closely related to the circulatory and lymphatic systems. These functions include: 1. The spleen serves as a reservoir for blood for use when the need arises. 2. The destruction of damaged red cells by cells known as macro/phages [large, to eat] (MAK-rō-faj-ez). This also includes red cells which have worn out and break up in the blood stream. These small fragments are called hemo/conia [blood, dust] (hē"mō-KŌ-nē-ah) or "blood dust." 3. The formation of lymphocytes by the lymphoid tissue of the spleen.

DISEASES AND ANOMALIES OF THE HEART AND BLOOD VESSELS

Heart disease may be due to a variety of causes, but the most frequent ones are infections, arterio/scler/osis [artery, hard] (ar-tē"rē-ō-skle-RŌ-sis), high blood pressure, congenital malformations, and nutritional deficiency. Emotion is a very frequent cause of functional disturbances of the heart.

The heart may be attacked by a large number of infectious agents, but the most common offenders are the spiro/chete [coil, hair] (SPĪ-rō-kēt) of syphilis and the organism responsible for rheumat/ic [a flux] (rū-MAT-ik) fever.

The two most important diseases of the arteries are arteriosclerosis and athero/scler/osis [gruel] (ath"er-ō-skle-RŌ-sis). In arteriosclerosis the vessels become hard, stiff and brittle owing to atrophy of the muscular and elastic tissues and their replacement by salts of lime. Atherosclerosis, also called ather/omatoses [tumors] (ath"er-Ō-mah-tō-sēz) or ather/oma (ath-er-Ō-mah), is a type of arterial degeneration caused by a breaking down of the arterial endothelium (tunica intima). Patches of endothelium break down and are replaced by a soft, fatty material in which lime salts are later deposited. This leads to a weakening of the arterial wall and is the cause of such vascular emergencies as cerebral hemorrhage (apoplexy) and coronary thrombosis. Syphilis may also cause disease of the arteries.

NORMAL ARTERY
ADVENTITIA
MEDIA
LUMEN
INTIMA

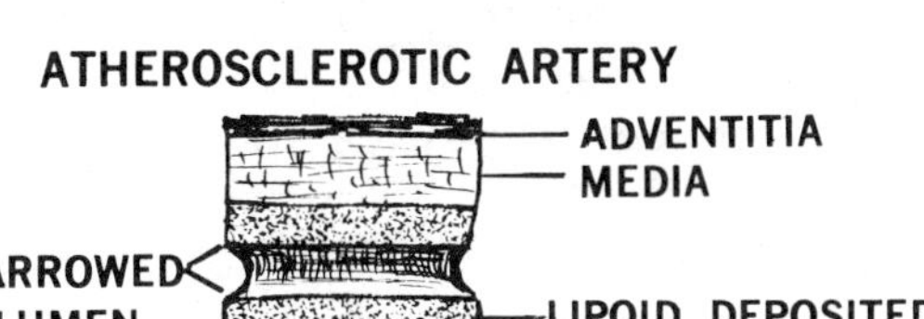

The principal causes of disease of the veins are infections due to pyo/ [pus] gen/ic [produce] (pī-ō-JEN-ik) bacteria. Trauma may result in wounds of the heart, arteries or veins.

Tumors of the heart are rare, and, when present, are nearly always meta/ [beyond] stat/ic [to stand] (met-ah-STAT-ik). Arteries are rarely invaded by primary tumors or metastatic tumors, but veins, though never the seat of primary tumors, are rather frequently invaded by cancerous growths originating in other structures.

Four factors are present in the diagnosis of heart disease: 1. the etio/ [cause] logic (ē"tē-ō-LOG-ik) diagnosis; 2. the anatomic diagnosis (anatomic lesions present); 3. the physiological diagnosis; 4. the functional diagnosis.

The most frequent etiologic types of heart disease are syphilit/ic (sif-i-LIT-ik) heart disease which occurs in middle aged persons; rheumatic heart disease which is predominantly a disease of children and young adults and which is caused by the presence of rheumatic fever resulting in an acute inflammation which involves the whole heart, the endocardium, myocardium and pericardium -- a pan/card/itis [all, heart] (pan-kar-DĪ-tis); arterio/sclerot/ic [hard] (ar-tē"rē-ō-skle-ROT-ik) heart disease which is due to sclerotic lesions of the coronary arteries and which predominates in elderly persons; congenital heart disease which may present any of these lesions: pulmonary sten/osis [hard] (ste-NŌ-sis), patency [open] (PĀ-ten-sē) of the septum between the ventricles, dextro/position [right] (deks-TROP-i-zish-en) of the aorta, patency of the ductus [passage] (DUK-tus) arteriosus [artery] (ar-tē-rē-Ō-sus), co/arct/ation [with, make tight] (kō-ark-TĀ-shun) of the aorta and dextro/card/ia (deks-trō-KAR-dē-ah).

The three important diseases of the pericardium are fibrin/ous (FĪ-brin-us) peri/card/itis [around] (per"ē-kar-DĪ-tis), pericardial ef/fusion [out, to pour] (i-FŪ-zhun) and adhesive pericarditis.

The most important diseases of the heart muscle are acute inflammation, called myo/card/itis [muscle] (mī"ō-kar-DĪ-tis); chronic degenerative changes, often called chronic myocarditis; hyper/trophy [above] (hī-PER-tro-fē); and dilat/ation [stretching] (dil-ah-TĀ-shun).

The only portions of the endocardium which are frequently diseased are those which cover the valves of the heart. Endo/cardi/al [within] (en-dō-KAR-dē-al) disease, or endo/card/itis (en"dō-kar-DĪ-tis), is practically synonymous with valvul/ar [valve] (VAL-vū-lar) disease.

Under normal circumstances the impulse for the heartbeat originates in the sinus node and the speed and regularity with which this node discharges impulses determine the rate and rhythm of the heart. In this situation, a sinus rhythm is said to be present. If a sinus rhythm is unusually rapid it is called sinus tachy/card/ia [rapid] (tak-ē-KAR-dē-ah); if it is unusually slow it is called sinus brady/card/ia [slow] (brā-dē-KAR-dē-ah); if it is irregular it is called sinus ar/rhythm/ia [not, rhythm] (ah-RITH-mē-ah). If, for one reason or another, some other portion of the heart muscle controls the heart's rate and rhythm, an ec/top/ic [out, place] (ek-TOP-ik) rhythm is said to exist. Under certain circumstances, even though the sinus node is controlling the heart's rhythm most of the time, another region will occasionally send out an impulse, causing the heart to beat ahead of time. Such a beat is called an ectopic or pre/mature [before, early; ripe] (pre-mah-TYO͞OR) beat. The most important ectopic rhythms are paroxysm/al [to irritate] (par-oks-IZ-mal) tachycardia, aur/icul/ar [ear, small] (aw-RIK-ū-lar) fibrillation[1] [the twitching of fibers] (fī-bre-LĀ-shun) and

1. This word may be pronounced with a long or a short i in the first syllable (fi).

auricular flutter. When the impulse from the sinus node fails to reach the ventricles, or is delayed in its passage, a condition known as heart block, or more properly, aur/iculo/ventr/icul/ar (aw-rik"ū-lō-ven-TRIK-ū-lar) block, occurs.

Congestive [to heap together] (kon-JES-tiv) failure may occur either in acute or chronic heart disease but more commonly in the latter. It may occur in heart disease of any cause, in conditions which affect the myocardium directly, such as diphtheria [membrane] (dif-THĒ-rē-ah) and coronary sclerosis, or indirectly, such as chronic valvular disease or hypertension.

Cardiac pain can occur under two sets of circumstances, coronary narrowing and coronary occlusion. Pain due to coronary narrowing is called angina [quinsy] (AN-ji-nah) pectoris [breast bone] (PEK-tō-ris). This condition is due to the heart muscle being inadequately supplied with oxygen. The commonest cause is arteriosclerosis.

Coronary thromb/osis [clot] (throm-BŌ-sis) is a complication of arteriosclerotic heart disease and its outstanding symptom is cardiac pain. It is the occurrence of a blood clot in one of the coronary arteries or in branches thereof, so that a smaller or larger area of the heart muscle is deprived entirely of blood. This region of the muscle undergoes death, giving rise to the formation of an infarct [to stuff in] (IN-farkt).

Substances that prevent coagulation of blood are called anti/coagulants [against, to clot] (an"te-kō-AG-ū-lants). Some of the substances used are hirudin[1] (hī-ROO-din), heparin [liver] (HEP-ah-rin), dicoumarin[2] (dī-KOO-mah-rin). Dicoumarin is used in the treatment of coronary thrombosis and other forms of intravascular clotting.

The most important and most common structural disease of the arteries is arteriosclerosis or hardening of the arteries.

Thrombosis and em/bol/ism [in, to throw] (EM-bō-lizm) refer to occlusion of a vessel by

1. A substance extracted from the salivary glands of the leech that has the property of preventing coagulation of the blood. An antithrombin. This term may also be pronounced HIR-ū-din.

2. From "coumaron" the native name in Guiana of the tonka bean.

foreign material; thrombosis is due to the formation of a blood clot within the vessel; embolism is due to obstruction by the lodging of some particle floating in the blood stream, when it reaches an artery whose lumen [light] (LŪ-men) is no larger than the object itself. Emboli [a plug] (EM-bō-lī) may consist of pieces of thrombi [a clot] (THROM-bī) from the heart, from arteries, or from veins; of small pieces of fat which have entered veins as a result of injury, or even bubbles of air or nitrogen.

Aneurysm[1] [widening] (AN-ū-rizm) refers to a localized dilatation of an artery. The most common aneurysm is that of the aorta. Dis/secting [apart / to cut] (dis-SEK-ting) aneurysm is a peculiar condition of the aorta in which blood suddenly escapes through a weakened portion of the intima and dissects its way between the coats of the vessel, separating them by its own pressure. Arterio/ven/ous [vein] (ar-tē-rē-ō-VĒ-nus) aneurysm connects both with an artery and a vein, so that blood continually flows through it in a shortcircuited path.

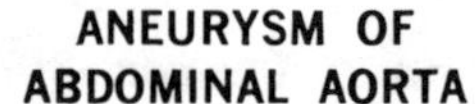
ANEURYSM OF ABDOMINAL AORTA

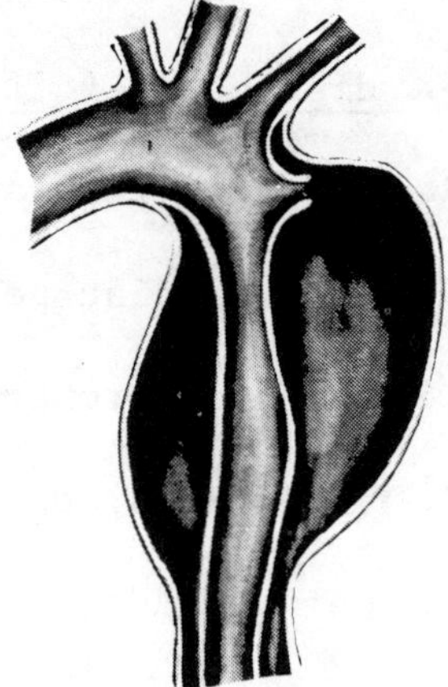
DISSECTING ANEURYSM OF THE DISTAL ARCH OF THE AORTA

Rare diseases of the arteries include thrombo/angi/itis [vessel] (throm"bō-an-jē-Ī-tis) obliterans [destroy] (ō-BLIT-er-anz) or Buerger's disease, Raynaud's disease, erythro/mel/algia [red / limb] (ē-rith"rō-mel-AL-jē-ah) or Weir (wēr) Mitchell's disease. Acro/cyan/osis [extremity / blue] (ak"rō-sī-ah-NŌ-sis) is a sort of focal type of Raynaud's disease. Peri/arter/itis (per"ē-ar-ter-Ī-tis) nodosa [nodes] (nō-DŌ-sah) is a rare inflammatory disease of the arteries, accompanied by thrombosis and the occurrence of numerous tiny aneurysms which give individual vessels a nodular appearance.

Hypertension or high blood pressure is a manifestation of many different diseases, which include various affections of the kidneys, lead poisoning,

1. This is the older spelling. The more modern spelling is "aneurism." Both are used, however.

<u>tox/emia</u> *poison* (toks-Ē-mē-ah) of pregnancy, and tumors of the adrenal glands. The most frequent type of hypertension is one in which it occurs without any known cause; this type is called essential hypertension.

Hypotension or low blood pressure, like hypertension, may occur in a variety of conditions, among which are hemorrhage, shock, weakened states due to various diseases, and Addison's disease.

The two most important primary or <u>in/trins/ic</u> *on the inside* (in-TRIN-sik) diseases of the veins are <u>varic/ose</u> *swollen vein* (VAR-i-kōs) veins and <u>thrombo/phleb/itis</u> *vein* (throm"bō-fle-BĪ-tis). Varicose veins (<u>varices</u>[1] [VAR-i-sēz]) consist of greatly dilated tortuous veins, most commonly of the legs, in which the pressure is elevated and the blood flow stagnant or even reversed. This is caused by defective venous valves which allow the pressure of an unbroken column of blood from the heart to distend the veins in the legs. Thrombophlebitis is inflammation of veins associated with thrombosis. <u>Phlebo/thromb/osis</u> (fleb"ō-throm-BŌ-sis) is the occurrence of venous thrombosis without antecedent inflammation.

DISEASES OF THE BLOOD

<u>An/emia</u> *without blood* (ah-NĒM-ē-ah) is a reduction either of the red cells per unit of circulating blood, of the hemoglobin, or of both.

Acute anemias due to blood loss are due to a single or to repeated large hemorrhages. Chronic anemia due to blood loss is due to continuous or intermittent slow bleeding.

Anemias due to defective formation of blood may be secondary or primary. Among the secondary anemias are those due to iron deficiency, to chemical poisons and bacterial toxins which depress the bone marrow, x-ray and radium which may injure the bone marrow and to organic diseases of the bone marrow. The primary anemias due to defective blood formation

ABNORMAL TYPES OF RED BLOOD CELLS FOUND IN ANEMIA

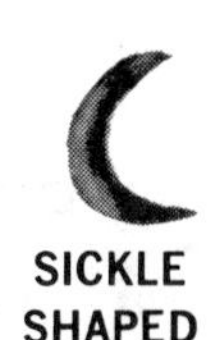

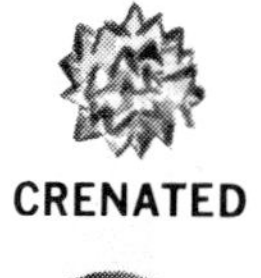

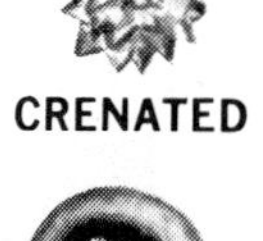

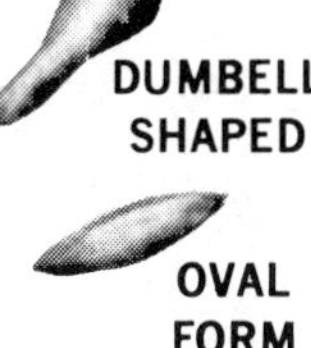

1. Plural of "varix" meaning "a dilated vein."

include per/nicious[1] [through slaughter] (per-NISH-us) anemia, primary a/plast/ic [not formed] (ā-PLAS-tik)[2] anemia, erythro/blast/ic [cell,germ] (ē-rith"rō-BLAS-tik) anemia, splen/ic [spleen] (SPLEN-ik) anemia, and congenital anemia of infancy.

Poly/cyt/hemia [many cell blood] (pol"ē-sī-THĒ-mē-ah) is an increase above normal of the number of erythrocytes per unit of circulating blood. It may be primary or secondary. Primary polycythemia is known as erythr/emia (er"i-THRĒ-mē-ah) or Osler's disease.

The leuk/emias [white] (lū-KĒ-mē-ahs) are diseases which are characterized by the presence of abnormal white cells in the blood and usually also by tremendous increase in the total white cell count.

The term granulo/cyto/penia [grain poverty,lack] (gran"ū-lō-sī-tō-PĒ-nē-ah) refers to a diminu/tion [small] (dim"i-NŪ-shun) of the number of granulocytes in the circulating blood. It is also referred to as a/granulo/cytosis [lack] (ā-gran"ū-lō-sī-TŌ-sis)[3] and neutro/penia [neutrophile] (nū-trō-PĒ-nē-ah).

Purpura [purple] (PUR-pū-rah) is a condition characterized by spontaneous bleeding into the skin and mucous membranes. Hemo/phil/ia [blood to love] (hē-mō-FIL-ē-ah) is a hereditary disease in which, because the blood clots very slowly, the patients bleed excessively from even trifling injuries. This disease affects only males, but only females can transmit it to their children. People affected with this disease are called "bleeders." Certain substances which hasten clotting are known as styptics [contraction] (STIP-tiks) or hemo/statics [to stop] (hē-mō-STAT-iks). Some of these are alum, ferric chloride, zinc chloride and silver nitrate. When bleeding is arrested by hastening coagulation of the blood or by constriction of the bleeding vessels it is called hemo/stasis (hē-mō-STĀ-sis).

DISEASES OF THE LYMPHATICS

The lymph vessels may be the site of inflammation due to bacterial invasion (lymph/ang/itis [water vessel] [limf-an-JĪ-tis]), may possess congenitally deficient valves, or fail to attain normal size, so that lymph is unable to be properly

1. Translates to "destructive"
2. Optional pronunciation ah-PLAS-tik
3. Optional pronunciation ah-gran"ū-lō-sī-TŌ-sis

drained from the tissues by them; they may be obstructed by parasites (filaria *(thread)* [fi-LĀ-rē-ah]), or by pressure of tumors, inflammatory swelling, or fibr/osis (fī-BRŌ-sis) of the tissues.

Lymphangitis or inflammation of the lymph vessels is nearly always of strepto/cocc/al *(twisted berry)* (strep-tō-KOK-al) origin, and is due to invasion of lymph vessels by organisms causing inflammation in the tissues.

Obstruction of the lymphatics gives rise to a characteristic hard swelling called lymph/edema *(swelling)* (limf-i-DĒ-mah). It differs from the edema due to venous stasis *(stop,halt)* (STĀ-sis) in that it is hard and does not pit on pressure. Edema may be quite local and form small, well-defined raised, pale areas in the skin. This may occur in persons who are susceptible to certain foods such as shell fish, strawberries, celery, etc. The condition is called urticaria *(nettle)* (ur-ti-KĀ-rē-ah) but is better known as "hives."

Elephantiasis *("elephant's disease")* (el"i-fan-TĪ-ah-sis) is a chronic swelling of a limb or other part of the body due to lymphatic obstruction.

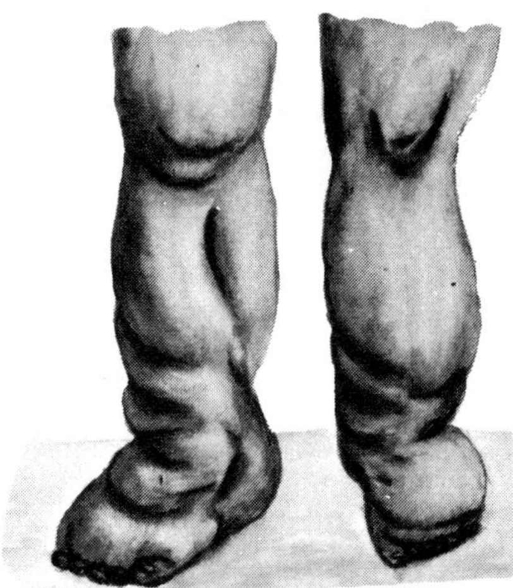

ELEPHANTIASIS OF LOWER EXTREMITIES

The lymph nodes are involved in a great variety of diseases. Organisms which enter the lymphatics are usually filtered out by the nearest lymph nodes, where the type of inflammation characteristic for the particular organism often occurs. Among the inflammatory diseases and conditions which are frequently complicated by inflammation of the lymph nodes are streptococcal infection of the tonsils, extremities, and other portions of the body, tuber/cul/osis *(node small)* (to͞o-ber-kū-LŌ-sis), syphilis, tularemia[1] *(a disease of rodents)* (to͞o-lah-RĒ-mē-ah), infectious *(to corrupt)* (in-FEK-shus) mono/nucle/osis *(single nucleus)* (mon"ō-nū-klē-ō-sis), chancr/oid *(cancer)* (SHANG-kroyd), and lympho/granul/oma (limf"ō-gran-ū-LŌ-mah) inguinale *(groin)* (ing-gwi-NAL-ē).

1. This disease is named after Tulare (lake and county in California) where the disease was first described.

Lymph/aden/itis [gland] (limf-ad-i-NĪ-tis) or inflammation of the lymph nodes may be acute or chronic. The symptoms vary with the severity of the inflammation and the location of the lymph nodes involved. The lymph nodes are also involved in other diseases: the leukemias, lympho/sarc/oma [flesh] (limf"ō-sar-KŌ-mah), and Hodgkin's[1] (HOJ-kinz) disease, for example. They are also frequently involved in cancer of the different organs of the body; cancer usually spreads first to the regional lymph nodes by way of the lymph vessels. In all of these conditions the principal local manifestation is enlargement of the nodes.

SURGERY OF THE HEART AND BLOOD VESSELS

Extra/corpore/al [outside, body] (eks"trah-kor-PŌ-rē-al) circulation is a by-passing of the heart by diverting the blood around the heart and lungs for the purpose of providing inflow diversion of blood around the heart. This enables the surgeon to operate on an almost bloodless heart under direct vision.

Various techniques are used to achieve extracorporeal circulation. They include:

1. Cardio/pulmon/ary [heart, lung] (kar"dē-ō-PUL-mō-nār-ē) by-pass
2. Left ventricular or partial by-pass using the patient's own lung for oxygenation. This is used for surgery on the descending aorta.
3. By-pass of heart combined with hypo/therm/ia[2] [below, heat] (hī-pō-THER-mē-ah). Use of heat exchange and pump oxygenator or heart-lung machine.

The most common types of oxygenators are:

1. Gibbon bubble oxygenator,
2. DeWald pump and bubble oxygenator,
3. Disc oxygenator,
4. Screen oxygenator,
5. Membrane oxygenator.

Cardiac a/sy/stole[3] [not, together, to send] (ā-SIS-to-le), cardiac arrest, and cardiac standstill

1. English physician, 1798-1866
2. Artificial reduction of body temperature in an effort to lower the metabolic requirements of the patient.
3. Optional pronunciation ah-SIS-tō-lē

are terms used interchangeably to designate cessation of heart action. Untreated arrest promptly terminates in death. Treatment consists of cardiac pulmonary re/suscit/ation [again / to raise up] (rē"sus-i-TĀ-shun) and cardiac massage in which the chest is not opened and immediate manual rhythmical compression of the chest is performed. This method is called "closed-chest heart massage." If this fails, open wound compression of the heart is sometimes undertaken. Ventricular fibrillation is the most serious arrhythmia encountered during any cardiac surgery.

Cardiac catheter/iz/ation [catheter / to treat] (kath"i-ter-i-ZĀ-shun) is a procedure of diagnostic value in detecting various cardiac defects and disease. A radi/opaque[1] [ray / shady] (rā-dē-ō-PĀK) cardiac catheter is inserted into an accessible vein and passed into the heart and vessels leading from the heart. It is performed from either the right or left sides of the body. Various techniques are used depending on the area to be studied.

Lesions of the heart amenable to surgery fall into two categories:

1. Acquired lesions which include mitral valvular stenosis, aortic valvular stenosis, tricuspid valvular stenosis, mitral regurgitation, constrictive pericarditis, coronary heart disease, aortic insufficiency, ventricular aneurysms and traumatic lesions of valves and septum.
2. Congenital lesions include severe pulmonary stenosis, transposition of the great vessels, tetra/logy [four] (te-TRAL-ō-jē) of Fallot[2] (fal-Ō), inter/atri/al [between / atrium] (in"ter-Ā-trē-al) sept/al [wall] (SEP-tal) defects, inter/ventricul/ar [ventricle] (in"ter-ven-TRIK-ū-lar) septal defects.

Patent [open] (PĀ-tent) ductus arteriosus is not a true congenital deformity. It is a developmental abnormality due to failure of involution and obliteration of an entirely normal fetal vascular channel, the ductus arteriosus. Surgical procedure is complete division of the ductus arteriosus. This is obliteration

1. Also spelled "radio-opaque"
2. Etienne-Louis A. Fallot, French physician, 1850-1911

of the ductus by dividing the ductus and suturing the cut ends.

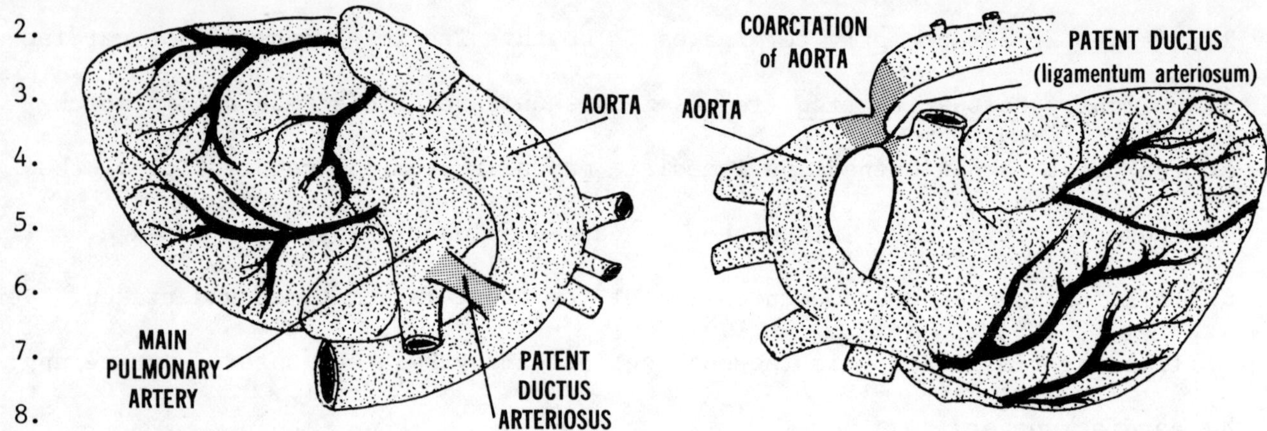

PATENT DUCTUS ARTERIOSUS **COARCTATION OF THE AORTA**

Coarctation of the aorta is a stricture or narrowing of some portion of the aorta most commonly located near the insertion of the ductus arteriosus. It causes a reduction of the circulation to the lower limbs, kidneys, etc. Various methods are employed in the surgical treatment of this condition. They consist of

1. resection of the stricture between clamps and end-to-end anastomosis of the aortic ends (aortic anastomosis),
2. plastic revision,
3. vascular grafts.

The esophagus *gullet* (ē-SOF-ah-gus) and/or trachea[1] *rough* (TRĀ-kē-ah) may be compressed by a double aortic arch, ab/errant *from to wander* (AB-er-ant) vessels (anomal/ous *irregular* [ah-NOM-ah-lus] origin of the in/nominate *no name* [in-NOM-in-āt] and/or left common carotid *to put to sleep* [kah-ROT-id] arteries), anomalous origin of the right subclavian artery. Ligation and surgical division of the compression vessels is performed.

Mitral stenosis, obstruction of the valve orifice between the left atrium and left ventricle, is nearly always caused by rheumatic disease. Com/missuro/tomy *together to join* (kom"i-sūr-OT-ō-me) (separation of the leaflets of the valve -- fused mitral com/missures [KOM-i-sūrs]) by mechanical dilatation is performed. This is also known as ventricular dilatation of mitral valve.

1. windpipe

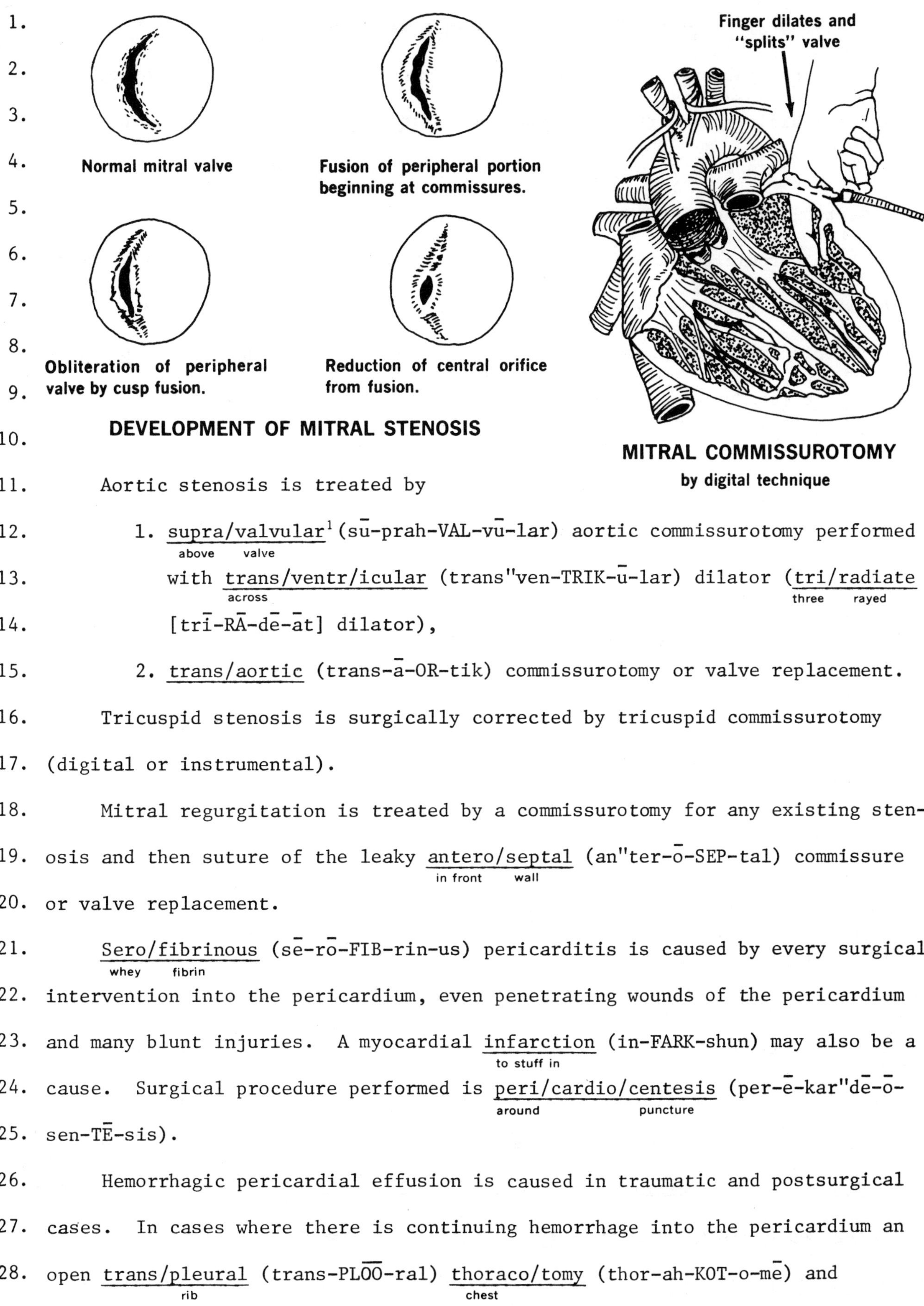
Normal mitral valve
Fusion of peripheral portion beginning at commissures.
Obliteration of peripheral valve by cusp fusion.
Reduction of central orifice from fusion.
Finger dilates and "splits" valve

DEVELOPMENT OF MITRAL STENOSIS

MITRAL COMMISSUROTOMY
by digital technique

Aortic stenosis is treated by

1. supra/valvular[1] *above valve* (sū-prah-VAL-vū-lar) aortic commissurotomy performed with trans/ventr/icular *across* (trans"ven-TRIK-ū-lar) dilator (tri/radiate *three rayed* [trī-RĀ-dē-āt] dilator),
2. trans/aortic (trans-ā-OR-tik) commissurotomy or valve replacement.

Tricuspid stenosis is surgically corrected by tricuspid commissurotomy (digital or instrumental).

Mitral regurgitation is treated by a commissurotomy for any existing stenosis and then suture of the leaky antero/septal *in front wall* (an"ter-ō-SEP-tal) commissure or valve replacement.

Sero/fibrinous *whey fibrin* (sē-rō-FIB-rin-us) pericarditis is caused by every surgical intervention into the pericardium, even penetrating wounds of the pericardium and many blunt injuries. A myocardial infarction *to stuff in* (in-FARK-shun) may also be a cause. Surgical procedure performed is peri/cardio/centesis *around puncture* (per-ē-kar"dē-ō-sen-TĒ-sis).

Hemorrhagic pericardial effusion is caused in traumatic and postsurgical cases. In cases where there is continuing hemorrhage into the pericardium an open trans/pleural *rib* (trans-PLOO-ral) thoraco/tomy *chest* (thor-ah-KOT-o-mē) and

1. From hereon the adjective endings will not be separated for translation as it is assumed they have been learned by this time.

peri/cardio/tomy (per″ē-kar-dē-OT-ō-me) is performed.

Sup/purative (SUP-ū-rah-tiv) pericarditis and infected serofibrinous pericarditis are treated by open peri/cardi/ectomy (per″ē-kar-dē-EK-tō-mē) with evacuation of ex/udate (EKS-ū-dāt), instillation of antibiotics and establishment of transpleural drainage.

below pus; out to sweat

Chronic constrictive pericarditis is caused by a constrictive, dense membrane surrounding part or all of the heart. Treatment consists of pericardiectomy and removal of the constriction by blunt dissection[1] (peri/cardio/lysis [per″ē-kar-dē-OL-i-sis]). Where the pericardium may be adherent a complete removal of the pericardium may be necessary (pericardiectomy).

Subacute or acute bacterial endocarditis is characterized by septic/emia (sep-ti-SĒ-mē-ah) and the growth of certain pyogenic organisms in vegetations developing upon the cardiac valves. Treatment consists of

decay

1. commissurotomy after bacterial invasion has been controlled by antibiotics,
2. com/missuro/rrhaphy (kom″i-sūr-OR-ah-fē) for "teardrop" stenotic and incompetent valve, the functionally insufficient valve and in cases of created (traumatic) insufficiency.

Coronary arterial disease is a condition in which, due to a disease process affecting the coronary arteries themselves, the effective coronary arterial blood flow has become diminished sufficiently to produce evidences of what has been designated as coronary insufficiency, coronary occlusion with or without thrombosis, or myocardial infarction. Surgical efforts are directed to improve the vascular/iz/ation (vas″kū-lar-i-ZĀ-shun) of the heart by adding a new source of blood to the myocardium or to enhance the benefits derived from some of the remaining existing sources of myocardial nutrition. Procedure is called cardio/peri/cardio/pexy (kar″dē-ō-per-ē-kar″dē-ō-PEK-sē) or surface re/vascular/ization (rē″vas-kū-lar-i-ZĀ-shun). Some procedures are:

vessel

1. Blunt dissection means the "teasing" or "breaking" of tissue (dissecting through the tissue planes) with the finger. It is the opposite of dissection with a sharp instrument such as a scalpel.

1. Intra/myo/cardial [inside muscle] (in-trah-mī-ō-KAR-dē-al) implantation of the left internal mammary artery and known as the Vineberg procedure.

2. Coronary end/arter/ectomy [within] (end-ar-ter-EK-tō-mē) which is the removal of the obstructing area within the lumen of the vessel.

Aortic regurgitation or insufficiency may be congenital or may be acquired as a result of luetic [syphilis] (lū-ET-ik), bacterial, or rheumatic valvul/itis (val-vū-LĪ-tis). As a result of the valvular lesion, blood leaks back into the ventricle during dia/stole [through to send] (dī-AS-tō-lē). Treatment surgically is by placement of the "butterfly" valve.

Pulmonic [lung] (pul-MON-ik) stenosis is a severe mechanical obstruction to the free flow of blood from the right ventricle into the pulmonary vascular tree. Surgical procedures performed include pulmonary valvulo/tomy (val-vū-LOT-ō-mē) and pulmonary valvulo/plasty (VAL-vū-lō-plas-tē).

Truncus [trunk] (TRUNG-kus) arteriosus (an extreme stage of aortic septal defect) with pulmonary stenosis is treated by any one of several procedures:

1. Blalock-Taussig operation (a type of shunt),
2. Potts-Smith operation (a type of shunt),
3. Direct anastomosis of the end of the pulmonary artery to the aorta for conditions in which the Blalock-Taussig or Potts-Smith procedures are not applicable. The pulmonic obstruction may be treated by valvulotomy for valvular stenosis and infundibul/ectomy [funnel] (in-fun-dib"ū-LEK-tō-mē) for infundibular (in-fun-DIB-ū-lar) stenosis.

TRUNCUS ARTERIOSUS COMMUNIS

Potts-Smith or Blalock anastomosis is performed for tricuspid a/tresia *(not a hole)* (ah-TRĒ-zē-ah) with hypo/plasia *(below formation)* (hī-pō-PLĀ-zē-ah) of right ventricles.

Tetralogy of Fallot is a grouping of congenital cardiac defects commonly found in adults, namely, pulmonic stenosis, interventricular septal defects, dextroposition of the aorta so that it receives blood from the right as well as the left ventricle, and hypertrophy of the right ventricle. Various procedures are performed consisting of pulmonary valvulotomy or valvuloplasty, dilatation of pulmonary arterial stricture, infundibulectomy, infundibulectomy and valvulotomy, and shunting operations: Blalock-Taussig anastomosis, Potts-Smith anastomosis; Brock's method under direct vision.

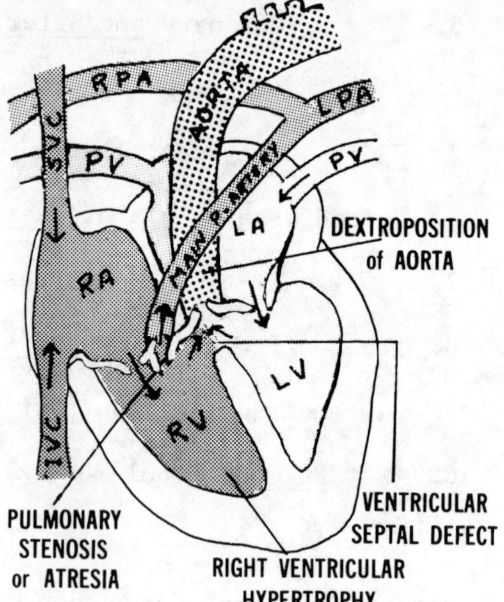

TETRALOGY OF FALLOT

Atrial septal defects and anomalous drainage of the pulmonary veins are the commonest of all congenital cardiac defects. Procedure used is the open method under direct vision in which the atrial septal defect is closed by suture. Lutembacher's *(French physician)* (LŌŌ-tem-bak-erz) syndrome *(a running together)* (SIN-drōm) known as mitral stenosis may accompany atrial septal defects in which case a mitral commissurotomy is also performed.

Similar procedures are performed for fenestrated *(having window-like openings)* (fen-is-TRĀ-ted) septum (the presence of several openings in close association. The defect is located inferiorly and just above the atrio/ventricular *(atrium ventricle)* [ā"trē-ō-ven-TRIK-ū-lar] valves).

Ventricular septal defects are repaired by open method under direct vision in which there is a direct suture of the defect.

Diverticul/ectomy *(to turn aside)* (dī-ver-tik"ū-LEK-tō-mē) is performed for diverticula (dī-ver-TIK-ū-lah) or aneurysms of the heart. They are usually of the ventricles.

Tumors of the heart can be classified as pericardial, cardiac and intracardiac. They are usually metastatic but some tumors are primary. Primary malignant tumors of the heart are much less common than benign tumors. Types of malignant tumors are rhabdo/myo/sarc/oma *a strip muscle flesh* (rab"dō-mī"ō-sar-KŌ-mah), leio/myo/sarc/oma *smooth* (lī"ō-mī"ō-sar-KŌ-mah), fibroma, fibro/myxo/sarc/oma *mucus* (fī"bro-mik-sō-sar-KŌ-mah), myxo/sarc/oma (mik"sō-sar-KŌ-mah), lipo/sarc/oma *fat* (lī"po-sar-KŌ-mah), meso/theli/oma *middle nipple* (mē-sō-thē-lē-Ō-mah), endo/thelio/sarc/oma *within* (en-dō-thē"lē-ō-sar-KŌ-mah), hem/angio/sarc/oma *blood vessel* (hē-man-jē-ō-sar-KŌ-mah), lymph/angio/sarc/oma (limf"an-jē-ō-sar-KŌ-mah). E/nucle/ation[1] *out kernel* (ē-nū-KLĒ-ā-shun) of the tumor is performed when possible.

An aneurysm is a relatively localized outpouching of the wall of an artery or of a cardiac ventricle due to disease. Types of aneurysms are dissecting, arteriosclerotic, cardiac, syphilitic arterial, traumatic arterial.

Types of surgical treatment performed:

1. Complete excision of the aneurysmal *widening* (an-ū-RIZ-mal) sac and suture repair of the aorta.
2. Partial excision of aneurysmal sac and reconstruction of a suitable blood passageway.
3. Resection of an aortic segment and replacement by a prosthetic tube (most common procedure today).
4. Resection of the entire descending thoracic aorta and replacement with an aortic homograft.

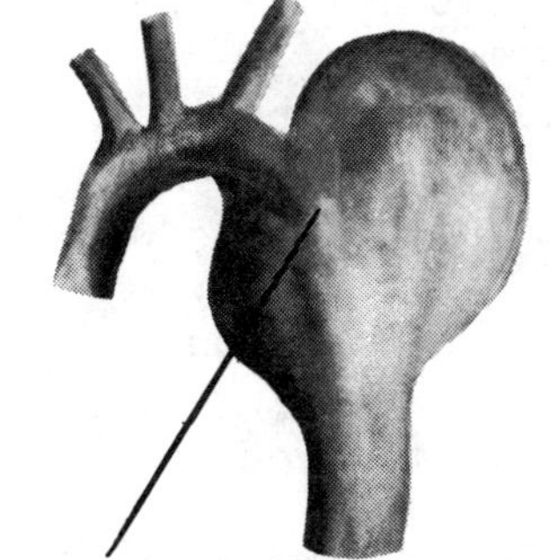
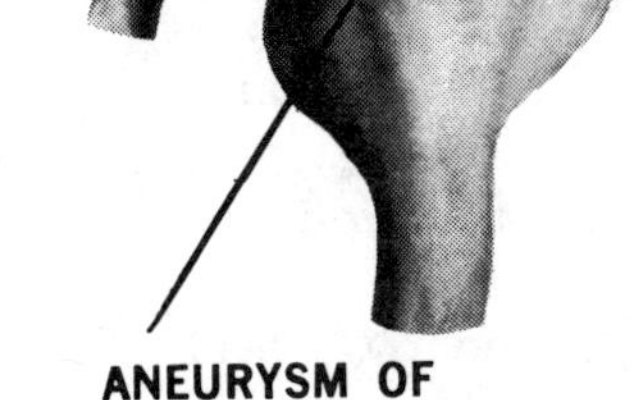

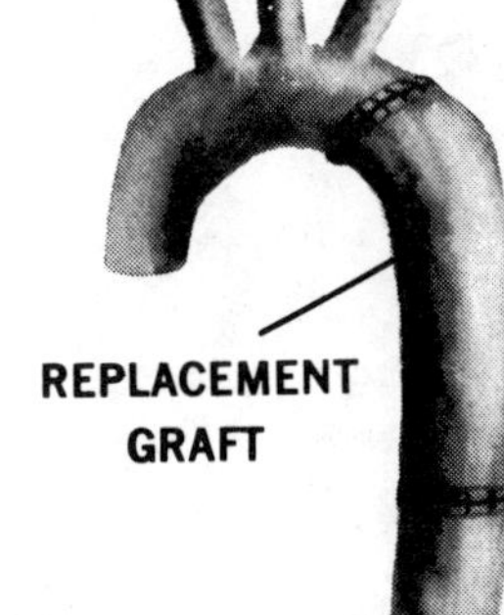

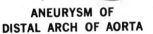

1. To shell out, like a nut

5. Resection of aneurysms involving the aortic arch.
6. Resection and transplantation of the entire thoracic aorta.
7. Aortic arch resection with the aid of the Gemeinhardt pump.

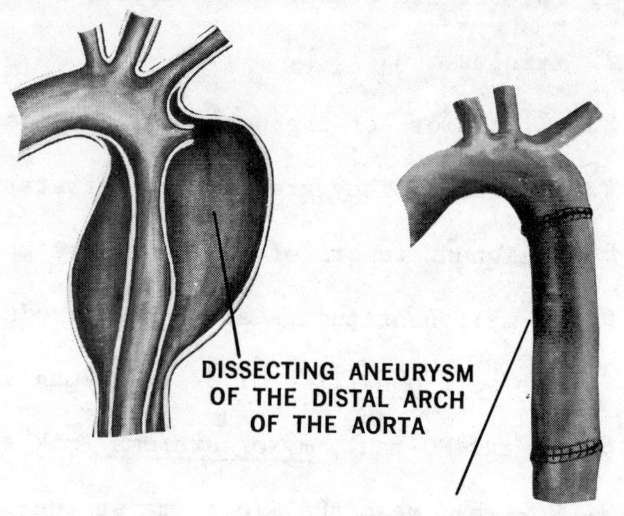

Obliterative disease (Leriche's [la-RĒSH-ez] syndrome) is treated by

1. Excision and end-to-end inter/pol/ation *(between pole)* (in-ter-pō-LĀ-shun) of graft or plastic prosthesis *(an addition)* (pros-THĒ-sis) (thrombotic [throm-BOT-ik] segment of terminal aorta removed and replaced by graft or prosthesis).
2. End-to-side by-pass with graft or plastic

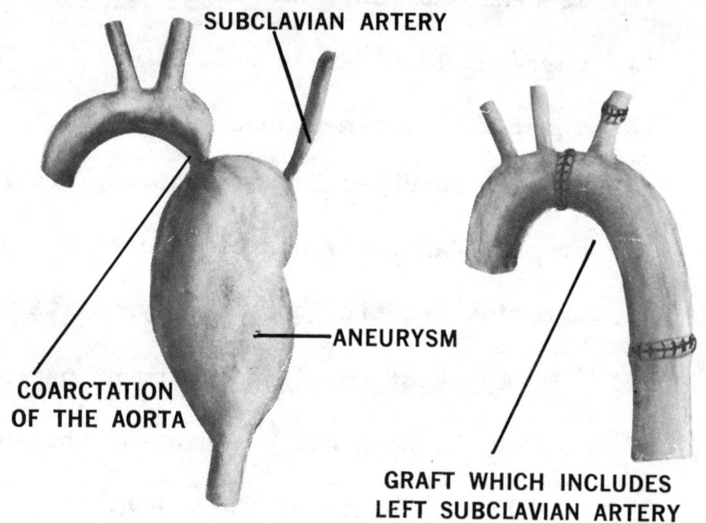

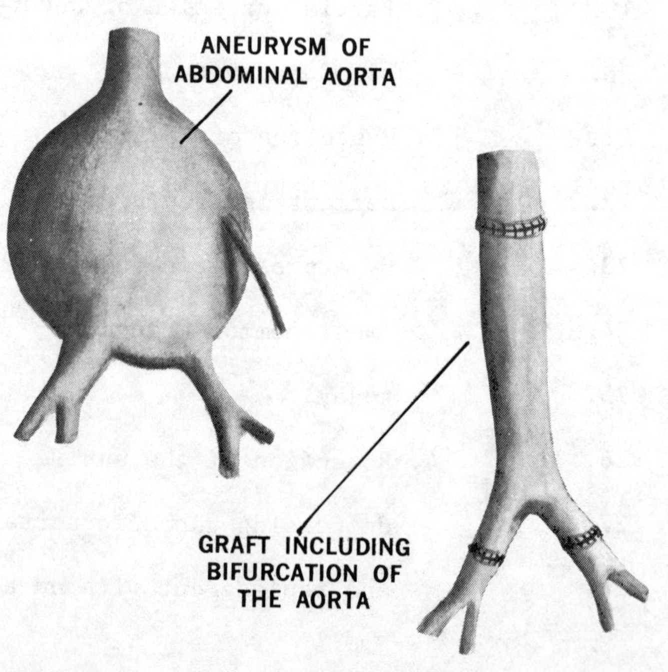

prosthesis (occluded segment left intact; plastic repair to restore continuity to aorta).

3. Thrombo/end/arter/ectomy (throm"bō-end-ar"ter-EK-tō-mē) which is the removal of clot and plaque from inside the artery.

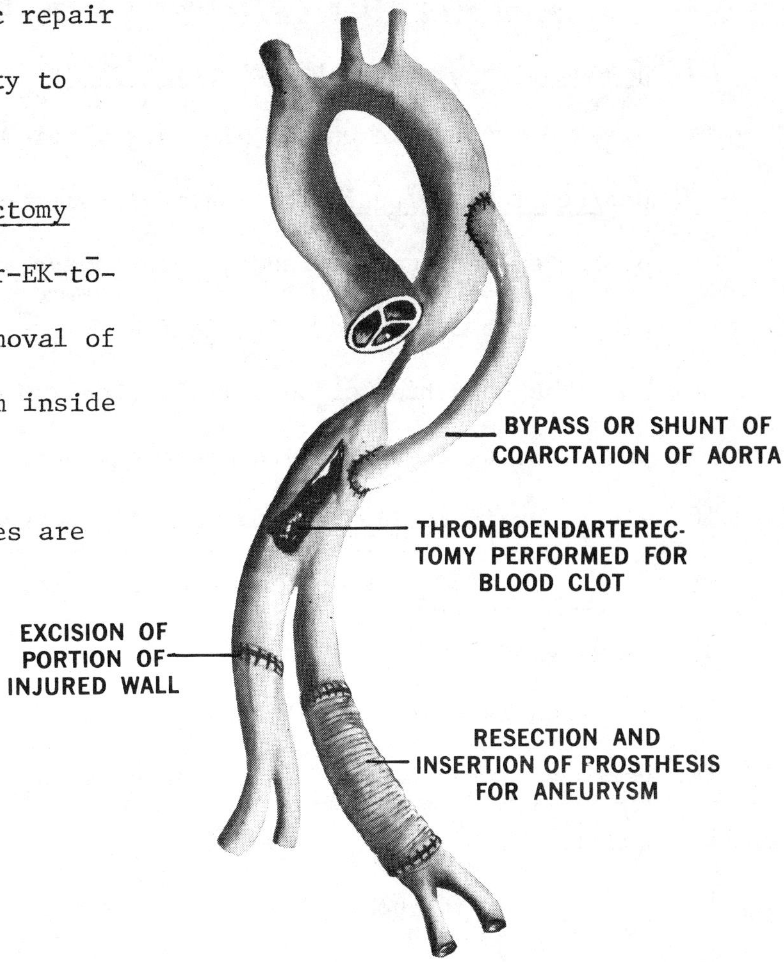

Several surgical procedures are performed for arteriovenous fistula (FIS-tū-lah). They include:

pipe

1. Repair of the arterial opening after removal of a portion of the vein.
2. Trans/venous (trans-VĒ-nus) closure of the opening.
3. Repair of the opening in both artery and vein.
4. Mass ligature of the fistula where the first four procedures cannot be carried out.

SURGICAL PROCEDURES PERFORMED ON THE AORTA

BYPASS OR SHUNT OF COARCTATION OF AORTA

THROMBOENDARTERECTOMY PERFORMED FOR BLOOD CLOT

EXCISION OF PORTION OF INJURED WALL

RESECTION AND INSERTION OF PROSTHESIS FOR ANEURYSM

Two basic surgical methods generally employed either alone or in combination for the treatment of varicose veins are

1. ligation of the varicose vein combined with varying degrees of resection (vein stripping),
2. obliteration by the injection of a sclerosing solution.

Phlebothrombosis is treated with proximal venous ligation if embol/iz/ation (em-bō-li-ZĀ-shun) has occurred.

a plugging

SURGERY OF THE LYMPHATIC SYSTEM

Splen/ectomy [spleen] (sple-NEK-tō-mē) is performed for hemo/lytic [solution] (hē-mō-LIT-ik) jaundice[1] [yellow] (JAWN-dis), thrombo/cyto/penic [poverty, lack] (throm"bō-sī-tō-PĒ-nik) purpura, Banti's disease or splenic anemia, Felty's syndrome, primary splenic neutropenia, splenic pan/hemato/cyto/penia [all] (pan-hē"ma-tō-sī-tō-PĒ-nē-ah), Gaucher's disease, rupture of the spleen due to trauma, spleno/megaly [large] (sple-nō-MEG-ah-lē), cirrhosis [orange yellow] (si-RŌ-sis) of the liver and mal/aria [bad air] (mah-LĀ-rē-ah).

The condition of portal hypertension may be produced by obstruction of the portal vein or some of its branches, before it reaches the liver, within the liver, or in the hepatic [liver] (hē-PAT-ik) vein or vena cava. Surgeries performed may be 1. porta/caval [portal vein vena cava] (por-tah-KĀ-val) shunt, 2. porto-renal [kidney] (por-tō-RĒ-nal) shunt or 3. splenectomy.

Complete or radical neck dissection is done for metastatic carcinoma of the cervical lymph nodes. It is not used for tuberculosis of the cervical lymph nodes.

Par/ot/id [beside ear condition] (pah-ROT-id) tumors are excised and the greatest danger is the possibility of severing the facial nerve when removing the tumor thus causing facial paralysis.

Salivary [saliva] (SAL-i-vā-rē) duct stones: small stones are "milked" out of the ducts and large stones are brought to the end of the duct in the same way and an incision is made over them and through the orifice thus allowing extraction of the stone.

Ranula[2] [tadpole] (RAN-ū-lah) is a cystic tumor beneath the tongue and is also known as sub/lingual [below tongue] (sub-LING-gwal) cyst. It is treated by

1. marsupial/iz/ation [pouch to treat] (mar-sū"pē-al-i-ZĀ-shun) which is used on rare occasions. This procedure consists of opening the cyst, emptying its contents and stretching its edges to the edges of the external excision. The interior of this sac suppurates and closes by granulation.

1. From Latin "icterus" and French "jaune" meaning "yellow"
2. Diminutive of "rana" meaning "frog"

2. excision which is the treatment most frequently used.

Adamantin/oma [very hard] (ad"ah-man-te-NŌ-mah), an epithelial tumor of the jaw, is excised.

Excision of the submaxillary salivary gland is done for tumor or stones.

Lateral cervical fistul/ectomy [pipe] (fis-tū-LEK-tō-mē) is performed for lateral cervical fistulae, which are long epithelial tubes present at birth. The entire tube is removed.

Branchial [gills] (BRANG-kē-al) sinus is resected. Branchial cleft cysts, of which there are two types, are excised. The first branchial cleft cyst is situated just in front of the top of the ear and just below the hair of the temple. The lower branchial cleft cysts are in the carotid sheath at about the level of the hyoid bone.

Hygr/omas [moist] (hī-GRŌ-mahs) are cavernous lymphangiomas of the neck and are usually first seen in infancy. They are excised.

In radical surgeries performed for cancer of the breast and in other areas where there is a large concentration of lymph nodes and vessels these nodes are removed for the purpose of halting the spread of the cancer.

INDEX
CHAPTER V

PAGE	LINE	
129	5	streptococcal
128	21	styptics
120	16	subclavian
140	24	sublingual
134	2	suppurative
133	12	supravalvular
136	19	syndrome
120	6	synovial
123	19	syphilitic
124	19	tachycardia
131	22	tetralogy of Fallot
133	28	thoracotomy
126	5	thrombi
126	19	thromboangiitis
118	5	thrombocytes
140	3	thrombocytopenic
139	5	thromboendarterectomy
127	8	thrombophlebitis
125	15	thrombosis
138	21	thrombotic
117	6	thyroid
121	20	tibial
127	1	toxemia
132	19	trachea
133	13	triradiate
133	15	transaortic
133	28	transpleural
139	18	transvenous
133	13	transventricular
114	7	tricuspid
135	14	truncus
121	13	tubercle
129	25	tuberculosis
129	26	tularemia
115	13	tunica
129	13	urticaria
124	14	valvular
135	6	valvulitis
135	13	valvuloplasty
135	12	valvulotomy
127	9	varices
127	8	varicose
115	10	vasa vasorum
134	24	vascularization
113	17	venae cavae
114	20	ventricular
113	18	ventriculum
113	4	venules
120	14	villi

GLANDS

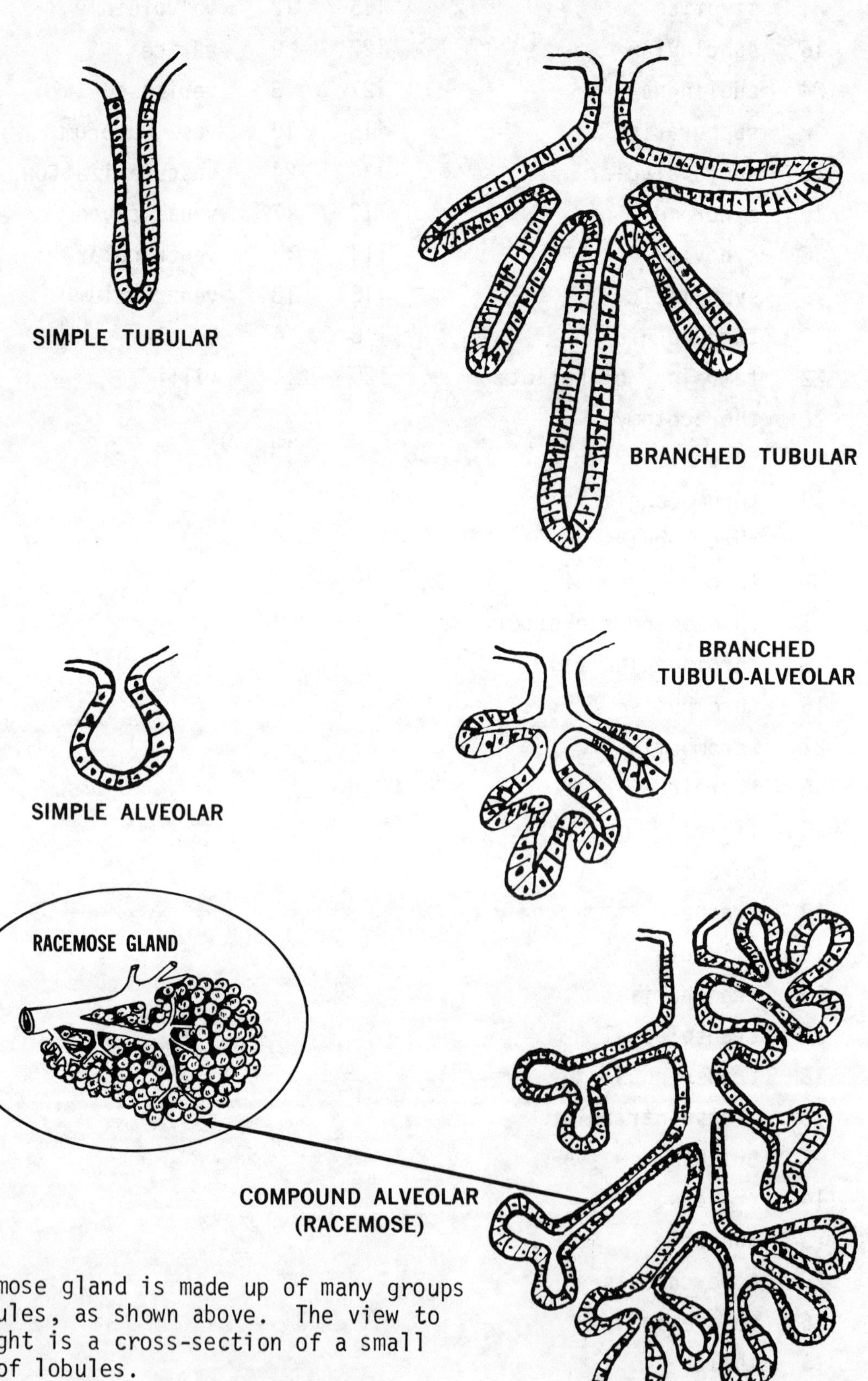

A racemose gland is made up of many groups of lobules, as shown above. The view to the right is a cross-section of a small group of lobules.

CHAPTER VI
THE ENDOCRINE SYSTEM

A gland is a secreting organ, or an organ which abstracts certain materials from the blood. It then takes these materials and makes of them a new substance. Glands may be classified according to structure and function. If classified according to structure, they are of two kinds, simple and compound.

The new substance, the product of a gland, elaborated from the blood by cell action, and intended for use in the body, is a secretion.

An excretion is a secretion, except that the excretion is generally formed to be thrown out of the body. It, therefore, follows that all excretions are first secretions, and, with the exception of urine, all excretions are made use of before they are eliminated, for example, the bile.

If classified according to function, glands are of two kinds, secretory *to separate* (se-KRĒ-ter-ē)[1] or those that form secretions and excretory *to separate out* (EKS-kre-tō-rē) or those that form excretions. The secretory glands are of two types, one type provided with ducts and a second type called ductless or endo/crine *within to separate* (EN-dō-krin) glands. Based on the difference in structure and mode of liberating their secretions, secretory glands are divided into two groups, those producing external secretions, and those producing internal secretions.

External secretions is used to designate those secretions of glandular tissues which are carried to their destination by a duct. The digestive fluids secreted (se-KRĒ-ted) by the salivary *spittle* (SAL-i-vā-rē), gastric *stomach* (GAS-trik), and intestinal glands, the pan/creas *all flesh*[2] (PAN-krē-as) and the liver, are external secretions. The secretions of the lacrimal *tear* (LAK-re-mal), tarsal *sole of the foot*[3] (TAHR-sal), ceruminous *wax* (se-RŪ-min-us), sebaceous *oily, fatty* (se-BĀ-shus) and sweat glands are also external secretions. All of these secretions are carried off from their

1. The most common pronunciation seems to be SĒ-kre-tō-rē despite the dictionary pronunciation used in the text.
2. From the Greek "kreas"
3. Translates as a "broad flat surface"

THE ENDOCRINE SYSTEM

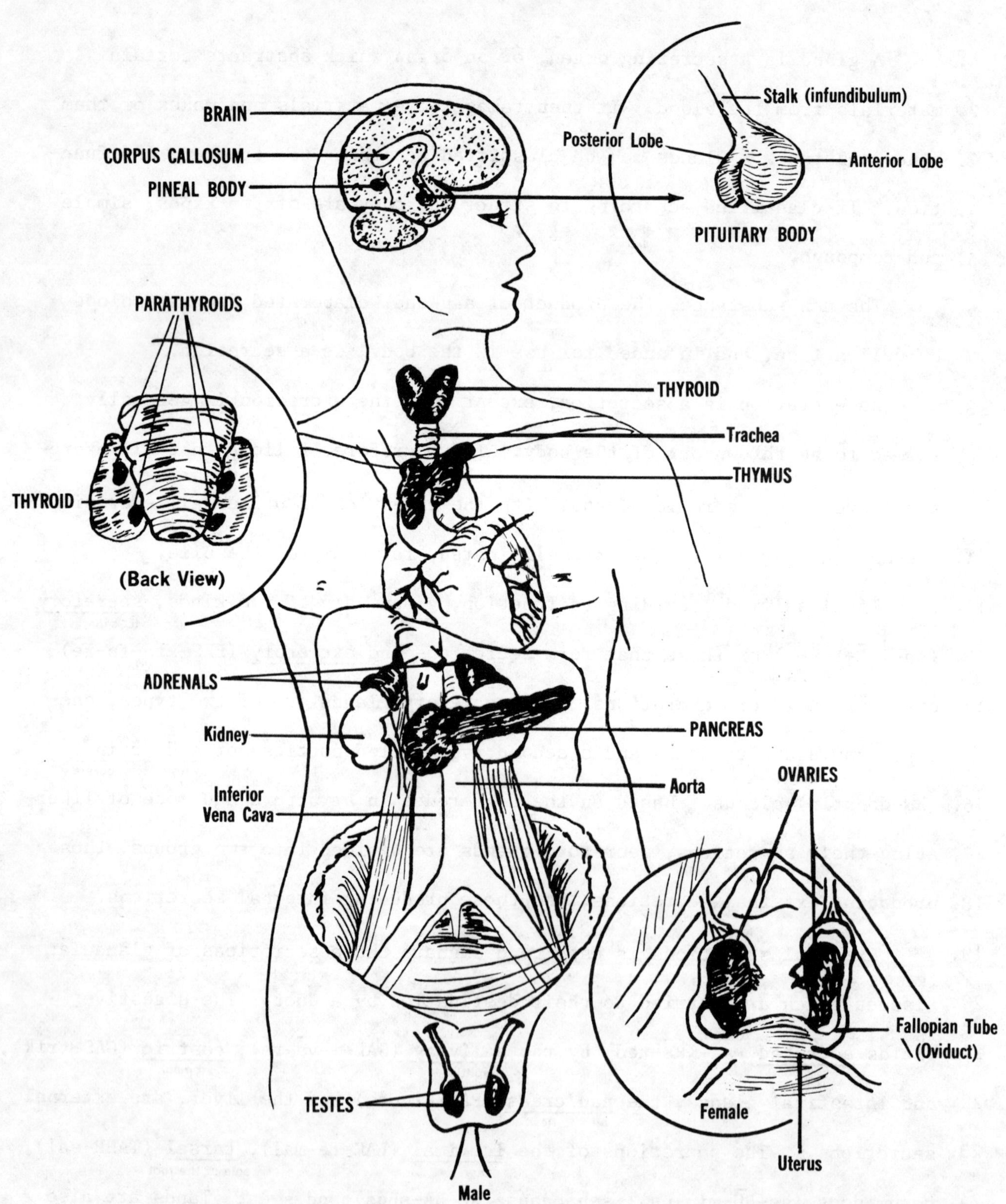

respective glands in which they are formed, by means of ducts.

The functions of these secretions vary. Those concerned with digestion promote chemical reactions: the lacrimal, tarsal, ceruminous, sebaceous and sweat glands moisten, lubricate and protect the surfaces upon which they are discharged; the per/spiration *through to breathe* (per-spi-RĀ-shun) helps in regulating body heat; the secretion of the mammary *breast* (MAM-mah-rē) glands furnishes nutritive material which is specially adapted to the needs of the young of the species.

The digestive fluids owe their power to promote chemical reactions to en/zymes *in to leaven, to ferment* (EN-zīms). Enzymes are complex organic substances which act as catalyzers *to dissolve* (KAT-ah-līz-ers).

The endocrine or ductless glands form a group of organs that produce secretions, called internal secretions, which leave the gland by the blood or lymph *water* (limf). Many of the glands that possess ducts and form an external secretion form an internal secretion as well, for example, the liver and pancreas.

There are seven ductless glands: the thyr/oid *shield* (THĪ-royd), the para/thyroids *beside* (par-ah-THĪ-royds), the thymus *excrescence*[1] (THĪ-mus), the supra/renal *above kidney* (sū-prah-RĒ-nal) glands or ad/renals *near* (ad-RĒ-nals), the pituitary *phlegm* (pi-TŪ-i-tār-ē) body or hypo/physis *below to grow* (hī-POF-i-sis), the pineal *pine cone*[2] (PIN-ē-al) body or epi/physis *on,upon* (ē-PIF-i-sis) and the gonads *from seed*[3] (GON-ads) (ovaries *egg bearer* [Ō-vah-rēz] and testes *shell (plural)* [TES-tēz]).

Special cells in the pancreas and liver, also portions of the lining membrane of the stomach and intestines function as ductless glands and furnish internal secretions.

The thyroid is a small, flat gland consisting of a right and left lobe placed on either side of the trachea *rough* (TRĀ-kē-ah), below the thyroid cartilage. The lobes are connected by a strand of their own substance, called the isthmus *a joining strip* (IS-mus), which stretches across the front of the

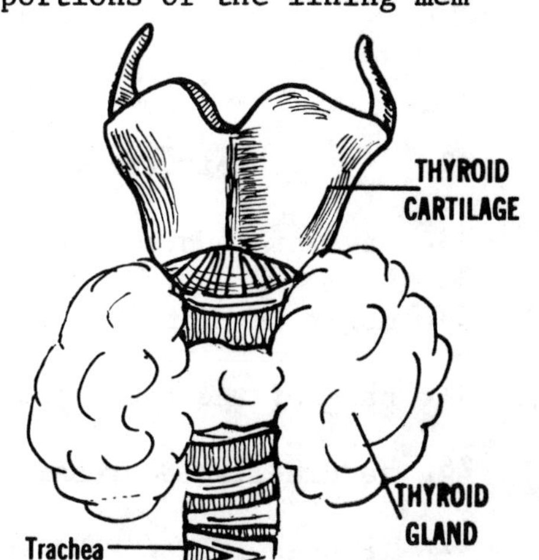

THYROID GLAND
(Front View)

1. Although the thymus gland is included here with the other endocrine glands no evidence of its action as such has been discovered. It is now listed in the lymphatic system.
2. The pineal body is included with the endocrine glands because it is ductless. However, its endocrine activity is not established.
3. Optional pronunciation GŌ-nads.

trachea. The thyroid gland furnishes thyroxin [a hormone] (thī-ROK-sin) which is absolutely essential to health. It contains as high as 65 percent of iodine [violet-like] (Ī-o-din). The general effect of the gland is to control the metabolic [change] (met-ah-BOL-ik) rate.

THYROID GLAND (Back View)

The parathyroids consist of four to six small glands usually located between the posterior borders of the lateral lobes of the thyroid gland and its capsule.

The thymus consists of two lateral lobes, which occasionally unite to form a single mass, or the two lobes may have an intermediate lobe between them. It is located beneath the breastbone. At birth the gland is larger than a baby's fist. It is a temporary organ, reaching its greatest size at the time of puberty [grown-up] (PŪ-ber-tē), when it gradually diminishes to about the size of a thumb.

The suprarenal glands or adrenals are two small, yellowish bodies placed above and in front of the upper end of each kidney. Each gland is surrounded by a thin capsule of fibrous [fiber] (FĪ-brus) tissue and consists of two parts known as the cortex [rind,bark] (KOR-teks) and the medulla [marrow,middle] (me-DUL-ah), which differ in origin and function. The medulla secretes a substance called epi/ [on,upon] nephrin [kidney][1] (ep-i-NEF-rin).

The pituitary body or hypophysis is a mass of reddish gray tissue about 1 centimeter in diameter. It is situated at the base of the brain and is lodged in a saddle-like depression, the sella turcica ["Turkish saddle"] (SEL-ah TUR-si-kah), of the sphen/oid [wedge] (SFĒ-noyd) bone. It consists of two lobes:

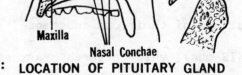

LOCATION OF PITUITARY GLAND

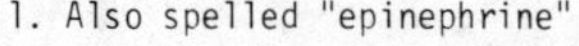
1. Also spelled "epinephrine"

the anterior lobe and the posterior lobe. A substance called pituitrin [phlegm] (pi-TŪ-i-trin) or hypo/physin [to grow] (hī-POF-is-in) is obtained from extracts of the posterior lobe. Pituitrin is used in obstetrics [midwife] (ob-STET-riks) to promote contractions of the uterus. It is also used in post/partum [after delivery] (pōst-PAR-tum) and pulmonary [lung] (PUL-mō-nār-ē) hemorrhage.

The pineal body or epiphysis is a small reddish gray body that develops as an outgrowth of the third ventricle of the brain and remains attached to the roof of the ventricle. It decreases in size after puberty.

The ovaries produce ova [egg] (Ō-vah) and two internal secretions. One secretion is formed by the vesicular [bladder] (ve-SIK-u-lar) follicles [little bag] (FOL-i-kls) and is called oestrin [estrogen] (ES-trin). A second internal secretion formed by the cells of the corpus [body] (KOR-pus) luteum [yellow] (LŪ-tē-um) is progestin (prō-JES-tin) or pro/ge/sterone [before pregnant steroid] (prō-JES-ter-ōn). This secretion prepares the uterus for the reception of the fertilized ovum.

The testes produce spermato/zoa [seed animal,life] (sper"mah-tō-ZŌ-ah) and the inter/stitial [between to set] (in-ter-STISH-al) cells produce an internal secretion, testo/sterone [shell,testicle steroid] (tes-TOS-ter-ōn).

In addition to other functions the liver forms two substances, glyco/gen [sweet,sugar to produce] (GLĪ-kō-jen) and urea [urine] (ū-RĒ-ah) from materials which it takes from the blood and which are subsequently returned to the blood.

The pancreas forms an external secretion, the pancreatic (pan-krē-AT-ik) fluid, but special groups of cells in the pancreas called the islands of Langerhans[1] (LAHNG-er-hanz) furnish an internal secretion containing insulin [island] (IN-sū-lin) which is essential for the normal course of sugar metabolism [change] (me-TAB-ō-lizm).

The mucous membrane lining the pyloric [gate] (pī-LOR-ik) end of the stomach contains some cells which secrete a hormone [to excite] (HOR-mōn) known as gastrin [a hormone] (GAS-trin).

1. German pathologist 1847-1888

The spleen (splēn)(lien [LĪ-ēn]) *spleen* is classed by some authorities as belonging with the ductless glands and by others as belonging with the lymph nodes. It is situated directly behind the diaphragm, behind and to the left of the stomach.

DISEASES AND ANOMALIES

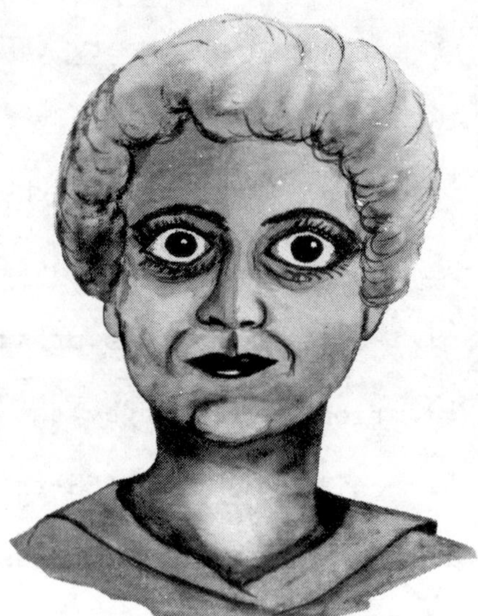

Exophthalmic goiter with staring eyes and enlargement of the thyroid.

Hypo/thyroidism (hī-pō-THĪ-royd-izm): Goiter *throat* (GOY-ter), cretinism *human being, not an animal* (KRĒ-tin-izm) and myx/edema *mucus swelling* (mik-se-DĒ-mah) are patho/logical *disease* (path-ō-LOJ-i-kal) conditions due to hypothyroidism. These conditions are caused by a decrease in the iodine content of the gland or as a result of a/trophy *lack* (AT-rō-fē) or removal of the thyroid.

Hyper/thyroidism *above* (hī-per-THĪ-royd-izm): Over-activity of the thyroid gland produces a condition called Graves'[1] disease or ex/ophthalmic *out eye* (ek-sof-THAL-mik) goiter.

Aden/oma *gland* (ad-i-NŌ-mah) of the thyroid (aden/omat/ous *tumor* [ad-i-NŌ-mah-tus] or nodular *node* [NOD-ū-lar] goiter) is a benign tumor consisting of cells like those of normal thyroid tissue. Cancer of the thyroid usually starts in an adenomatous goiter.

Thyroid/itis (thī-royd-Ī-tis) or inflammation of the thyroid gland is quite rare.

The parathyroids secrete a hormone which brings about the release of calcium *lime* (KAL-sē-um) from bones and its liberation into the blood stream. The purpose of these glands is the maintenance of a constant amount of calcium in the blood, the calcium being concerned in the metabolism of nervous and muscular tissue. Hyper/parathyroidism (hī"per-par-ah-THĪ-royd-izm) is most often due to adenoma (benign tumor) of one of the parathyroids. Large cysts often form within the bones (osteitis *bone* [os-tē-Ī-tis] fibrosa *fiber* [FĪ-brō-sah] cystica *sac,bladder* [SIS-tik-ah]), and patho/

1. Robert J. Graves, Irish physician, 1796-1853

logic (path-ō-LOJ-ik) fractures may occur. Hypo/parathyroidism (hī"pō-par-ah-THĪ-royd-izm) is caused by a lack of parathyroid secretion which results most commonly from accidental injury or removal of the parathyroid glands during thyroid/ectomy (thī-royd-EK-tō-mē).

Hypersecretion of the adrenal cortex produces different syndromes in children than in adults, and in males than in females. In children it leads to premature sexual development (precocious *ripe before time* [prē-KŌ-shus] puberty). In girls, male characteristics may develop. In adult females it is manifested by the development of male characteristics. Additionally, a peculiar obesity *fat* (ō-BĒ-si-tē) limited to the face, neck and trunk may develop, and marked hypertension may be present. This combination of symptoms constitutes Cushing's[1] (KOOSH-ings) syndrome. Cortical hyperfunction is rare in adult males, and the symptoms apparently vary in different cases; in some, increased masculinity; in others, feminism, with or without obesity, and hypertension is said to develop. Hyperfunction of the adrenal medulla causes hypertension, together with other symptoms of excessive secretion of adrenalin *a hormone* (ad-REN-ah-lin): tachy/cardia *fast heart* (tak-ē-KAR-dē-ah), tremor of the hands, and blanching of the skin. Hypofunction of the adrenal cortex leads to a syndrome called Addison's[2] (AD-i-sonz) disease.

Primary tumors of the adrenals may arise in the cortex or medulla and may be malignant or benign. In medullary *marrow, middle* (MED-ū-lār-ē) tumors two primary tumors are encountered, the neuro/blast/oma *nerve germ, cell* (nū"rō-blas-TŌ-mah) and the para/gangli/oma *beside swelling* (par"ah-gang-glē-Ō-mah) (pheo/chromo/cyt/omas *dark color cell* [fē-ō-krō"mō-sī-TŌ-mahs]).

The male gonads or testes secrete a hormone, testosterone, which causes the development of the male sex characteristics. It also has to do with muscular strength.

In young boys, hypersecretion of the testes leads to precocious puberty,

1. Harvey Cushing, Boston surgeon, 1869-1939
2. Thomas Addison, English physician, 1793-1860

with early development of secondary sex characteristics. In grown men, hyperfunction of the testes causes more rapid growth of beard, increase in body hair, and increase in muscular strength.

In young boys, hypofunction or hyposecretion of the testes causes delayed or retarded development of male characteristics. In adults, cessation of testicular *[testis]* (tes-TIK-ū-lar) function is followed by variable recession of male characteristics but not always to a great degree. The principal effects of lack of testicular secretion are decrease of strength, vigor and ambition.

Diseases of the testes are concerned chiefly with hypersecretion which is most commonly due to tumors of the secretory cells, and hyposecretion which may be due to congenitally poor development of the testes, to lack of descent of the testes into the scrotum *[bag]* (SKRŌ-tum) (crypt/orchid/ism *[hide,conceal / testicle]*[1] [krip-TOR-kid-izm]), to degeneration secondary to inflammation, vascular disease, trauma or to castration *[to deprive of generative power]* (kas-TRĀ-shun).

A/meno/rrhea *[lack / month]* (ā-men-ō-RĒ-ah)[2] may be primary, consisting of a failure of establishment of the menses *[month]* (MEN-sēz) in young girls in their teens; or, it may be secondary, in which the menses, which have been previously established, suddenly cease.

During the meno/pause *[month / cessation]* (MEN-ō-pawz), or, as it is often called, "the change of life," certain unpleasant symptoms occur which may be considered as normal. In some women these symptoms are extraordinarily severe or prolonged. Marked emotional disturbances or even psychoses *[mind]* (sī-KŌ-sēz) may occur. Hypertension may also appear at this time of life. Meno/pausal (men-ō-PAW-zal) symptoms are usually more severe if the menopause has been induced artificially by removal or ir/radiation *[into / to emit rays]* (ir-rā"dē-Ā-shun) of the ovaries. Estrin or other substances with estro/genic *[estrin / to produce]* (es-trō-JEN-ik) effects (stilbestrol *[synthetic female hormone]* [stil-BES-trol], estradiol *[female hormone]* [es-trah-DĪ-ol]) are used to give relief from menopausal symptoms.

Osteo/porosis *[bone / callus]* (os"tē-ō-pō-RŌ-sis) also known as porosis (pō-RŌ-sis) of

1. Also spelled "cryptorchism"
2. Optional pronunciation ah"men-ō-RĒ-ah

the bones (particularly those of the spine) may occur from ten to twenty years after the menopause, whether the menopause was natural or artificially induced.

Functional uterine[1] [uterus] (Ū-ter-in) bleeding is abnormal bleeding from the uterus. It may be due to organic disease of the uterus, to cancer, benign tumors, inflammation, or from certain tumors of the ovary.

Ovarian (ō-VĀ-rē-an) neo/plasms [new formation] (NĒ-ō-plazms) may secrete follicular (fō-LIK-ū-lar) hormone, luteal [yellow] (LŪ-tē-al) hormone, or abnormal hormones which have effects like testicular or adrenal cortex hormones. These neoplasms may be malignant or benign. Granulosa [granules] (gran-ū-LŌ-sah)cell tumors arise from follicular cells and secrete estrin in large amounts. Corpus luteum tumors are rare, and occur during the childbearing period. Arrheno/blast/omas [male germ,cell] (ah-rē"nō-blas-TŌ-mahs) are malignant tumors believed to arise from rests of testicular cells in the ovary. Their secretion has a masculinizing effect.

Hypersecretion of the eosino/phile [dawn to love] (ē-ō-SĪN-ō-fil) cells of the pituitary gland may result in a condition known as gigantism [giant] (JĪ-gan-tizm). This occurs if the hypersecretion begins before or around the age of twenty-two and causes growth to an abnormally great height. After the age of twenty-five when the epi/physes [on,upon to grow] (ē-PIF-i-sēz) have united, growth in the length of bones is no longer possible. As the bones are unable to grow in length they become thicker and heavier which results in a condition called acro/megaly [extremity large] (ak-rō-MEG-ah-lē). If the hypersecretion begins before union of the epiphyses and persists after their closure the result is a giant with acro/megalic (ak-rō-me-GAL-ik) features.

The syndrome which describes the hypersecretion of the baso/phile [base] (BĀ-sō-fil) cells of the pituitary body is called pituitary baso/philism (bā-SOF-i-lizm).

Deficiency of anterior lobe secretion in children is manifested by re/tardation [back,again delay,hindrance] (rē-tar-DĀ-shun) of growth and sexual development. In severe cases

1. Optional pronunciation Ū-ter-īn

it is accompanied by signs of adrenal hypofunction as well. It thus produces infantile or pituitary dwarfs. In adults, the manifestations are due largely to deficient production of the hormones of the gonads, thyroid, and adrenals due to lack of stimulation.

In adults severe hypo/pituitarism (hī"pō-pe-TŪ-i-tār-izm) produces a syndrome called Simmond's disease or pituitary cac/hexia [ill / to be] (kah-KEK-sē-ah).

Deficiency of the posterior lobe hormone results in tremendous increase of the output of urine and excessive thirst. This syndrome is called dia/betes [through / to go] (dī-ah-BĒ-tēz) insipidus [tasteless] (in-SIP-i-dus).

Tumors of the pituitary are nearly always benign but commonly cause death because of their location. They compress important structures and cause increase in the pressure within the skull by interfering with the flow of cerebro/spinal [brain / spine] (ser"i-brō-SPĪ-nal) fluid. There are four types of pituitary tumors which occur fairly commonly. These are the chromo/phobe [color / fear] (KRŌ-mō-fōb) adenoma, the eosinophile adenoma, the basophile adenoma, and the cranio/pharyngi/oma [skull / pharynx] (kra"nē-ō-fah-rin-jē-Ō-mah).

Tumors of the pineal gland are uncommon and are particularly rare in women.

Diabetes mellitus [sweetened with honey] (mel-LĪ-tus)[1] is a disease in which the ability of the body cells to utilize gluc/ose [sweet] (GLOO-kōs) is diminished or lost. Glucose must be converted into glycogen to be used. For the transformation of glucose into glycogen, a hormone (insulin) secreted by the islands of Langerhans of the pancreas is required. The classical symptoms of severe diabetes are poly/dipsia [much, many / thirst] (pol-ē-DIP-sē-ah) (excessive thirst), poly/phagia [to eat] (pol-ē-FĀ-jē-ah) (increased appetite in spite of which great loss of weight may occur), poly/uria [urine] (pol-ē-Ū-rē-ah) (the secretion of excessive amounts of urine), glucos/uria (gloo-kō-SŪ-rē-ah) (the presence of sugar in the urine), hyper/glyc/emia (hī"per-glī-SĒ-mē-ah) (an abnormally high concentration of sugar in the blood).

1. Frequently pronounced MEL-i-tus probably to eliminate confusion with "itis" suffix meaning "inflammation."

The treatment of diabetes, in general, consists of the regulation of diet and the administration of insulin (orally or by injection).

Spontaneous hypo/glyc/emia (hī"pō-glī-SĒ-mē-ah) refers to a condition which may be considered the reverse of diabetes mellitus. In these cases excessive secretion of insulin produces abnormally rapid combustion of glucose and causes manifestations due to hypoglycemia. This condition, also called hyper/insulin-ism (hī-per-IN-sū-lin-izm) is most commonly due to adenoma (benign tumor) of the secretory cells of the islands of Langerhans.

DISEASES OF METABOLISM

The term metabolism applies to the chemical changes that take place within the cells and tissues of the body as it carries on its life processes.

Acid/osis [sour] (as-i-DŌ-sis) refers to a shift of the reaction of the body fluids toward the acid side.

Alkal/osis [alkaline] (al-kah-LŌ-sis) is the reverse of acidosis. It is the state in which the ability to cope with alkalis [potash] (AL-kah-līz) is reduced.

Obesity is the presence of an excessive amount of fatty tissue in the body. In normal persons obesity results from excessive caloric intake or from limitation of physical activity.

Hemo/chromat/osis [blood color] (hē"mō-krō-mah-TŌ-sis) or bronze diabetes is a disease characterized by a bronzing of the skin due to the deposition of an iron containing pigment (hemo/siderin [iron] [hē-mō-SID-er-in]).

Ochron/osis [yellow] (ō-krō-NŌ-sis) is a condition characterized by pigmentation of the skin due to the deposition of an unidentified black pigment which is also deposited in the cartilaginous [gristle] (kar-ti-LAJ-i-nus) tissue of the body resulting, in the case of the joints, in arthritis.

Porphyrins [purple] (POR-fi-rins) are organic pigments which normally exist in the body in small amounts. When excessive quantities of these pigments are formed a condition known as porphyria[1] (por-FIR-ē-ah) occurs. Two forms of this con-

1. Optional pronunciation por-FĪ-rē-ah

dition are recognized: congenital porphyria which is usually present from birth and is characterized by the passage of urine which turns dark or almost black on exposure to sunlight, erythema [redness,flush] (er-i-THĒ-mah) and blistering of the skin which occurs upon only slight exposure with death resulting if such "burns" cover a considerable portion of the body; and acute porphyria which usually occurs in women between thirty and fifty years of age.

Gout [a drop][1] (gowt) is a disorder of purine [pure + urine] (PYO͞OR-ēn) metabolism characterized by inflammation of the joints and sometimes by the deposition of sodium [an element] (SŌ-dē-um) urate [salt of uric acid] (Ū-rāt) in the sub/cutaneous [below skin] (sub-kyo͞o-TĀ-nē-us) tissues.

Amyl/oid/osis [starch] (am-i-loy-DŌ-sis) is the deposition of an unidentified substance called amyl/oid (AM-i-loyd) in the organs and tissues. It sometimes occurs in cases of long standing sup/puration [under pus] (sup-ū-RĀ-shun) such as chronic em/pyema [in pus] (em-pī-Ē-mah), osteo/myel/itis [bone marrow] (os"tē-ō-mī-i-LĪ-tis), or lung abscess, rarely in other diseases, such as syphilis, widespread carcinoma and rheumat/oid [a flux] (RŪ-mah-toyd) arthritis.

The xanth/omatoses [yellow tumors] (zan-thō-mah-TŌ-sēz) are diseases characterized by obscure disturbances of fat and lip/oid [fat] (LĪ-poyd)[2] metabolism in which lipoid substances are deposited in cells of various organs. They occur only in children and are known by the names of the men who first described them or who added to our knowledge of them: Gaucher's[3] (gō-SHĀZ) disease is characterized principally by progressive enlargement of the spleen; Tay-Sach's[4] disease is also known as amaurot/ic [darkening] (am-aw-ROT-ik) family idiocy [peculiar] (ID-ē-ō-sē); Niemann-Pick's[5] disease is characterized by the deposit of lecithin [egg yolk] (LES-i-thin) in many organs and tissues; Hand-Christian's[6] disease is a condition in which there is an accumulation of large cells containing chole/ster/ol [bile solid oil] (kō-LES-ter-ol) in the bones, in the orbits behind the eyes, and along the floor of the cranial cavity. All of these diseases are invariably fatal.

1. Comes from Latin "gutta" meaning "a drop"
2. Optional pronunciation LIP-oyd
3. Phillipe Gaucher, French physician, 1854-1918
4. Warren Tay, English physician, 1843-1927; Bernard Sachs, New York neurologist, 1858-1944
5. Albert Niemann, German physician, 1880-1921; Ludwig Pick, German physician, 1868-1935
6. Alfred Hand, American pediatrician, 1868-1949; Henry Asbury Christian, Boston internist, 1876-1951

SURGERY OF THE ENDOCRINE SYSTEM

Subtotal and total thyroidectomy are performed for the following indications: diffuse colloid [glutinous] (KOL-oyd) goiter, adenomatous goiter with and without toxicity, hyperplastic goiter, tracheal constriction caused by chronic thyroiditis, and malignant lesions consisting of papillary adeno/carcinoma [gland cancer] (ad"i-nō-kar-si-NŌ-mah), adenocarcinoma in an adenoma or malignant adenoma, and diffuse adenocarcinoma.

Parathyroid surgery is indicated in cases of hyperparathyroidism which results from either an adenoma or an adenocarcinoma developing in one or more of the parathyroid glands and from generalized primary hyperplasia which involves all of the parathyroid tissue. Operative procedure is excision of parathyroid adenoma.

Surgeries of the adrenal glands include unilateral ad/renal/ectomy [near kidney] (ad-ren al-EK-tō-mē) with excision of neoplasm for adenoma of the adrenal cortex; nephro-adrenalectomy [kidney] (nef"rō-ad-ren-al-EK-tō-mē) for large tumors; subtotal adrenalectomy or bilateral adrenalectomy for Cushing's syndrome associated with psychosis, multiple bone fracture and severe diabetes, and bilateral adrenalectomy for metastatic cancer of the breast.

INDEX
CHAPTER VI

CHAPTER VII
THE RESPIRATORY SYSTEM

All chemical changes in the tissue cells are dependent upon oxygen. Because of this constant need of oxygen it is necessary to furnish a continual supply. One of the products of these same chemical changes is carbon dioxide which necessitates the need for continual elimination. In the human the blood, which circulates in the body, is brought into contact with the air in the lungs. It is here that the blood takes up oxygen and releases carbon dioxide. As the blood circulates to the tissues and then to the cells it gives up the oxygen and takes on carbon dioxide. This exchange is a continuous function and is known as re/spiration [back,again / to breathe] (res-pe-RĀ-shun). To be effective it is dependent upon the proper functioning of the specific organs which make up the re/spiratory (RES-pir-ah-tō-rē)[1] system. Thus, the lungs are placed in communication with the nose and mouth by means of the bronchi [windpipe] (BRONG-kī), trachea [rough] (TRĀ-kē-ah), and larynx [windpipe] (LAR-inks).

The nose not only possesses an area specialized to register the sense of smell but also serves as a passage for air going to and from the lungs. As air is breathed in it is filtered, warmed and moistened as it passes through the nose. This is also an aid to phonation.

The nose is composed of two parts: the external nose and the internal cavity, the nasal fossae [ditch] (FOS-ē). The external nose is largely triangular in shape. It is composed of a framework of bone and cartilage, covered by skin and lined by mucous membrane. The nostrils or anterior nares [nostril] (NAR-ēz) are the external openings of the nasal cavities. The lateral wall of each external opening is called the ala [wing] (Ā-lah) of the nose. The nasal cavities are separated by the nasal septum. The margins of the nostrils are usually provided with a number of hairs.

1. Optional pronunciation re-SPĪ-rah-tō-rē

Attached to the lateral wall of each nasal cavity are three scroll-like processes of bone called the nasal conchae [shell] (KONG-kē) or turbinates [shaped like a top] (TER-bin-āts). The arrangement of the conchae makes the upper part of the nasal passage very narrow. Because of this arrangement breathing (under normal conditions) should take place through the nose as these passages are thickly lined and freely supplied with blood vessels. This keeps the temperature relatively high and even in the coldest weather it is possible to moisten and warm the

UPPER RESPIRATORY TRACT

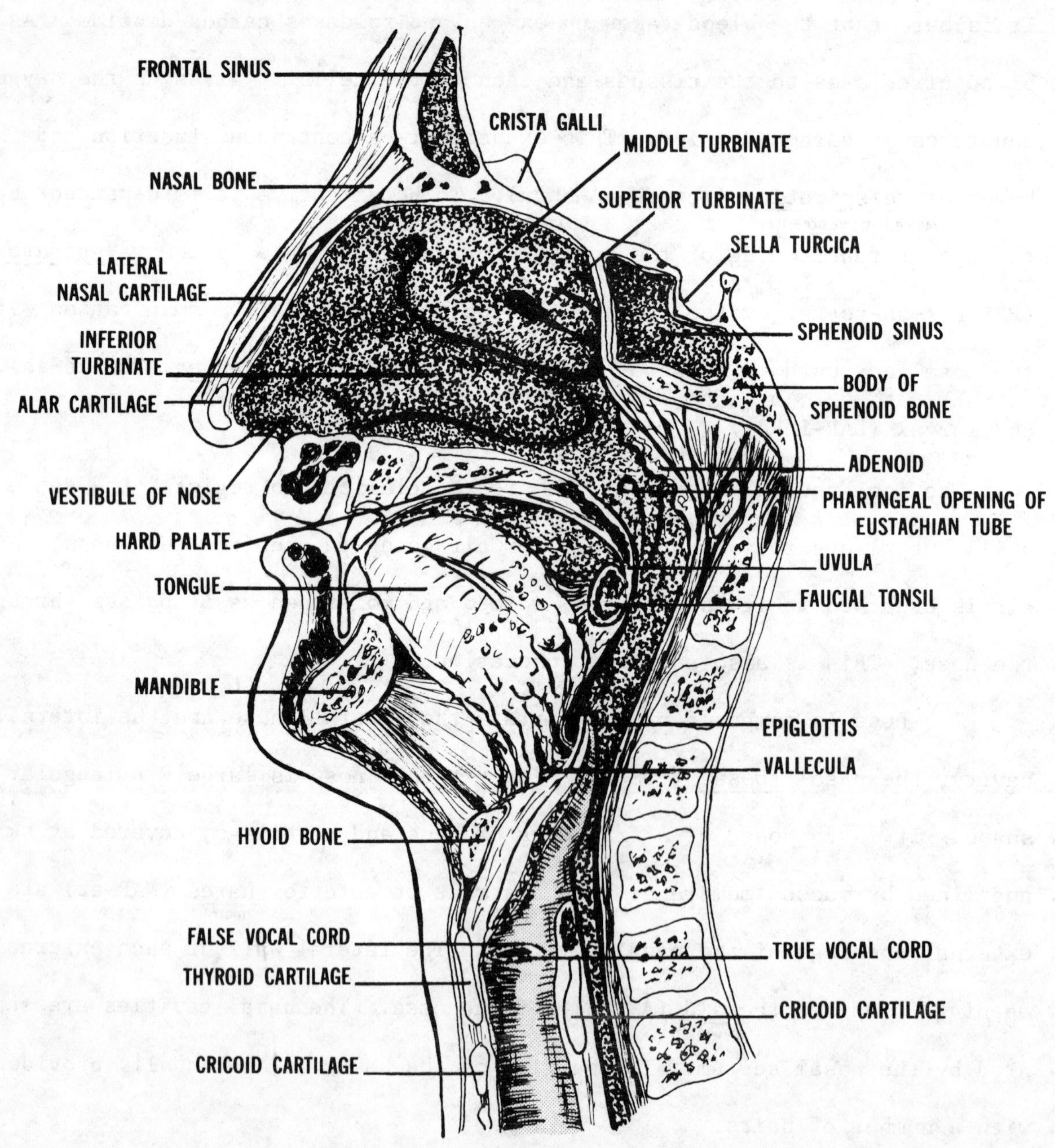

air before it reaches the lungs. In addition, the presence of hairs at the entrance to the nostrils and the cilia [hair] (SIL-ē-ah) of the epi/thelium [on,upon, nipple] (ep-i-THĒ-lē-um) serve as filters to prevent the passage of dust and other foreign substances which might be carried in with the inspired air.

The mouth serves as a secondary passage for air if the nasal passages are blocked. The pharynx[1] [throat] (FAR-inks) transmits the air from the nose or mouth to the larynx.[1]

The larynx or voice box lies in the upper and front part of the neck, between the root of the tongue and the trachea. Behind it lies the lower part of the pharynx leading to the esophagus [gullet] (ē-SOF-ah-gus). The great vessels of the neck and the vagus [wandering] (VĀ-gus) nerve lie on each side. The larynx is made up of nine pieces of fibro/cartilage [fiber gristle] (fī-brō-KAR-ti-lij) united by extrinsic [from without] (eks-TRIN-sik) and intrinsic [on the inside] (in-TRIN-sik) ligaments and moved by numerous muscles. There are three single cartilages (thyroid, cric/oid [a ring] [KRĪ-koyd], and epi/glottis [mouth of windpipe] [ep-i-GLOT-is]) and three paired cartilages (aryten/oid [ladle] [ar-i-TE-noyd], corniculate [shaped like a small horn] [kor-NIK-ū-lāt], and cunei/form [wedge] [kyōō-NĒ-i-form]). The thyroid resembles a shield and is the largest. It rests upon the cricoid and consists of two square plates or laminae [thin,flat plate or layer] (LAM-i-nē) which are joined at an acute angle in the middle line in front and form by their union the laryngeal [windpipe] (lah-RIN-jē-al) prominence known as the "Adam's apple."

The trachea or windpipe is cylindrical in shape. It is a membranous [a skin] (MEM-brah-nus) and cartilaginous tube. It lies in front of the esophagus and extends from the larynx on the level of the 6th cervical [neck] (SER-vi-kal) vertebra [to turn] (VER-te-brah) to opposite the upper border of the 5th thoracic vertebra where it divides into two tubes, the bronchi, one for each lung.

The bronchi which connect the trachea with the lungs and which are formed by the division of the trachea, differ slightly. The right bronchus is shorter, wider and more vertical in direction than the left, which is longer and narrower.

1. "pharynx" and "larynx" are often incorrectly pronounced as "pharnyx" and "larnyx." To overcome this think of "ice rinks." This association will make proper pronunciation easier.

THE RESPIRATORY SYSTEM

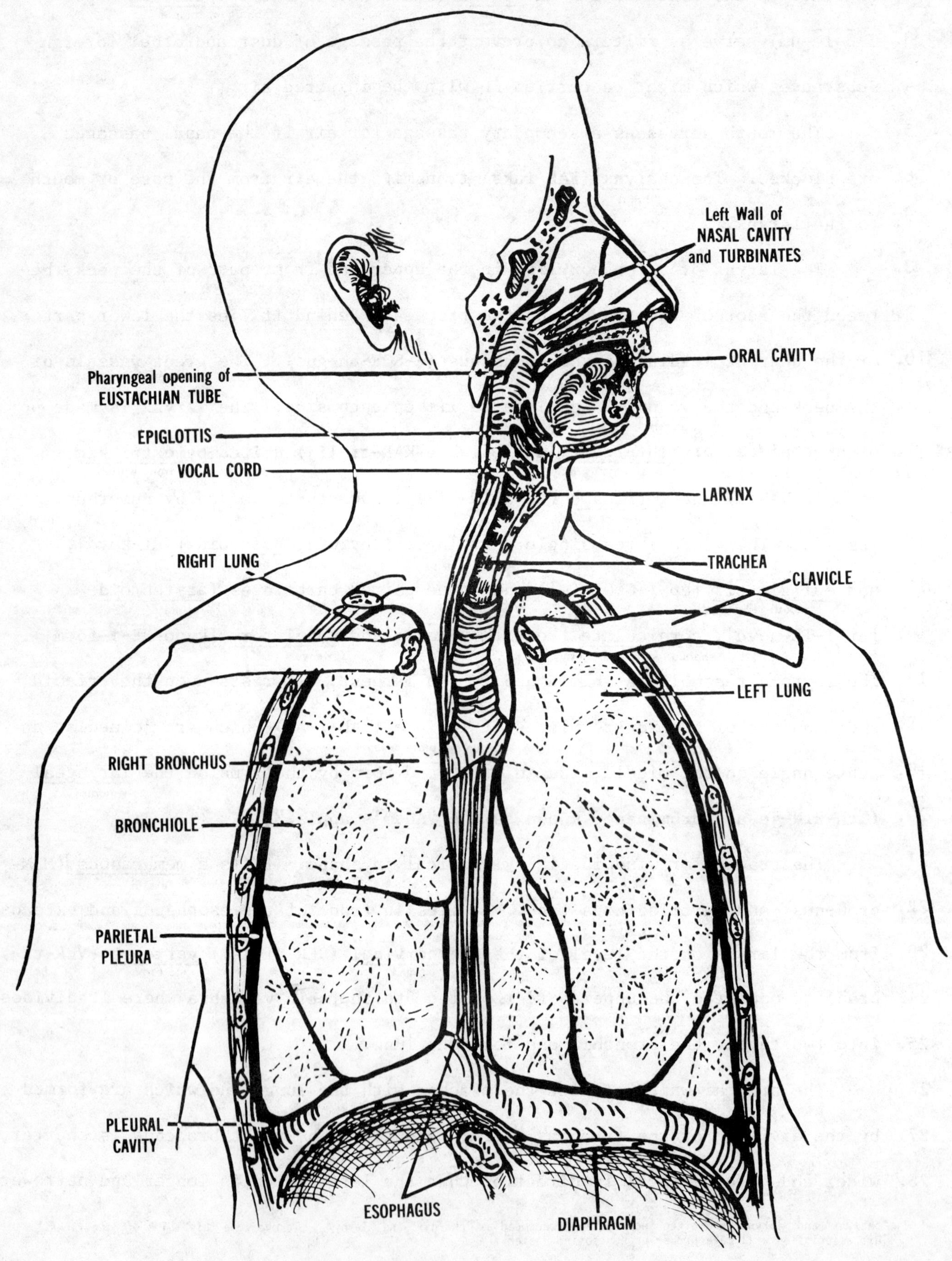

Left Wall of
NASAL CAVITY
and TURBINATES
ORAL CAVITY
Pharyngeal opening of
EUSTACHIAN TUBE
EPIGLOTTIS
VOCAL CORD
LARYNX
RIGHT LUNG
TRACHEA
CLAVICLE
LEFT LUNG
RIGHT BRONCHUS
BRONCHIOLE
PARIETAL
PLEURA
PLEURAL
CAVITY
ESOPHAGUS
DIAPHRAGM

After they enter the lungs the bronchi break up into smaller branches which are called bronchial [windpipe] (BRONG-kē-al) tubes or bronchi/oles [bronchus / small] (BRONG-kē-ōls). Each bronchiole ends in a small duct or atrium [entrance hall] (Ā-trē-um). On the atrium are small, irregular projections, the alveoli [cavity] (al-VĒ-ō-lī) or air cells.

The thoracic cavity, which is separated from the abdominal cavity by a sheet of muscle called the dia/phragm [through / wall] (DĪ-ah-fram), encloses the two pleural [rib,side] (PLO͞OR-al) cavities, each containing a lung. The pleural cavities are completely separated from each other by the media/stinum [middle / septum] (mē"dē-as-TĪ-num)[1]. The mediastinum contains the heart, the pericardium surrounding the heart, the pulmonary trunk and arteries, the venae [veins] cavae [hollows] (VĒ-nē KĀ-vē), the thoracic aorta and its branches, the trachea and part of the bronchi, the esophagus, the vagus nerves, the phrenic [diaphragm,mind] (FREN-ik) nerves, the thoracic duct, many lymph nodes and lymph vessels, the a/zygos [not / a yoke] (AZ-ig-os) vein, and the thymus gland or its fibrous remainder.

The pleura [rib] (PLO͞OR-ah) are serous sacs which enclose each lung. There are two layers of pleura: one layer is closely adherent to the walls of the chest and diaphragm and is known as the parietal [wall] (pah-RĪ-i-tal) pleura; the other layer known as the visceral [organ] (VIS-er-al) or pulmonary pleura closely covers the lung. The two layers move easily upon one another and friction is avoided because of the serum between them which keeps them moistened. If, however, the surface of the pleura becomes roughened, which may occur in inflammation or or pleurisy [rib,the side] (PLO͞OR-i-sē), a certain amount of friction results and the sounds produced by this friction can be heard by listening with the ear against the chest. In pleurisy the normally small amount of fluid secreted is considerably increased. This amount may be sufficient to separate the two layers of the pleura and change what is a potential pleural cavity into an actual pleural cavity. This condition is known as pleurisy with ef/fusion [out / to pour] (ef-Ū-zhun). If this effusion suppurates the condition is then called em/pyema [in / pus] (em-pī-Ē-mah).

1. Optional pronunciations mē"dē-ah-STĪ-num or mē"dē-AS-ti-num

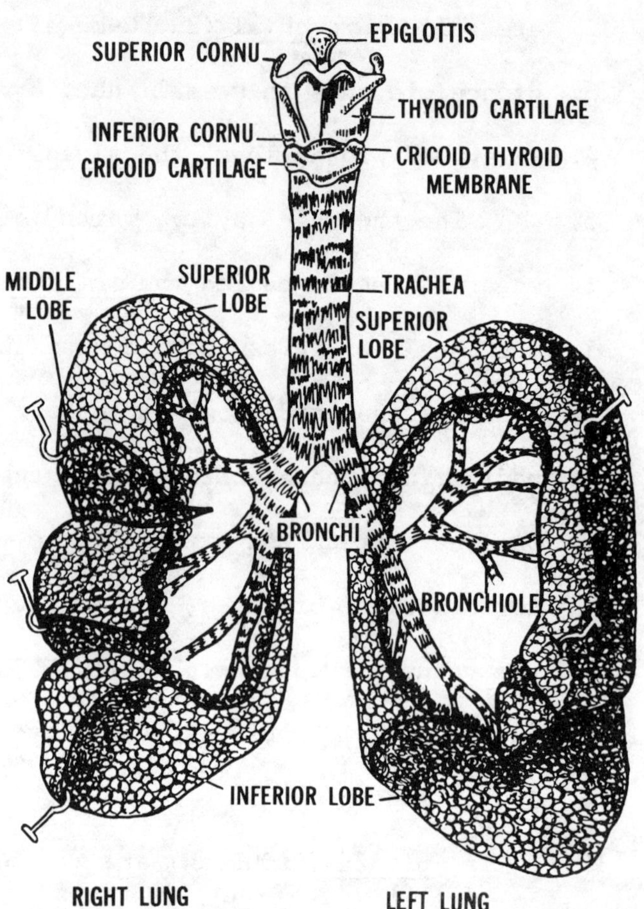

The lungs occupy the two lateral chambers of the thoracic cavity and are separated from each other by the mediastinum and its contents including the heart. The lungs, which are cone-shaped, each present a blunt, rounded apex or upper end which projects into the base of the neck above the first rib. The base of the lung is concave and rests on the diaphragm. Each lung is connected to the heart and trachea by the pulmonary artery, pulmonary vein, bronchial arteries and veins, the bronchus, plexuses of nerves, lymphatics, lymph nodes, and areolar *(small area)* (ah-RĒ-ō-lar) tissue which are covered by the pleura and constitute the root of the lung. These structures enter the lung substance through the hilum *(a small bit or trifle)* (HĪ-lum) which is a wedge-shaped area on the inner surface of the lung. Below and in front of the hilum is the cardiac impression to accommodate the heart. It is larger and deeper on the left than on the right lung because the heart projects farther into the left side.

The left lung has two lobes, an upper and a lower lobe. The right lung has three lobes, an upper, middle and lower lobe. The right lung is shorter, wider and slightly larger than the left.

In a healthy individual the lungs are spongy in consistency and porous. Because of the presence of air the lung tissue crepitates *(to crackle, to rattle)* (KREP-i-tāts) when handled and floats in water.

Each lobe of the lung is composed of many lob/ules *lobe small* (LOB-ūls). A bronchiole enters into each lobule and terminates into a series of air cells or alveoli. Venous blood to be aerated (the taking on of oxygen and release of carbon dioxide) is brought to the lungs by branches of the pulmonary artery. Branches of the bronchial arteries bring the arterial blood required to nourish the substance of the lung itself.

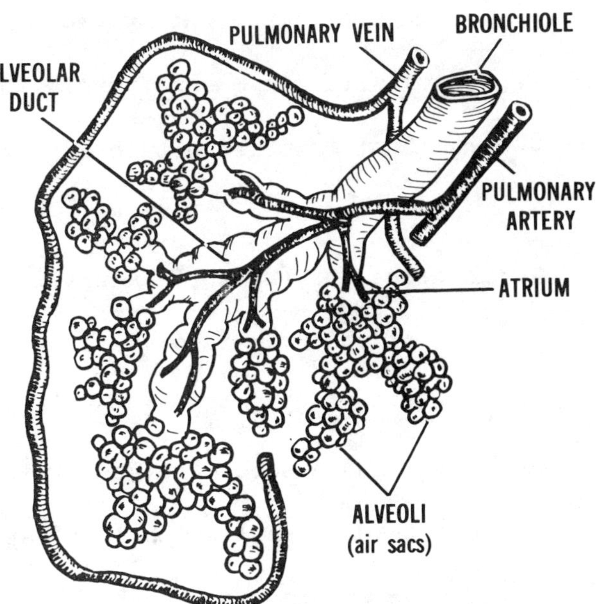

PRIMARY LOBULE OF THE LUNG

DISEASES AND ANOMALIES

Diseases of the respiratory system are most commonly caused by infection. In some of the specific infectious diseases, the respiratory organs are the principal or only organs involved (lobar *lobe* [LŌ-bar] pneumon/ia *lung* [nū-MŌ-nē-ah], tuberc/ulosis *nodes small* [tū-ber-kū-LŌ-sis], influenza *influènce(Italian)* [in-flū-EN-zah], common cold, whooping cough), while in others, such as measles[1] (MĒ-zelz) and typh/oid *stupor* (TĪ-foyd) fever, involvement of the respiratory system invariably occurs, together with lesions of other organs.

The respiratory organs are frequently invaded by malignant tumors. Primary cancers usually arise in the larynx or in the bronchi, and metastatic growths from cancers in other organs, such as the breast, are of common occurrence. Benign tumors, except of the larynx, are rare in this system.

The principal physical agents which cause respiratory disease are foreign bodies which may be aspirated into the upper respiratory tree and the inhalation of chemical agents such as silica *flint* (SIL-i-kah) dust and irritating gases. Allergies may also cause respiratory manifestations such as hay fever and asthma *panting* (AS-mah).

1. From the Dutch word "maselen." The Latin word for "measles" is "morbilli" which means "disease." The "morb" comes from "morbus" meaning "disease" and the "illi" means "small."

The most important symptoms of respiratory disease are cough, the raising of sputum [to spit] (SPŪ-tum), hemo/ptysis [blood spitting] (hē-MOP-tis-is), dys/pnea [difficult breathing] (disp-NĒ-ah), and pain in the chest associated with respiration.

Examination of the respiratory system consists of inspection of the nose, the naso/pharynx [nose throat] (nā-zō-FAR-inks), and the larynx with special instruments; of the rest of the respiratory system by examination of the chest through inspection, palpation [to touch, to stroke] (pal-PĀ-shun), percussion [to beat] (per-KUSH-un), and auscultation [to listen to] (aws-kul-TĀ-shun), and also by the use of the broncho/scope [to view] (BRONG-kō-skop) for broncho/scopy (brong-KOS-kō-pē) which is of special value in the detection of new growths arising within the bronchi.

Rhin/itis [nose] (rī-NĪ-tis) is an acute inflammation of the nose and occurs most commonly as part of the pathology to specific infectious diseases due to filtrable [to strain] (FIL-tra-bl) viruses [poison] (VĪ-ru-sez) or bacteria, and of the allergic disease, hay fever. Various types of rhinitis include vaso/motor [vessel mover] (vā-sō-MŌ-tor) rhinitis, hyper/trophic [excessive nourishment] (hī-per-TRŌ-fik) rhinitis, a/trophic [lack] (ā-TRŌ-fik) rhinitis (ozena [to smell] [ō-ZĒ-nah]), and chronic rhinitis.

Nasal polyps[1] [many + foot] (POL-ips) are rounded, hyper/emic [blood] (hī-per-Ē-mik), pedunc/ulated[2] [foot small] (pe-DUNG-kyo͞o-lāt-ed) benign tumors attached to the lateral walls of the nose. Polyps may also form in the para/nasal [beside nose] (par-ah-NĀ-zal) sinuses [hollow] (SĪ-nu-sez).

Malformations and deformities of the nose:

Congenital deformities: cleft nose, atresia [without opening] (ah-TRĒ-zē-ah) of the anterior nares, collapse of the nostrils, fistulae [pipe] (FIS-tū-lē) and epi/theli/al [on nipple] (ep-i-THĒ-lē-al)-lined cysts of the nasal dorsum.

Acquired deformities: This type results from trauma or disease and includes rhino/phyma [nose growth] (rī-nō-FĪ-mah) in which the nose becomes enlarged, atrophic changes (lupus [wolf] [LŪ-pus]) in which it shrinks, fracture, bridge sag from abscess or syphilis, partial or complete destruction of the nose due to trauma, syphilis, tuberculosis, nomah [a spreading] (NŌ-mah).

1. This word is a contraction of "polypous" and translates to "many + foot."
2. This word actually means "having a stalk or stem."

Most of the malformations and deformities of the nose (congenital or acquired) require surgery for treatment as well as for cosmesis *an adorning* (koz-MĒ-sis).

Inflammatory conditions of the nose may be acute (erysi/pelas *red skin*[1] [er-i-SIP-i-las], vestibul/itis *an entrance court* [ves-tib-ū-LĪ-tis], furuncul/osis *a petty thief* [fu"rung-kyo͞o-LŌ-sis], frostbite, burns, peri/chondr/itis *around cartilage* [per-ē-kon-DRĪ-tis], fracture and noma); or chronic, including vestibulitis, sebo/rrheic *suet flow* (seb-ō-RĒ-ik) dermat/itis *skin* (der-mah-TI-tis), acne[2] (AK-nē) rosacea *rosy* (rō-ZĀ-sē-ah), acne vulgaris *a crowd*[3] (vul-GĀ-ris), tuberculosis and lupus, syphilis, scler/oma *hard* (skle-RŌ-mah), leprosy *scaly* (LEP-rō-sē), glanders[4] (GLAN-derz), blasto/myc/osis *germ mucus* (blas-tō-mī-KŌ-sis).

The external nose is frequently the site of many types of benign and malignant neo/plasms *new formation* (NĒ-ō-plazms). Benign neoplasms include angi/oma *vessel* (an-jē-Ō-mah), papilloma, derm/oid *skin* (DER-moyd), aden/oma *gland* (ad-i-NŌ-mah), lip/oma *fat* (lī-PŌ-mah), chondr/oma *cartilage* (kon-DRŌ-mah), lymph/oma *water* (lim-FŌ-mah), fibr/oma *fiber* (fī-BRŌ-mah), my/oma *muscle* (mī-Ō-mah), verruca *wart* (ver-O͞OH-kah), oste/oma *bone* (os-tē-Ō-mah). Malignant neoplasms are carcinoma, sarc/oma *flesh* (sar-KŌ-mah), hem/angio/endo/theli/oma *blood vessel within nipple* (hē-man"jē-ō-en-dō-thē-lē-Ō-mah), lymph/angio/endo/theli/oma (limf-an"jē-ō-en-dō-thē-lē-Ō-mah), cylindr/oma *cylinder* (sil-in-DRŌ-mah).

Sinus/itis (sī-ne-SĪ-tis) is inflammation of the mucous membrane of the paranasal sinuses and occurs along with many or most cases of acute rhinitis.

Pharyng/itis (far-in-JĪ-tis) (acute inflammation of the pharynx) is commonly associated with acute rhinitis. In acute tonsill/itis *a stake* (ton-si-LĪ-tis), hyper/emia (hī-per-Ē-mē-ah) of the pharynx may be present, and in diphtheria *leather, membrane* (dif-THĒ-rē-ah), the membrane covers a fairly large area of the wall of the thorax.

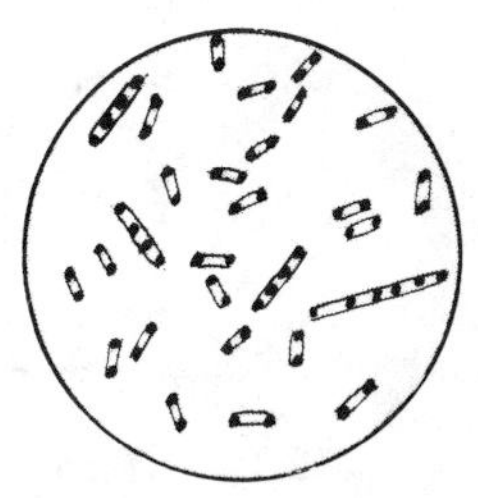

DIPHTHERIA BACILLI

Acute tonsillitis in its typical form is a specific disease caused by the hemo/lytic *to dissolve* (hē-mō-LIT-ik) strepto/coccus *twist berry,seed* (strep-tō-KOK-us); a/typical *not conforming* (ā-TIP-i-kl) or milder forms may occur in the absence of detectable patho/genic *disease to produce* (path-ō-JEN-ik) organisms, in infectious mono/nucle/osis *single nucleus* (mon"ō-nū-klē-Ō-sis), and

1. Also called "St. Anthony's fire."
2. Probably an early copying error of a Greek word meaning "a point" or a corruption of another Greek word meaning "chaff."
3. The definition of this word means "ordinary or common."
4. A disease of horses and some members of the cat family transmitted to man.

Vincent's stomat/itis [mouth] (stō-mah-TĪ-tis). The tonsils are involved in most cases of diphtheria. Peri/tonsillar (per-i-TON-si-lar) abscess or quinsy[1] [sore throat] (KWIN-zē) is a severe acute inflammation of the soft tissues of the palate adjacent to the tonsil, resulting in abscess formation.

Acute laryng/itis [windpipe] (lar-in-JĪ-tis) is usually secondary to infection of other portions of the upper respiratory tract. Chronic laryngitis results from long continued irritation from smoking, from the inhalation of irritating vapors, from continuous overuse of the voice, and from the aspiration of mucus into the larynx in persons with chronic catarrhal [to flow down] (kah-TAHR-al) conditions of the nose. Benign tumors of the larynx give rise to persistent hoarseness and paroxysmal [to irritate,to sharpen] (par-ok-SIZ-mal) cough. Cancer of the larynx is a very serious lesion since it tends to meta/stasize [in the midst of a placing] (me-TAS-tah-sīz) early to the neighboring lymph nodes and since it is often impossible to excise the tumor without removing the whole larynx. Obstruction caused by acute swelling or edema[2] [swelling] (i-DĒ-mah) of the tissues may occur in acute laryngitis due to any cause. It especially occurs in laryngitis secondary to strepto/coccal (strep-tō-KOK-al) infections of the throat and in those forms due to the accidental aspiration into the larynx of irritant chemicals or to the inhalation of hot smoke or flames. Foreign bodies which lodge in the larynx are usually caught above the vocal cords or are wedged between them; if a foreign body passes the vocal cords it nearly always passes down as far as the bifurcation [forked] (bī-fur-KĀ-shun) of the trachea.

Trache/itis (trā-kē-Ī-tis) is nearly always accompanied by laryngitis or bronch/itis (brong-KĪ-tis) or both as the trachea, itself, is not very often the seat of primary disease. Obstruction of the trachea is more often due to compression by media/stinal (me"dē-AS-ti-nal)[3] tumors (especially aneurysms) than to intrinsic disease.

Acute and chronic bronchitis, bronchi/ectasis [stretching] (brong-kē-EK-tah-sis) and bronchial obstruction are the most important diseases of the bronchi. Cancer

1. This term comes from the Greek "kynanchē" translating to "dog + to throttle." In Latin the word is "cynanche" and is pronounced "sin-ANG-kē."
2. Optional pronunciation ē-DĒ-mah
3. Optional pronunciation mē-dē-ah-STĪ-nal

of the lung nearly always arises from the epithelium of the bronchi and collapse of the lung is due in many cases to obstruction of these tubes.

While pneumonia is usually infectious it can be caused by inhalation or aspiration of chemical agents such as carbolic acid and various types of mineral dusts. Pneumo/cocci (lung / berry,seed) (nū-mō-KOK-sī) and strepto/cocci (strep-tō-KOK-sī) are the cause of acute pneumonia. However, it may be due to other organisms such as Friedlander's (FRĒD-len-derz) bacillus (staff or rod) (bah-SIL-us), the tubercle bacillus or to filtrable viruses. A lung abscess is an area of pneumonia in which the inflamed tissue undergoes death, destruction and conversion into pus. Carcinoma of the lung may be primary or metastatic. Atel/ectasis (imperfect) (at-i-LEK-tah-sis) is the collapse of the lung so that the air sacs become smaller in size. Emphysema (to inflate) (em-fi-SĒ-mah) of the lungs is overdistention of the air sacs. It is the reverse of atelectasis. The term pneumo/coni/osis (lung / dust) (nū"mō-kon-ē-Ō-sis) refers to chronic changes in the lungs which result from continued inhalation of certain mineral dusts. The most important of these is silica dust which causes the pulmonary disease known as silic/osis (silica) (sil-i-KŌ-sis). Primary coccidioido/mycosis (a form of fungus / fungus) (kok-sid-ē-oy"dō-mī-KŌ-sis) also known as valley fever, desert fever or San Joaquin valley fever is a disease common in the San Joaquin Valley of California and in some areas in the Southwest. It is caused by inhalation of the spores of the fungus Coccidioides (kok-sid-ē-OY-dēz) which results in acute symptoms resembling pneumonia or pulmonary tuberculosis.

There are three principal diseases of the pleura:

1. inflammation or pleurisy, of which there are three varieties:
   a. acute fibrinous pleurisy,
   b. pleurisy with effusion,
   c. chronic adhesive pleurisy;
2. the accumulation of fluid within the pleural sac (pleural effusion) which may result from inflammation, tumor or other causes;

3. the accumulation of air within the pleural sac known as <u>pneumo/thorax</u> [chest] (nū-mō-THŌ-raks).

With the exception of diseases of the individual organs of the mediastinum (the heart, the great vessels, lymph nodes, etc.) there are only a few diseases of the mediastinum which are of importance. They are inflammation or <u>media/stin/itis</u> (mē"dē-as-ti-NĪ-tis), tumors and emphysema of the mediastinum.

SURGERY

Nasal deformities including rhinophyma are corrected by <u>rhino/plasty</u> (RĪ-nō-plas-tē) and grafting where necessary.

Nasal polyps and <u>polyp/osis</u> (pol-i-PŌ-sis): Polyps occur singly or in numbers and are pedunculated or <u>sessile</u> [low growing] (SES-il). They may be <u>edematous</u> [swelling] (ē-DEM-ah-tus), fibrous, <u>angi/ectatic</u> [vessel stretching] (an-jē-ek-TAT-ik), glandular and cystic. Surgical procedures, which depend on the number of polyps and if there is sinus involvement, include <u>sub/mucous</u> [below] (sub-MŪ-kus) resection (SMR) or <u>polyp/ectomy</u> (pol-i-PEK-tō-mē).

Surgical treatment of tumors of the nasal cavity depends on the extent and type of neoplasm and ranges from simple excision to radical excision with grafting and postoperative irradiation.

Deviations of the nasal septum may be horizontal, vertical, oblique, or sigmoid. They are often associated with spurs, crests or external deformity. Surgical procedure is submucous resection of septum (SMR).

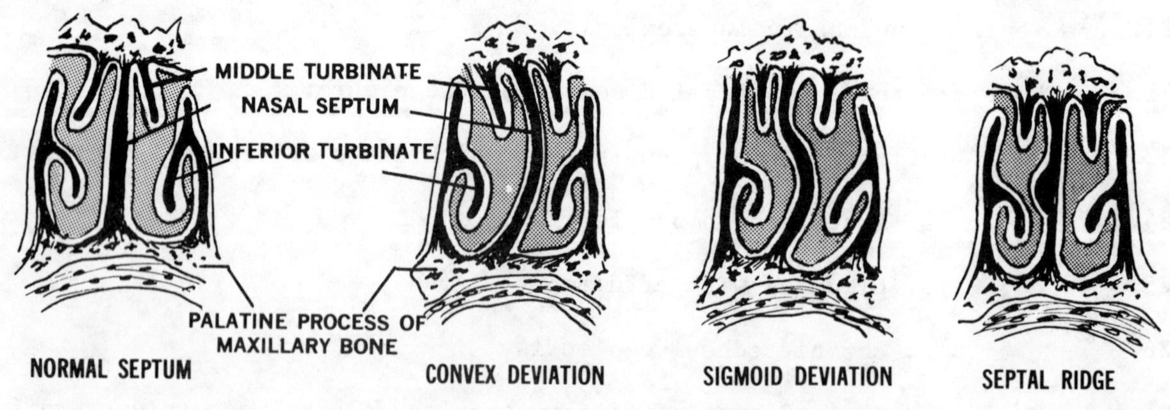

DEVIATED SEPTUM

The nasal accessory sinuses, maxillary (antrum *(a cave)* [AN-trum] of Highmore), frontal, ethm/oidal *(sieve)* (eth-MOYD-al) (anterior or posterior cells) and sphen/oidal *(wedge)* (sfē-NOYD-al), are often sites of chronic and acute disease. Chronic inflammation of the mucous membrane of the sinus (known as chronic sinusitis, hypertrophic sinusitis, chronic rhinitis, hypertrophic rhinitis or chronic catarrh *(to flow down)* [kah-TAHR]) is classified as edematous, in/filtrative *(into filter)* (in-FIL-trah-tiv), fibrotic, cystic and degenerative. The treatment of nasal sinus disease consists essentially of measures to improve ventilation and drainage. When conservative measures fail and surgery is required various procedures may be employed including SMR, polypectomy, turbin/ectomy (ter-bi-NEK-tō-mē). The maxillary sinus may be approached by a window beneath the inferior turbinate in the lateral nasal wall or by the subnasal route with removal of the lining membrane of the sinus. The frontal, ethmoid and sphenoid sinuses may be approached intra/nasally *(inside)* (in-trah-NĀ-sah-lē) or externally. Two procedures commonly performed are the Killian[1] (KIL-ē-an) frontal sinus operation which is done under general anesthesia, and the Caldwell-Luc[2] (KALD-wel-lūk) operation which is the most frequently used radical operation upon the antrum at this time.

Intranasal frontal sinus or external frontal sinus operations are performed for chronic frontal sinusitis. Ex/enteration *(out intestine(bowel))* (eks-en-ter-Ā-shun) of ethmoidal cells is performed for acute and chronic ethmoid/itis (eth-moyd-Ī-tis).

Fibroma and papill/oma *(nipple)* (pap-i-LŌ-mah) are the most common forms of benign neoplasms of the tongue. They may be removed by surgical or electro/surgical *(electricity)* (ē-lek-trō-SURJ-ik-al) excision and electro/coagulation *(to curdle or clot)* (ē-lek"trō-kō-ag-ū-LĀ-shun). Removal of hemangioma and lymphangioma of the tongue depends on the size and location of the neoplasm. They may be removed by electrosurgery and sometimes by excision of small wedges of tissue until the tongue is reduced to its normal size.

Thyro/glossal[3] *(shield tongue)* (thī-rō-GLOS-al) cysts require surgical excision.

1. Gustav Killian, German laryngologist, 1860-1921
2. George W. Caldwell, American physician, 1834-1918; Henry Luc, French laryngologist, 1855-1925
3. Relates to the thyroid gland and the tongue

Acute peritonsillar abscess (quinsy, phlegmonous *inflammation* [FLEG-mo-nus] tonsillitis) is treated by incision and drainage (I & D).

Tonsill/ectomy (ton-si-LEK-tō-mē) is performed for chronic tonsillitis, muco/purulent *mucus pus* (myo͞o"kō-PYO͞OR-e-lent) rhinitis, pathological tonsillitis, recurrent peritonsillar abscess, cystic or focal infection, chronic oto/rrhea *ear* (ō-tō-RĒ-ah), repeated attacks of serous ot/itis *ear* (ō-TĪ-tis) media, recurrent or persistent cervical adeno/pathy *gland* (ad-i-NOP-ah-thē).

Aden/oid/ectomy (ad-i-noy-DEK-tō-mē) is performed for hyper/plasia (hī-per-PLĀ-zē-ah) of the pharyngeal tonsil (the growth of normal adenoid tissue in the pharyngeal vault). In children tonsillectomy and adenoidectomy (T & A) are usually performed together.

Endo/laryngeal *within* (en-dō-lah-RIN-jē-al) and extra/laryngeal *outside* (eks-trah-lah-RIN-jē-al) surgical procedures performed for tuberculosis of the larynx include endo/scopic (en-dō-SKOP-ik) removal of granulomas, tracheotomy, plastic repair, resection, thyro/tomy (thī-ROT-ō-mē), laryngo/tomy (lar-ing-GOT-ō-mē), and, rarely, hemi/laryng/ectomy *half* (hem"ē-lar-in-JEK-tō-mē) and laryng/ectomy (lar-in-JEK-tō-mē).

Laryngo/scopy (lar-ing-GOS-kō-pē) (suspension, indirect or direct) is used with surgical removal by snare, followed by cauter/ization *to burn to treat* (kaw"ter-i-ZĀ-shun), or electro/dis/section *apart to cut* (ē"lek-trō-dis-SEK-shun) of benign tumor, evacuation and reduction of cysts by igni/puncture *fire pierce* (IG-nē-pungk-cher).

Surgical treatment of malignant growths of the larynx depends on the extent of the growth, the type of malignancy, and the area of the larynx involved. Thus, several types of procedures may be used: electrosurgery, radical surgery with electrocoagulation, electrodissection, and, in advanced cases, laryngectomy.

Acute laryngeal distress due to some form of obstruction of the larynx requires immediate treatment for relief. Indications for tracheotomy include foreign bodies in the larynx, diphtheritic *leather* (dif-ther-IT-ik) laryngitis, obstruction in the larynx, stenotic conditions, tumors, strictures, acute blockage of the upper respiratory tract caused by fracture, paralysis, croup *cry aloud* (kro͞op) and epi/glott/itis (ep-i-glo-TĪ-tis).

Laryngo/fissure *to split*[1] (lah-ring"gō-FISH-ūr) or thyrotomy is performed to remove tumors from the larynx that are not accessible by direct means and to extirpate *to root out* (EK-ster-pāt) intrinsic malignant neoplasms that do not necessitate removal of the entire larynx.

Hemilaryngectomy is a more extensive operation than laryngofissure. It is used when malignant growths are limited to one side and when it is suspected that the cartilaginous and deep structures are involved in the process.

Total laryngectomy is performed for infiltrating and intrinsic malignancies of the larynx. Patients who receive this surgery must learn to speak without a larynx (develop a pseudo/voice *false* [SŪ-dō-voys]).

Bronchoscopy is indicated for the following conditions:

1. tracheal or bronchial obstruction
2. to obtain uncontaminated secretions for culture purposes
3. to search for the source of unexplained hemoptysis
4. asthma
5. obscure thoracic disease
6. unexplained cough
7. to secure tissue for biopsy
8. for the extraction of foreign bodies
9. to promote endo/bronchial *within* (en-dō-BRONG-kē-al) drainage
10. aspiration of purulent secretions
11. dilatation of bronchial stenosis
12. electrocoagulation of endobronchial tumors
13. local application of medication
14. preliminary to tracheo/tomy (trā-kē-OT-ō-mē)

1. Also known as "laryngotomy"

15. bronchial lavage *(to wash)* (lah-VAHZH) for collection of specimens for tumor cells, infective organisms or germs and to help clear atelectasis.

Thora/centesis *(chest / puncture)*[1] (thō"rah-sen-TĒ-sis) is the introduction of a needle through the chest wall for purposes of diagnosis or therapy. Indications include:

1. tension pneumothorax (caused by injury to the lung)
2. hemo/thorax *(blood)* (hē-mō-THŌ-raks) -- hemorrhage into the pleural spaces from two places of origin: the systemic or pulmonary circuits
3. empyema
4. needle biopsy of mass lesions (tumor, cancer, abscess of lung or chest)

Thoraco/stomy (thō-rah-KOS-tō-mē) is performed for acute empyema and to control persistent formations of pleural fluid.

Phrenic nerve interruption is used in collapse therapy of pulmonary tuberculosis. Another procedure used is that of plombage *(filling in)* (plom-BAHZH) which is the partial collapse of the lung achieved by stripping the parietal pleura from the thorax and packing the space between chest wall and lung with foreign material such as paraffin[2] (PAR-ah-fin) or lucite *(a translucent resin)* (LŪ-sīt) balls.

Extra/pleural *(outside)* (eks-trah-PLŪ-ral) thoraco/plasty (THŌ-rah-kō-plas-tē) is performed for tuberculosis with cavitation *(formation of a cavity)* (kav-i-TĀ-shun) which is moderately or far advanced, mostly confined to one lung and productive in character. It produces collapse of the chest wall and, therefore, of underlying pulmonary tuberculous lesions. It is a permanent or irrevocable procedure and consists of resection of ribs, usually 5 to 7 ribs.

Operations for chronic empyema consist of drainage by the use of an intercostal air-tight tube or by resection of the thoracic cage overlying the cavity.

Open thoraco/tomy (thō-rah-KOT-ō-mē) is done for de/cortic/ation *(from / bark)*[3] (dē"kor-ti-KĀ-shun) following hemothorax, for fibrosis caused by hemothorax, for chronic empyema either tubercular or non-tubercular and for open lung tumor, pleural or

1. Also used as thoracocentesis
2. Comes from Latin "parum" meaning "little" and "affinis" meaning "neighboring, akin." Probably received this combination of word components because of its slight tendency to chemical reaction.
3. Means literally "to deprive of bark"

peri/cardial [around heart] (per-ē-KAR-dē-al) biopsy.

Chronic airway obstructive disease (C.A.O.), cor [heart] pulmonale [lung][1] (kor pul-mō-NAH-le), chronic obstructive lung disease (C.O.L.D.) or chronic obstructive pulmonary emphysema (C.O.P.E.) are treated by the use of intermittent positive pressure breathing (I.P.P.B.) for 1. more effective cough, 2. medication in bronchial tube, 3. adequate ventilation and 4. to help clear atelectasis.

Pulmonary resection:

1. Lob/ectomy [lobe] (lō-BEK-tō-mē) is performed in pulmonary infections such as bronchiectasis, lung abscess, suppurative pneumon/itis (nū-mō-NĪ-tis) and, in recent years, tuberculous processes and carcinoma.
2. Segmental pulmonary resection is the excision of one or two segments of a pulmonary lobe
3. Wedge resection is used for granuloma and for biopsy of the lung
4. Pneumon/ectomy (nū-mō-NEK-tō-mē) is the total extirpation [to root out] (ek-ster-PĀ-shun) of a lung and may be indicated for primary neo/plastic [new formation] (nē-ō-PLAS-tik) processes such as bronchio/genic [to produce] (brong-kē-ō-JEN-ik) carcinoma, for diffuse infections rendering a lung useless as from bronchiectasis or multiple abscesses, for carefully selected tuberculous lesions, as a sequel to trauma as in war injuries.

Dia/phragmatic [through partition] (dī"ah-frag-MAT-ik) hernia (HER-nē-ah): the most frequently encountered type is esophageal [gullet][2] (ē-sof"ah-JĒ-al) hiatus [an opening(aperture)] (hī-Ā-tus) hernia and the type found in infants and children is that of congenital diaphragmatic hernia. Both are corrected surgically by hernio/rrhaphy [hernia] (her-nē-OR-ah-fē).

1. Heart failure due to blood vessel blockage or to advanced lung disease. The blood vessels of the lung narrow and the heart is unable to pump blood through them adequately.
2. Optional pronunciation (used primarily in Europe) is es-ō-FĀ-jē-al

INDEX
CHAPTER VII

THE GASTRO-INTESTINAL SYSTEM

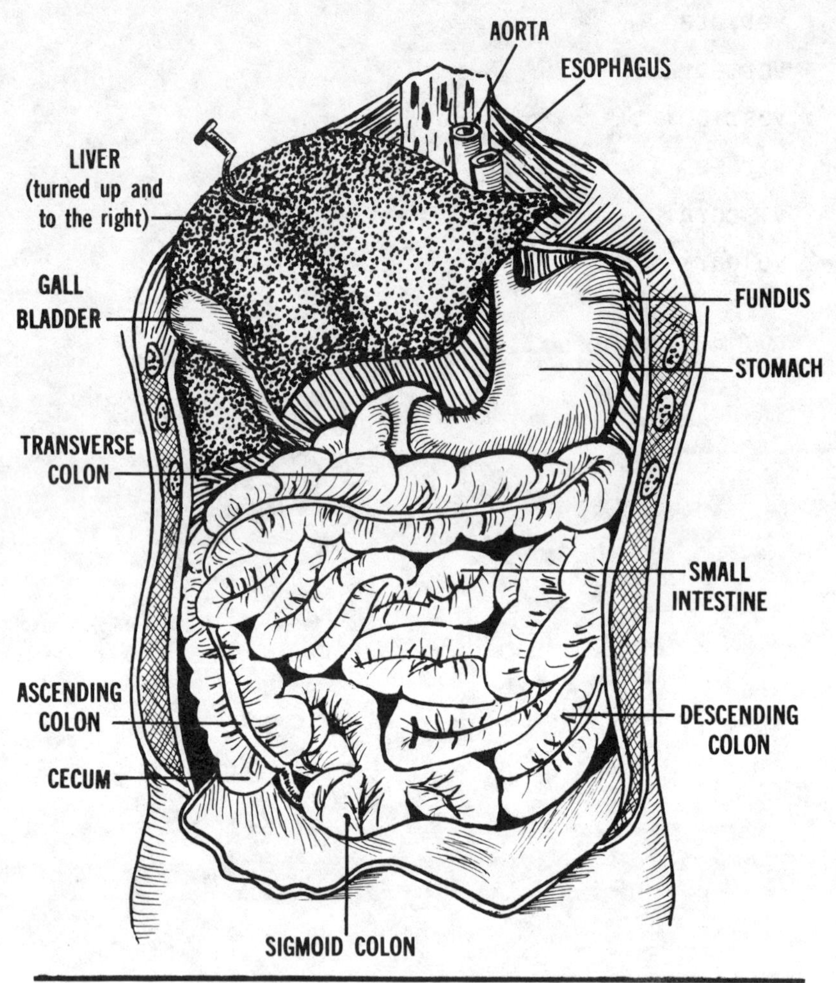
AORTA
ESOPHAGUS
LIVER
(turned up and
to the right)
GALL
BLADDER
FUNDUS
STOMACH
TRANSVERSE
COLON
SMALL
INTESTINE
ASCENDING
COLON
DESCENDING
COLON
CECUM
SIGMOID COLON

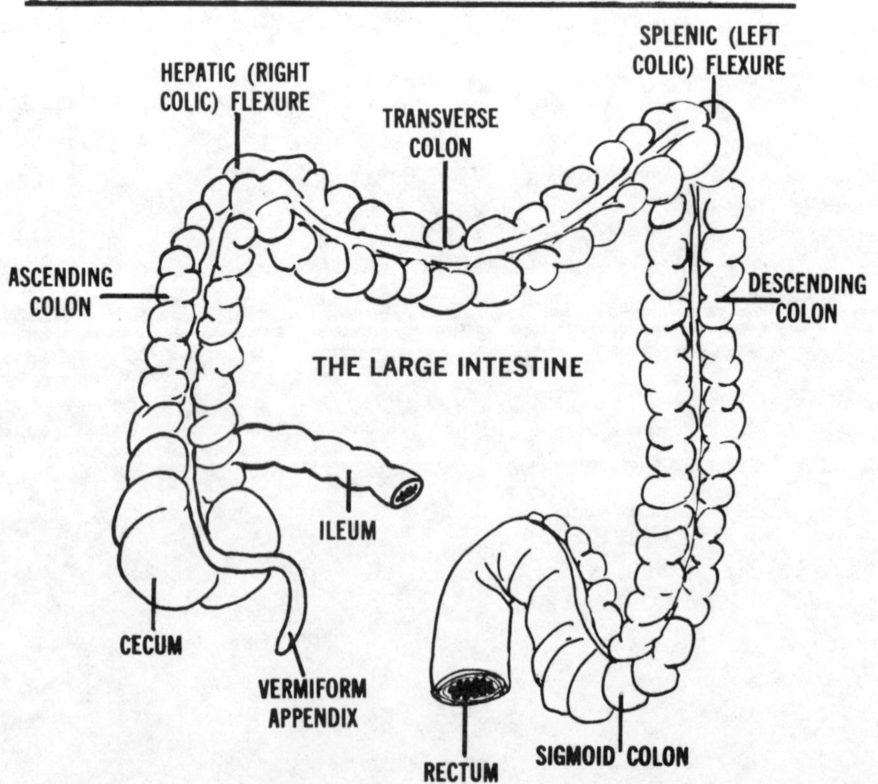
SPLENIC (LEFT
COLIC) FLEXURE
HEPATIC (RIGHT
COLIC) FLEXURE
TRANSVERSE
COLON
ASCENDING
COLON
DESCENDING
COLON
THE LARGE INTESTINE
ILEUM
CECUM
VERMIFORM
APPENDIX
RECTUM
SIGMOID COLON

CHAPTER VIII
THE GASTRO-INTESTINAL SYSTEM

The alimentary canal, the tongue, teeth, saliv/ary *spittle* (SAL-i-vā-rē) glands, pancreas and liver make up the di/gestive *apart to carry* (dī-JES-tiv) system.

The alimentary canal, which extends from the mouth to the anus, is a continuous tube about 30 feet long.

The esophagus *gullet(to carry food)* (ē-SOF-ah-gus), which connects with the pharynx at its upper end and with the stomach at its lower end, has four coats. Where the esophagus extends below the diaphragm the fourth coat is the peri/toneum *around to stretch* (per"i-to-NĒ-um). The peritoneum is the largest serous membrane in the body. The omentum *membrane enclosing bowels* (ō-MEN-tum) which hangs like a curtain in front of the stomach and the intestines is one of the important folds of the peritoneum. Another important fold of the peritoneum is the mes/entery *middle intestine* (MES-en-ter-ē) which attaches the small and much of the large intestine to the posterior abdominal wall.

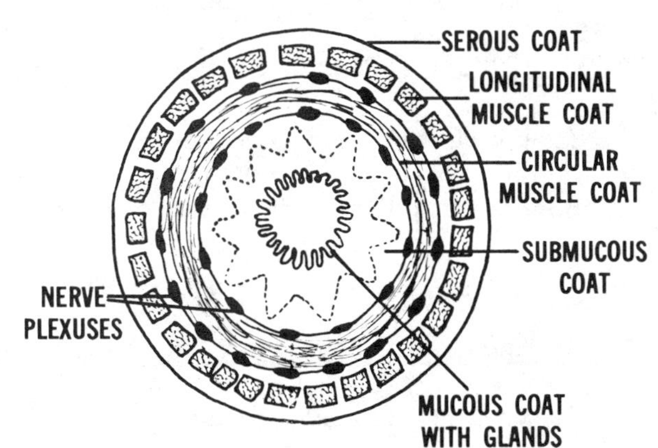

Cross Section Showing
COATS OF ALIMENTARY CANAL

The alimentary canal is divided into distinct areas: 1. the mouth, which contains the tongue, the openings of the ducts of the salivary glands, and the teeth; 2. the pharynx; 3. the esophagus; 4. the stomach; 5. the small or thin intestine which is divided into the duodenum *twelve*[1] (dū-ō-DĒ-num), jejunum *empty* (jē-JŪ-num)[2] and ileum *to roll up, twist* (IL-ē-um); 6. the large or thick intestine which is divided into the cecum *blind* (SĒ-kum) and colon; 7. the rectum; 8. the anal canal. The colon is subdivided into the ascending, transverse or mesial, descending and sig/moid *letter 'S'* (SIG-moyd) colon.

1. Optional pronunciation dū-OD-i-num. The translation "twelve" refers to its length.
2. Optional pronunciation jeh-JŪ-num

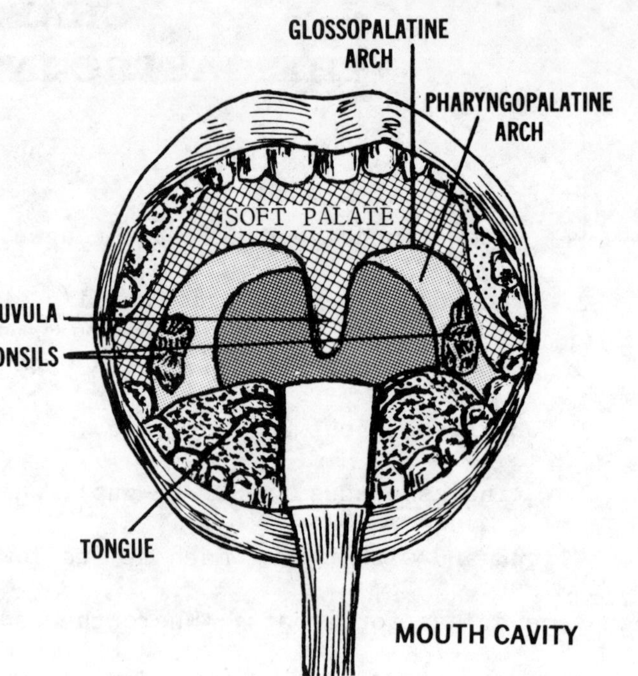

MOUTH CAVITY

The mouth (also called the oral or bucc/al *cheek* [BŪK-al] cavity) is an oval-shaped cavity enclosed on the sides by the cheeks and in front by the lips while behind it communicates with the pharynx. The hard and soft palate *roof of mouth* (PAL-at) form the roof of the mouth and the tongue forms the greater part of the floor of the mouth.

The processes of the maxillae *jawbone* (mak-SIL-ē) and palatine *palate* (PAL-ah-tīn) bones form the hard front portion of the palate. These processes are covered by peri/osteum *around bone* (per-ē-OS-tē-um) and mucous membrane. Hanging from the middle of the lower border of the palate is a small process called the palatine uvula *grape* (Ū-vu-lah) (little grape).

The fauces *throat* (FAW-sēz) refers to the aperture *an opening* (AP-er-chūr) leading from the mouth into the pharynx or throat cavity. The two arches which form on both sides of the uvula are called the glosso/palatine *tongue* (glos"ō-PAL-ah-tīn) arch or the anterior pillars of the fauces and the pharyngo/palatine *pharynx* (fah-ring"gō-PAL-al-tīn) arch or the posterior pillars of the fauces.

Situated in the triangular space between these arches are two masses of lymph/oid *water* (LIM-foyd) tissue, one on either side, called the palatine tonsils (commonly shortened to tonsils). Just below the tongue are masses of lymphoid tissue called the lingu/al *tongue* (LING-gwal) tonsils.

The tongue is the special organ of the sense of taste and assists in mastication *to gnash teeth* (mas-ti-KĀ-shun), deglutition *to swallow* (dē-glū-TISH-un) and digestion.

There are many minute glands in the mucous membrane which lines the mouth. These glands pour their secretion into the mouth. The chief secretion is that supplied by the salivary glands which are three pair of compound saccular (sac,bag) (SAK-ū-lar) glands called the par/otid (beside ear) (pah-ROT-id), sub/maxill/ary (below) (sub-MAK-si-lār-ē) and sub/lingu/al (sub-LING-gwal). The secretion which these glands release mixes with the secretions of the small glands of the mouth to form saliva (sah-LĪ-vah).

The maxillae and the mandible contain sockets in which the teeth are lodged. These sockets are known as alveoli (cavities) (al-VĒ-ō-lī) and are found in the alveol/ar (al-VĒ-ō-lar) process of the jaw bones.

There are two sets of teeth which develop during life. The first set is

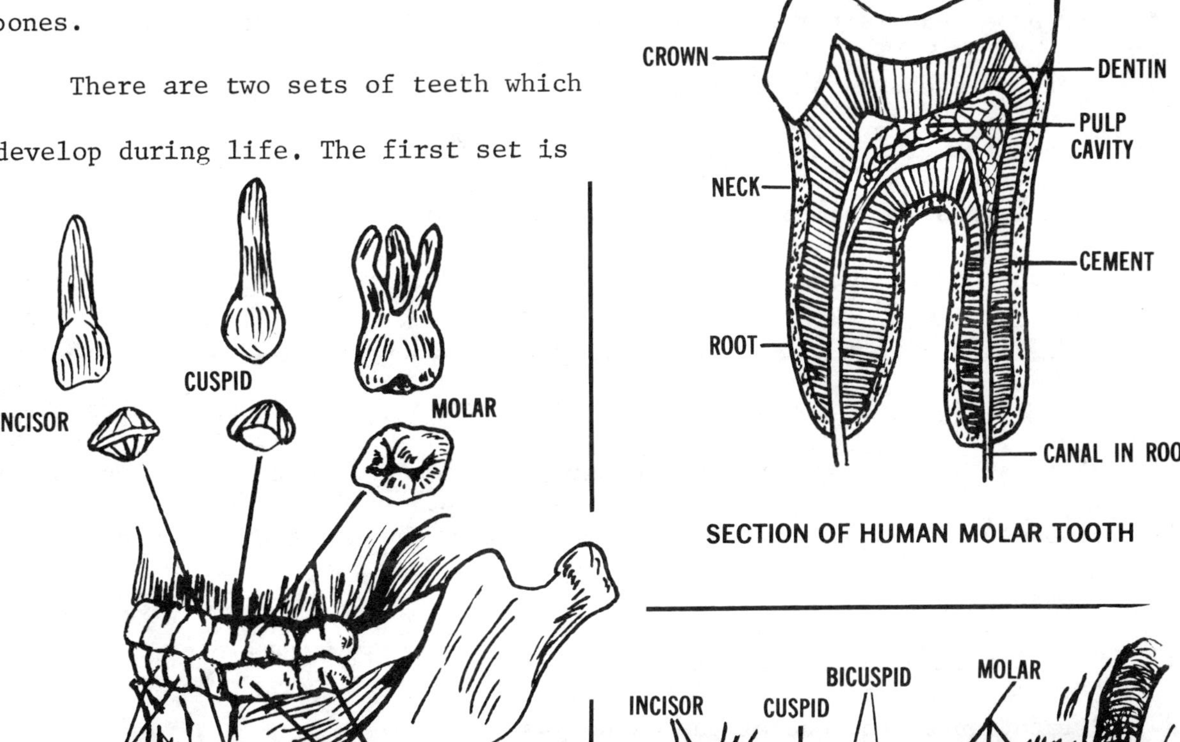

SECTION OF HUMAN MOLAR TOOTH

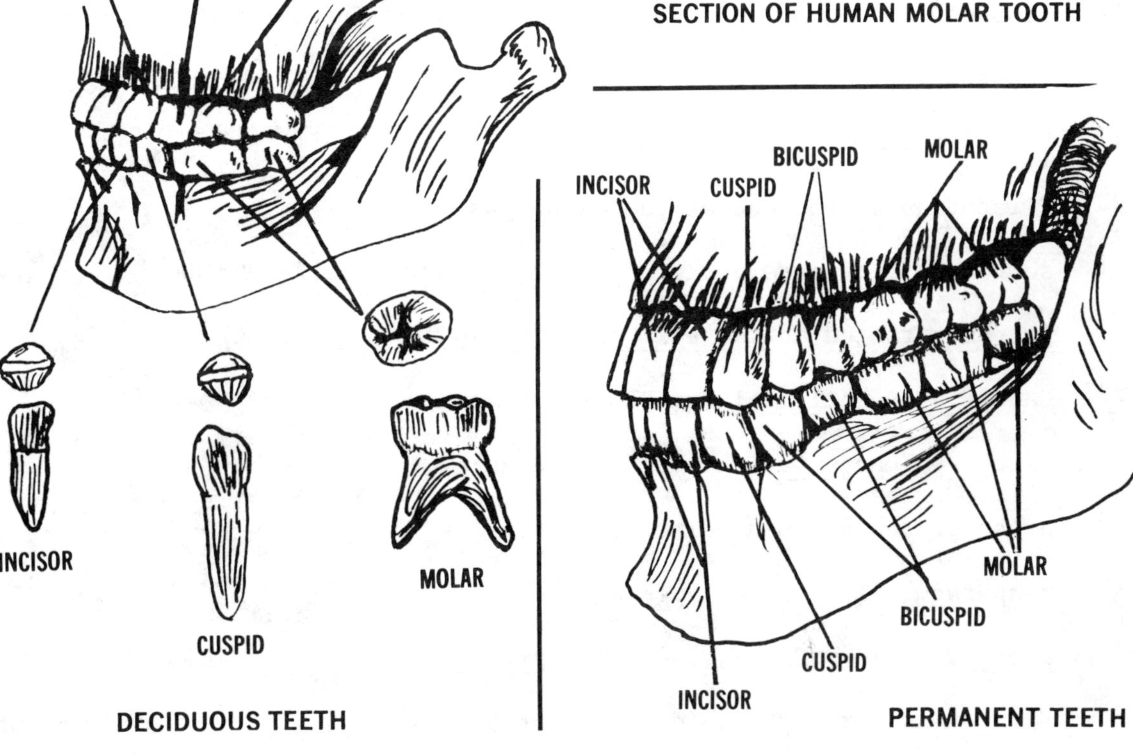

DECIDUOUS TEETH

PERMANENT TEETH

deciduous [to fall off] (dē-SID-ū-us) or milk teeth which are 20 in number, 10 in each jaw: four incisors [to cut into] (in-SĪ-zors), two canines [dog] (KĀ-nīns), and four molars [mass] (MŌ-lars). The second set of teeth are called the permanent teeth and they replace the deciduous teeth. There are 32 permanent teeth, 16 in each jaw: four incisors, two canines, four pre/molars [before] (prē-MŌ-lars) or bi/cuspids [two points] (bī-KUS-pids), and six molars.

The cone-shaped musculo/membranous [muscle] (mus"kyo͞o-lō-MEM-brah-nus) tube which connects the mouth to the esophagus is called the pharynx or throat cavity. Its broad end is turned upward and its constricted end is turned downward where it ends in the esophagus. The pharynx is divided into three parts: the nasal, the oral and the larynge/al [larynx] (lah-RIN-jē-al). The pharynge/al [pharynx] (fah-RIN-jē-al) tonsils, commonly called aden/oids [gland] (AD-i-noyds), are a mass of lymphoid tissue located about the center of the posterior wall of the naso/pharynx [nose throat] (nā-zō-FAR-inks).

Beginning at the lower end of the pharynx, just behind the trachea, is a muscular tube about nine to ten inches long known as the esophagus or gullet. It passes through the diaphragm and ends in the upper or cardiac end of the stomach.

The stomach is a collapsible, sac-like dilatation at the end of the esophagus and serves as a temporary receptacle for food. It is situated in the epi/gastr/ic [on stomach] (ep-i-GAS-trik), umbilic/al [navel] (um-BIL-i-kal) and left hypo/chondriac[1] [below cartilage] (hī-pō-KON-drē-ak) areas of the abdomen, directly under the diaphragm. It has two openings, the esophageal [gullet] (ē-SOF-ah-jē-al) and pylor/ic [gate,orifice] (pī-LOR-ik) orifices which are guarded by

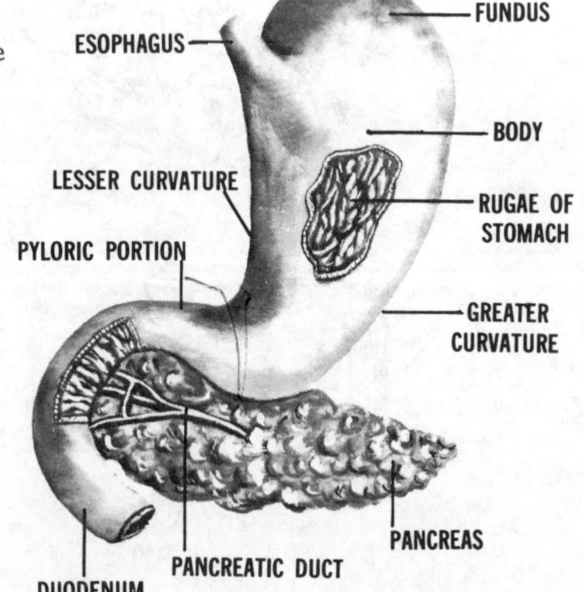

THE STOMACH

1. Pertains to the hypochondrium (hī"pō-KON-drē-um) (below the ribs) and to hypochondriasis (hī"pō-kon-DRĪ-ah-sis). An individual with hypochondriasis was called a hypochondriac because it was believed the hypochondrium and the spleen were the seat of this disorder. The current definition of "hypochondriasis" is "an unfounded belief that one is suffering from some disease."

<u>sphincter</u> *to bind fast* (SFINK-ter) muscles; and two borders or curvatures called the lesser and greater curvatures. The <u>fundus</u>[1] *bottom* (FUN-dus) of the stomach is the blind, rounded part above the entrance of the esophagus. The smaller or opposite end is called the pyloric portion. The portion between the fundus and pyloric regions is called the body.

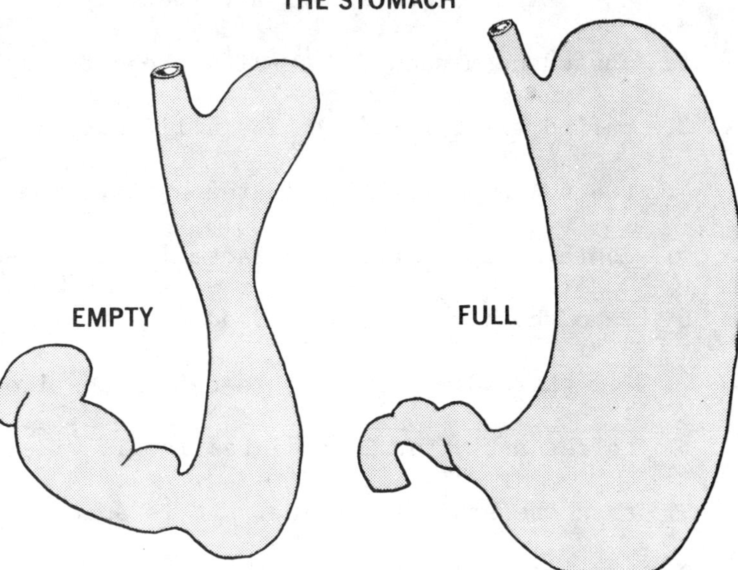

Extending from the pylorus to the colic valve is a <u>con/voluted</u> *together rolled* (KON-vō-lū-ted) tube about 23 feet in length known as the small or thin intestine. It is located in the central and lower part of the abdominal cavity and is divided into the duodenum, jejunum and ileum.

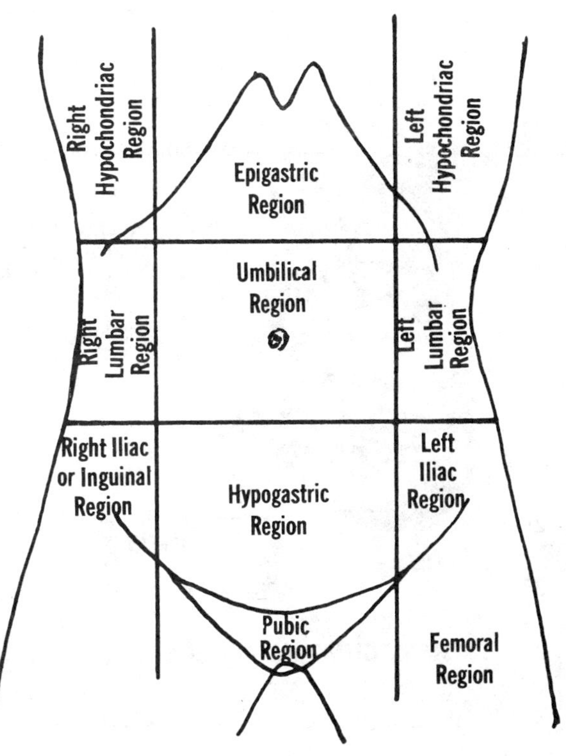

The duodenum, which is the shortest and broadest part, is about 10 inches long and extends from the pyloric end of the stomach to the jejunum.

The jejunum is about 7½ feet long and extends from the duodenum to the ileum. The ileum extends from the jejunum to the large intestine which it joins at a right angle. The orifice of the ileum is guarded by a sphincter muscle known as the colic or <u>ileo/cecal</u> *ileum cecum* (il"ē-ō-SĒ-kal) valve. This valve prevents the return of material that has been discharged into the large bowel. The mucous membrane of the entire length of

1. Means "farthest from the opening of an organ"

the small intestine has a velvety appearance caused by minute finger-like projections called villi[1] *tuft of hair* (VIL-lī). The villi number between 4 and 5 million in the human. They contain capillaries and lacteals *milk* (LAK-tē-als) into which the digested food passes.

VILLUS

Extending for five feet from the ileum to the anus, the large intestine is wider than the small intestine. It is about 2½ inches wide at the cecum. The large intestine is divided into four parts: 1. the cecum with the vermi/form *worm* (VER-mi-form) appendix *to hang upon* (ah-PEN-diks); 2. the colon which is subdivided into the ascending, transverse or mesial, descending and sigmoid colon; 3. the rectum; 4. the anal canal.

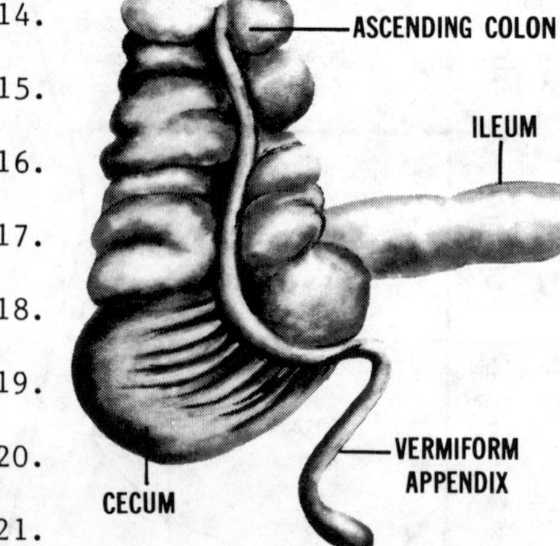

THE CECUM AND APPENDIX

The cecum is a large blind pouch at the beginning of the large intestine. The small intestine opens into the side wall of the large intestine about 2½ inches above the beginning of the large intestine. This two and one-half inch area forms the cul-de-sac *bottom of the bag* (KUL-dē-sak) known as the cecum. Attached to the end of the cecum is a narrow, worm-like tube, the vermiform appendix. The average length of the appendix is about three inches but length, diameter, direction and other relations of the appendix are variable.

The rectum is continuous with the sigmoid colon and is about five inches long. It terminates in the anal canal which is about one inch or one and one-half inch in length. The external opening, called the anus, is guarded by an internal and external sphincter. The condition known as piles or hemo/rrhoids *blood / to flow*

1. Also translates to "shaggy hair of beasts"

(HEM-ō-royds) is caused by enlargement of the veins of the anal canal.

The largest gland in the body is the liver. Ordinarily it weighs from 42 to 56 ounces. Located in the right hypochondriac and epigastric areas of the abdomen the liver frequently extends into the left hypochondriac region. It is connected to the under surface of the diaphragm and the anterior walls of the abdomen by five ligaments: the falci/form *sickle* (FAL-si-form), the coronary, the two lateral ligaments. The first, or round ligament, is a fibrous cord caused by atrophy of the umbilical vein of intra/uterine *inside uterus* (in-trah-Ū-ter-in)[1] life. The liver has four lobes which are separated by fossae or fissures. Some of these fissures are the sagitt/al *arrow* (SAJ-i-tal), the portal (or transverse), the fossa for the gall bladder (also called the gall bladder bed), and the fossa for the inferior vena cava. The lobes formed by these fissures or fossae are the right (the largest), the left (the smaller and wedge-shaped), the quadr/ate *four* (KWOD-rāt) (square), and the caud/ate *tail* (KAW-dāt) (tail-like). There are five sets of hepatic *liver* (hē-PAT-ik) vessels: 1. branches of the portal tubes; 2. bile ducts; 3. branches of the hepatic artery; 4. hepatic veins; 5. the lymphatics.

The numerous bile ducts spread throughout the liver unite and form larger and larger ducts until two main ducts unite in the portal fossa and form the hepatic duct. The hepatic duct passes downward and joins at an acute angle the duct from the gall bladder, the cystic *sac,bladder* (SIS-tik) duct. The hepatic and cystic ducts join together and form the common bile duct (the chole/dochus *bile receptacle* [kō-le-DŌ-kus])[2] which passes downward for about three inches and then enters the duodenum about three inches below the pylorus.

The chief bile pigment is called bili/rubin *bile red* (bil-i-RO̅O̅-bin). The main function of the bile is the digestion and absorption of fat. The chamber formed by the joining of the common bile duct and the pancreatic duct is known as the ampulla *small jar* (am-PŪL-ah) of Vater[3] (FAH-ter). The opening of this chamber is

1. Optional pronunciation in-trah-Ū-ter-īn
2. Optional pronunciation kō-LED-ō-kus
3. Abraham Vater, German anatomist, 1684-1751

guarded by a ring of muscle called the sphincter of Oddi (OD-dī).[1]

Glisson's[2] (GLIS-unz) capsule is a fibrous tissue capsule which invests the liver.

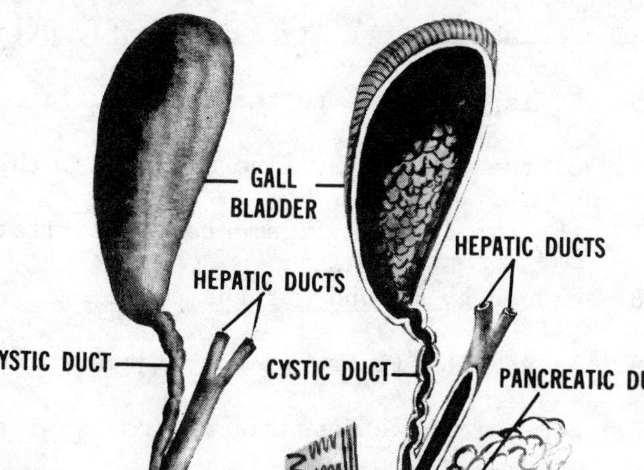

GALL BLADDER

The gall bladder, which is about three to four inches long and one inch wide, is a pear-shaped sac. It is lodged in the gall bladder fossa on the under surface of the liver. The gall bladder serves as a reservoir for bile.

The pancreas is divided into head, body and tail. In shape it somewhat resembles a hammer. It is a soft, reddish or yellowish-gray gland and lies in front of the first and second lumbar vertebrae and behind the stomach. It weighs about two to three ounces and is about five inches long and two inches wide. In structure the pancreas is composed of many lobules and is, therefore, known as a racemose (full of clusters) (RAS-i-mōs) gland. Each lobule contains one of the branches of the main duct which terminates in a group of pouches or alveoli. It is between these alveoli that small groups of cells are found which are called the islands of Langerhans[3] (LAHNG-er-hanz). These cells furnish the internal secretion of the pancreas from which insulin is extracted.

1. Optional pronunciation OD-dē; Ruggero Oddi, Italian physician of the 19th century.
2. Francis Glisson, English physician and anatomist, 1597-1677
3. Paul Langerhans, German pathologist, 1847-1888

PANCREAS AND DUODENUM

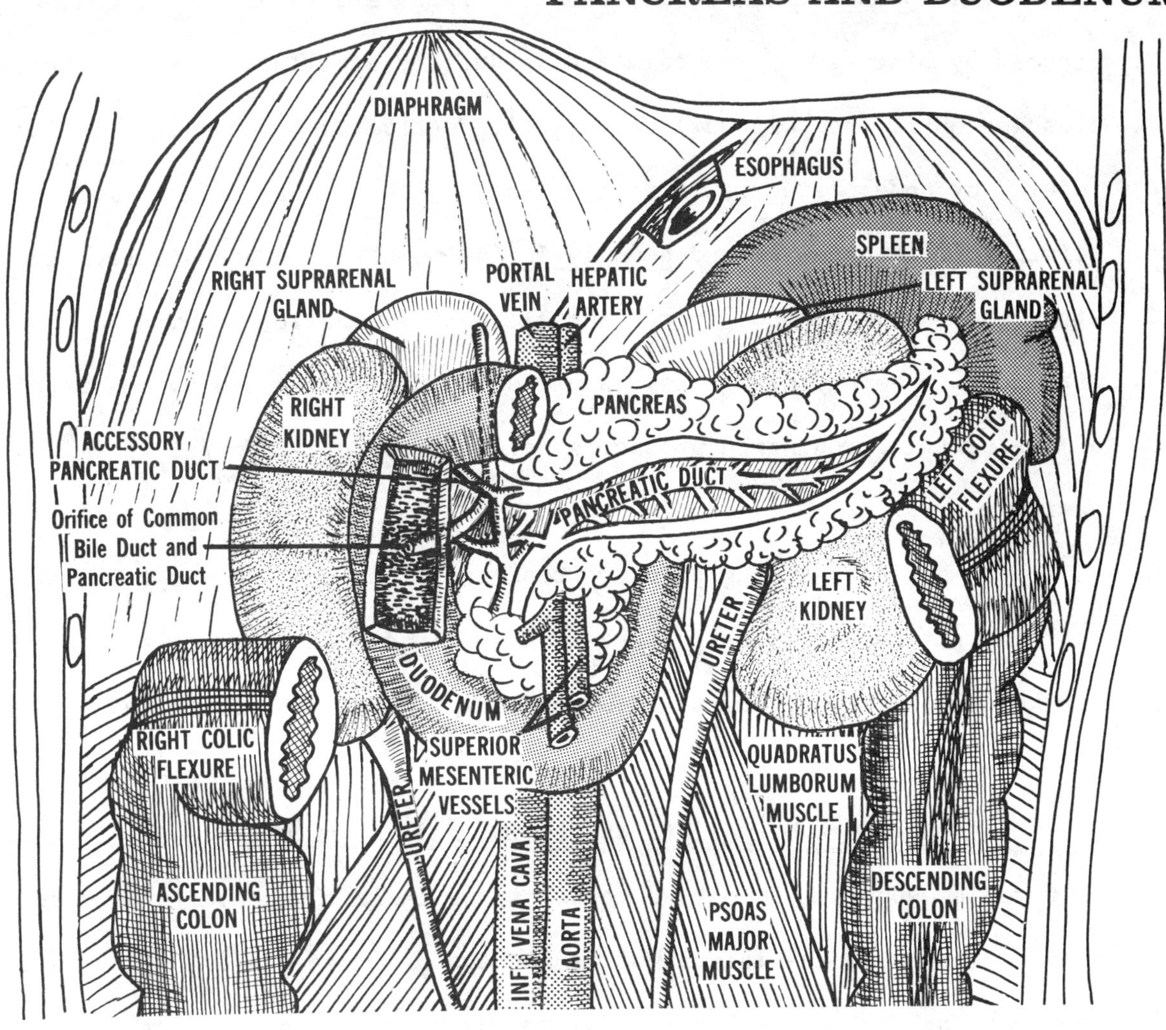

DISEASES AND ANOMALIES

Symptoms of digestive diseases are indicative of certain conditions. Some of these symptoms and the areas in which they occur are listed below:

Esophagus: re/gurgitation *(back / to flood)* (rē-gur-ji-TĀ-shun) of food.

Stomach: abdominal pain, vomiting, hemat/emesis *(blood / to vomit)* (hem-at-EM-i-sis)[1] (vomiting of blood), melena *(black)* (mel-Ē-nah)[2] (blood in the stools), dys/pepsia *(bad / digestion)* (dis-PEP-sē-ah).

Small intestine: vomiting, intermittent crampy pain in the abdomen, distension[3] of the abdomen with gas, painful spasm, dia/rrhea *(through)* (dī-ah-RĒ-ah).

Large intestine: pain, diarrhea, con/stipation *(together / a crowding)* (kon-ste-PĀ-shun).

1. Optional pronunciation hē"mat-EM-i-sis
2. Optional pronunciation MEL-i-nah. This term applies to bleeding from the stomach. The blood passing through the intestinal tract becomes dark and is termed "altered" or "occult" blood. This results in "tarry" stools.
3. Optional spelling "distention"

Liver: jaundice [yellow] (JAWN-dis) of which there are three types: obstructive (caused by blockage of the common bile duct by a gallstone or by a tumor pressing on it from without); toxic or infective where the liver cells are injured by some poison or infective process, thus decreasing their ability to eliminate bile pigment; and hemo/lytic [to dissolve] (hē-mō-LIT-ik) which is seen in conditions such as pernicious [destruction] (per-NISH-us) anemia, hemolytic anemia, and poisoning with certain hemolytic agents. Ascites [a bag] (ah-SĪ-tēz) caused by an obstruction of the portal circulation producing serum in the peri/tone/al [to stretch] (per-i-to-NĒ-al) cavity.

Gall bladder: aching pain and tenderness beneath the margin of the ribs on the right side; severe colicky[1] [colic] (KOL-ik-ē) pain in the same region due to blockage of the cystic duct (as by a stone); dyspepsia caused when fatty foods are eaten.

Pancreas: loss of weight, dyspepsia, and the occurrence of frequent large soft yellow stools caused by disease of the cells that have to do with digestion. Disease of the islands of Langerhans produces dia/betes [through to go] (dī-ah-BĒ-tez) mellitus [to sweeten] (MEL-i-tus)[2] or hyper/insulin/ism [above] (hī-per-IN-sul-in-izm).

Peritoneum: abdominal pain, tenderness, rigidity of the abdominal muscles and often distension of the intestines with gas, ascites (in some types of peritoneal disease).

The digestive system is susceptible to various types of inflammatory diseases. The following are the most common gastro-intestinal inflammations.

Stomat/itis [mouth] (stō-mah-TĪ-tis) or inflammation of the mouth may be diffuse or localized. It may affect only the gums (gingiv/itis [gums] [jin-je-VĪ-tis]) or the tongue (gloss/itis [tongue] [glos-Ī-tis]).

Esophag/itis [gullet] (ē-sof-ah-JĪ-tis) is usually due to the action of caust/ic [to burn] (KAWS-tik) chemicals.

Gastr/itis [stomach] (gas-TRĪ-tis) in an acute form is often due to chemical agents.

1. Sick with colic (acute abdominal pain)
2. Optional pronunciation me-LĪ-tis

It may also be infectious in nature, due to organisms contained in contaminated food (so-called food poisoning). Chronic gastritis refers to chronic inflammation of the stomach from other conditions such as cancer and ulcer of the stomach, cirrhosis[1] [tawny] (sir-Ō-sis) of the liver and pell/agra [skin rough] (pel-LAG-rah).

Enter/itis [intestine] (en-ter-Ī-tis) occurs in cases of food poisoning, bi/chloride [two chlorine] (bī-KLŌ-rīd) of mercury [metallic element] (MER-kū-rē) poisoning, and in some of the specific infectious diseases such as typh/oid [stupor] (TĪ-foyd) fever, Asiatic cholera [bile] (KOL-er-ah), tuberc/ul/osis [node small] (tū-ber-kū-LŌ-sis) of the intestine, and sometimes in bacill/ary [bacillus] (BAS-i-lā-rē) dys/entery [bad intestine] (DIS-en-ter-ē).

Col/itis [colon] (kō-LĪ-tis) may be due to all of the conditions which cause inflammation of the small intestine. The most frequent specific infections of the colon are ameb/ic [ameba] (ah-ME-bik) and bacillary dysentery. Colitis may also occur in ur/emia [urine blood] (ū-RĒ-mē-ah), or may be secondary to cancer or diverticulosis [to turn aside] (dī"ver-tik-ū-LŌ-sis) of the colon. Chronic ulcerative [a sore] (UL-ser-ah-tiv) colitis is an inflammatory colitis of unknown cause with alternating periods of re/mission [back to send] (rē-MISH-un) and exacerbation[2] [to increase] (eks-as-er-BĀ-shun).

Proct/itis [anus,rectum] (prok-TĪ-tis) besides occurring with inflammation of other portions of the large intestine, may be due to lympho/granul/oma [water grains] (lim"fō-gran-ū-LŌ-mah) venereum[3] (ve-NĒ-rē-um), tuberculosis, and other infectious diseases.

Appendic/itis [appendix] (ah-pen-di-SĪ-tis) is perhaps the most important inflammatory disease of the digestive system. It is considered a surgical disease.

The most common benign tumors of the digestive tract are polyps (POL-ips). Often there are numerous closely placed smaller tumors in a single region, a condition called polyp/osis [many + foot] (pol-i-PŌ-sis). Polyps are common in the stomach and colon, rare in the esophagus and small bowel. In some instances they undergo malignant change and become cancerous.

Pept/ic [digest] (PEP-tik) ulcer: an ulcer consists of localized destruction of tissue on a cutaneous [skin] (kyōō-TĀ-nē-us) or mucous surface. A peptic ulcer is an

1. Refers to the color of the cirrhotic (sir-OT-ik) liver.
2. A more current translation is "very bitter or harsh."
3. Pertains to Venus, goddess of love.

ulcer occurring in that portion of the digestive tube exposed to the action of the acid gastric juice. Peptic ulcers occur most commonly in the first portion of the duodenum, next most frequently in the stomach, and rarely in the lower portion of the esophagus. They may be acute or chronic; acute ulcers are more common in the stomach and chronic ulcers in the duodenum.

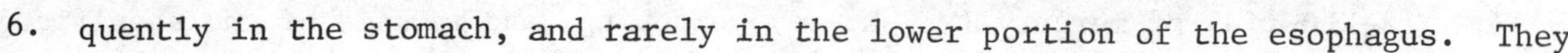

CONGENITAL ABNORMALITIES OF THE ESOPHAGUS

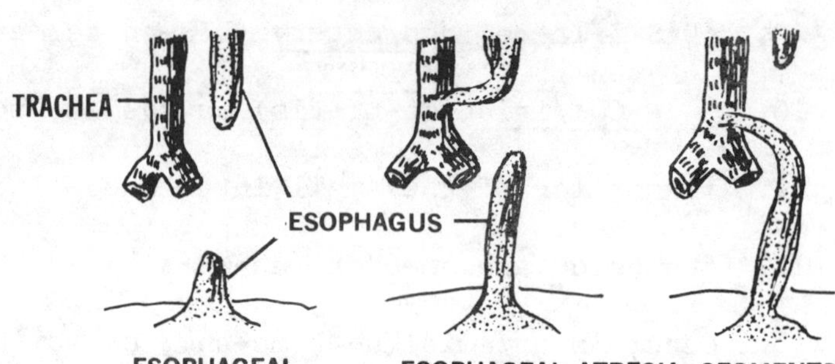

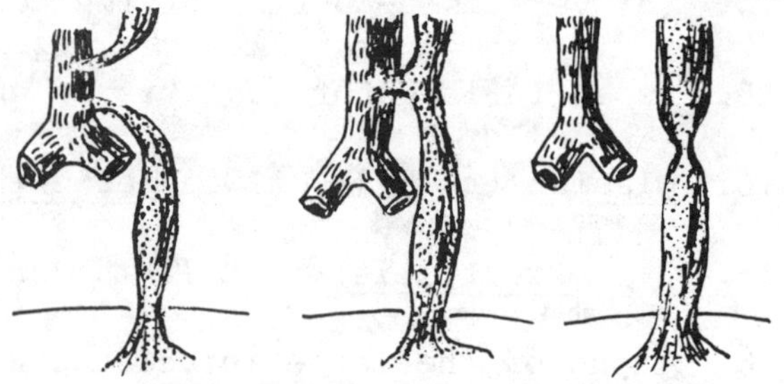

ANAL AND RECTAL ABNORMALITIES

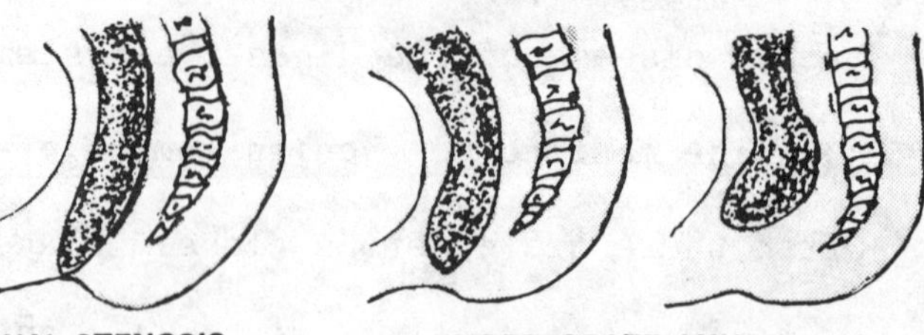

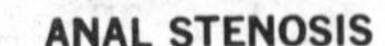

Con/genital (with / to begin) (kon-JEN-i-tal) malformations or defects of the digestive tube are not common, and many of them are incompatible with life. The esophagus may end in a blind pouch (atresia (without opening) [ah-TRĒ-zē-ah]) or open into the trachea; the rectum may be completely occluded at or near the anus (im/perforate (not perforated) [im-PER-fo-rat] anus); the lumen (light) (LŪ-men) of the small intestine may be lacking in several places. These anomalies are usually recognized during the first few days of life; their treatment is entirely surgical.

A diverticulum (to turn aside) (dī-ver-TIK-ū-lum) is a pouch or pocket leading off from a main cavity or tube. Diverticula (plural) (dī-ver-TIK-ū-lah) of the digestive tube are of fairly frequent occurrence and may be present in any portion of the tract.

Meckel's[1] (MEK-elz) diverticulum is a congenital anomaly, a persistence of a duct which, in the fetus (offspring) (FĒ-tus), extends from the ileum to the umbilicus (the navel) (um-BIL-i-kis).[2] It causes no symptoms unless it becomes inflamed, in which case symptoms and signs much like those of appendicitis develop; the only difference is that bloody stools are sometimes present in cases of Meckel's diverticul/itis (dī-ver-tik-ū-LĪ-tis). Surgical removal of the inflamed diverticulum is usually required.

The most common type of displacement of the digestive organs is falling or prolapse, known as viscero/ptosis (organ) (vis"er-op-TŌ-sis), in which case the viscera (VIS-er-ah) occupy an unusually or abnormally low position in the abdomen. Usually all of the abdominal organs, not a single one, are prolapsed. Diaphragm/atic (dī"ah-frag-MAT-ik) hernia is a displacement of individual organs of the digestive system which may be due to the presence of large tumors, to paralysis of either side of the diaphragm, or to hernias. In some cases, the stomach may herniate through the normal opening (hiatus (an opening) [hī-Ā-tus]) in the diaphragm through which the esophagus enters the abdomen; this is known as peri/esophage/al (per"ē-ē-SOF-ah-jē-al) or hiat/al (hī-Ā-tal) hernia.

Hirschsprung's[3] (HIRSH-sproongz) disease is a chronic dilatation of the colon of unknown cause. It occurs in children and is usually fatal.

Pyloric stenosis is an obstruction of the stomach which occurs in infants. It is corrected by surgery.

Obstructions of the intestine may be caused by strangul/ation (to choke) (strang-gū-LĀ-shun) of the bowel in hernias, or by peritoneal adhesions or malformation; foreign bodies; intus/susception (within / to receive) (in"tus-sus-SEP-shun); volvulus (to roll) (VOL-vū-lus), a knotting or twisting of the bowel.

The most important diseases of the liver are acute catarrh/al (to flow down) (kah-TAHR-al) jaundice, yellow atrophy, cirrhoses, abscess and cancer. This organ may also be involved in a number of specific infectious diseases, such as pneumonia (lung)

1. Johann F. Meckel (junior) German comparative anatomist and embryologist, 1781-1833
2. This is the most commonly used pronunciation. The optional pronunciation is um-bi-LĪ-kis.
3. Harold Hirschsprung, Danish physician from Copenhagen, 1830-1916

(nū-MŌ-nē-ah), septic/emia [decay] (sep-ti-SĒ-mē-ah), syphilis, tuberculosis, and Weil's (vilz) disease; in some of the poisonings, in such conditions as leuk/emia [white] (lū-KĒ-mē-ah) and amyl/oid [starch] (AM-i-loyd) disease.

Infectious hepat/itis [liver] (hep-ah-TĪ-tis) is an acute disease, the outstanding symptom of which is jaundice. It usually runs a benign course of four to six weeks.

The bile ducts or gall bladder or both may be the site of acute or chronic inflammation due to the ordinary organisms which cause infection. Infection is often aided by stasis [to halt] (STĀ-sis) resulting from the presence of stones in the gall bladder. Inflammation of the bile ducts is called chol/ang/itis [bile vessel] (kō-lan-JĪ-tis); of the gall bladder, chole/cyst/itis [gall bladder] (kō"le-sis-TĪ-tis). Chole/lith/iasis [gall stone] (kō"le-lith-Ī-ah-sis) refers to the presence of stones in the gall bladder or bile ducts.

SURGERY

Congenital malformations of the esophagus and their correction:

1. atresia of the esophagus: ligation of the tracheo-esophageal [trachea] (trā"kē-ō-ē-SOF-ah-jē-al) fistula and exteriorization [bringing outside of the body] (eks-tē"rē-or-i-ZĀ-shun) of the blind esophageal stump or ligation of the tracheo-esophageal fistula and anastomosis [make an opening] (ah-nas-tō-MŌ-sis) of the upper esophageal segment with the mobilized lower end of the esophagus.
2. congenital short esophagus: phrenico-exeresis [phrenic nerve removal] (fren"i-kō-ek-SER-ē-sis) (a/vulsion [away to pull] [ah-VUL-shun] of the phrenic nerve).

Injuries of the esophagus may occur from instrumentation, the swallowing of a foreign body or caustic substances, or through injuries of the chest. Surgical procedure is incision and drainage of infection (I & D) and closure of laceration.

Diverticul/ectomy (dī-ver-tik-ū-LEK-tō-mē) is performed for diverticula of the esophagus.

Benign obstruction of the esophagus may be produced by a number of non-malignant lesions. These include stenosis following the swallowing of lye or other caustic matters, cicatricial [scar] (sik-ah-TRISH-al) stenosis of the lower esophagus following esophagitis from repeated regurgitation of gastric juice, and idio/pathic [peculiar disease] (id-ē-ō-PATH-ik) stenosis of the esophagus commonly designated as a/chalasia [no relaxation] (ā-kah-LĀ-zē-ah)[1] or cardio/spasm [heart contraction] (KAR-dē-ō-spazm). Some of the strictures can be treated by repeated dilatation. The surgical procedure for cicatricial stenosis and cardiospasm is a lateral anastomosis between the esophagus and fundus of the stomach known as thoraco-esophago-gastro/stomy [thorax] (thō"rah-kō-ē-sof"ah-gō-gas-TROS-tō-mē). Other procedures used are cardio/plasty (KAR-dē-ō-plas-tē) and esophago/stomy (ē-sof-ah-JOS-tō-mē) and the Heller operation.

The large majority of tumors arising in the esophagus are carcin/omata [cancer tumors] (kar-sin-Ō-mah-tah). A trans/thoracic [across] (trans-thō-RAS-ik) approach is used for carcinoma of the cervical esophagus with excision of tumor and radical resection if necessary. Esophago/gastric (ē-sof"ah-gō-GAS-trik) anastomosis is performed for carcinoma of the middle third of the esophagus.

Benign lesions of the stomach (benign gastric tumors may be single or multiple), polyps (potentially malignant so require removal), fibroma, my/oma [muscle] (mī-Ō-mah), neuro/fibr/oma [nerve fiber] (nū"rō-fī-BRŌ-mah) require segmental resection of the stomach.

Diverticula of the stomach are rare but when they do occur the procedures performed are diverticulectomy or wedge resection.

Tuberculosis of the stomach is exceedingly rare but when it does occur a partial gastr/ectomy (gas-TREK-tō-mē) is performed.

Gastric syphilis may produce digestive symptoms simulating those of malignant disease. Differential diagnosis is made by x-ray. Procedure is anti/syphilitic [against]

1. Optional pronunciation ah-kah-LĀ-zē-ah

(an"te-sif-i-LIT-ik) treatment and in advanced cases of obstruction partial gastrectomy or gastro/entero/stomy (intestine) (gas"trō-en-ter-OS-tō-mē).

Types of surgery performed for gastric ulcer:

1. Hemi/gastr/ectomy (half) (hem-ē-gas-TREK-tō-mē) and vago/tomy (vagus nerve) (vā-GOT-ō-mē) followed by anastomosis of stomach and duodenum (Billroth[1] I [BIL-rōth] or modifications of Billroth I), or of stomach and jejunum (Polya[2]-Balfour [POL-yah-BAL-fur]), or Billroth II.
2. Excision of a portion of the stomach containing the gastric ulcer and vagotomy in some cases combined with pyloro/plasty (pylorus) (pī-LŌ-rō-plas-tē) or gastroenterostomy.
3. Trans/gastric (trans-GAS-trik) excision of the ulcer from the posterior wall of the stomach.
4. Sleeve resection of the stomach.

Types of operation performed for duodenal ulcer:

1. Pyloroplasty and gastro/duodeno/stomy (duodenum) (gas"trō-dū-o-de-NOS-tō-mē) with vag/ectomy (vā-GEK-tō-mē)
2. Vagectomy with gastroenterostomy
3. Hemigastrectomy, Billroth I (gastroduodenostomy) or Billroth II (gastroenterostomy) with vagectomy.

A variety of anastomosis procedures have been developed, anyone of which may be used following the subtotal or total gastrectomy performed for malignant lesions of the stomach. Some of these anastomosis procedures are: (Most of these procedures have been named for the men who developed them.)

Billroth I-von Haberer method, Mayo method, Horsley's modification of the Billroth I method, Finney-von Haberer method, Billroth I-Mayo method, Billroth I-Schoemaker modification. In the Polya operation, Hofmeister and Finsterer modification of Billroth II, Balfour-Polya modification, the procedure is a gastro/jejuno/stomy (gas"trō-jeh-jū-NOS-tō-mē) and

1. Albert Theodor Billroth, Vienna surgeon, 1829-1894, often called "the father of visceral surgery."
2. Eugene Polya, Budapest surgeon, 1876-1944

the cut end of the duodenum is always closed and the gastro-intestinal continuity is reestablished by joining the remaining portion of the stomach to the jejunum.

Transthoracic resection of the cardia and esophagus is performed for lesions of the cardia and the lower portion of the esophagus. Other procedures performed for lesions of the stomach include:

1. Posterior gastroenterostomy for pyloric obstruction;
2. Anterior gastroenterostomy when it is not preferable to do a posterior gastroenterostomy;
3. Gastro/stomy (gas-TROS-tō-mē) (used in a limited number of cases) for feeding purposes. Witzel[1] (VIT-zel) type of operation is done.
4. Jejuno/stomy (jeh-jū-NOS-tō-mē) is an exclusion operation for certain fixed irremovable malignant lesions of the lower end of the stomach. It is not often done.

Vagectomy or division of the vagus nerve to the stomach is done for relief of ulcer distress and acid production. It is occasionally performed by the transthoracic approach but more frequently is performed by the trans/abdominal (trans-abd-DOM-i-nal) approach.

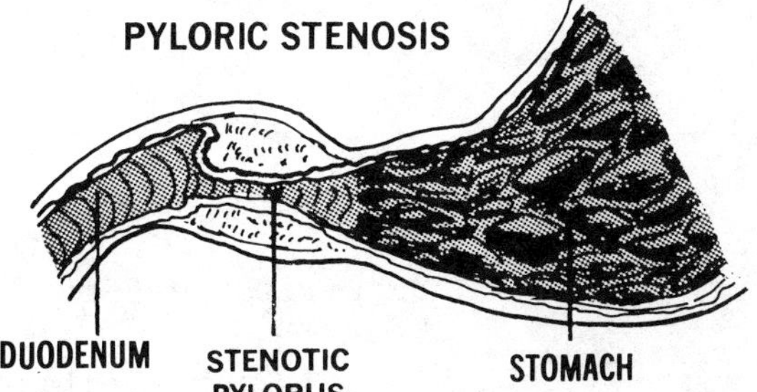

Pyloro/myo/tomy (muscle) (pī-lō"rō-mī-OT-ō-mē) is performed for stenosis of the pylorus. Also known as Fredet-Ramstedt[2] (fre-DĀ -RAHM-stet) operation.

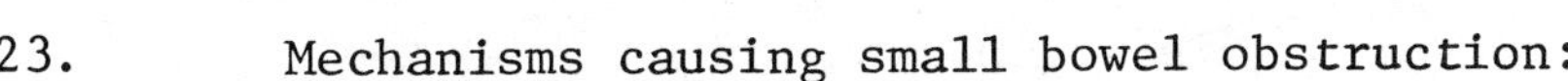

Mechanisms causing small bowel obstruction:

1. external hernia
2. adhesions of bowel to other loops or to the parietal peritoneum
3. adhesive bands
4. intussusception (enteric (intestine) [en-TER-ik], ileocolic, ileocecal, colic)

1. Friederich Oscar Witzel, German surgeon, 1856-1935
2. Pierre Fredet, French surgeon, 1870-1946; Conrad Ramstadt, German surgeon, born 1867.

5. foreign body or obturation obstruction usually due to a gall stone which has sloughed through both the gall bladder and intestinal walls
6. mesenteric (mesentery) (mes-en-TER-ik) venous (vein) (VĒ-nus) thromb/osis (clot) (throm-BŌ-sis); arterial thrombosis
7. congenital atresia and bands
8. volvulus
9. neo/plasms (new formation) (NĒ-ō-plazms) (primary neoplasms in the small bowel are fairly rare)
10. internal hernias are very rarely a cause of obstruction.

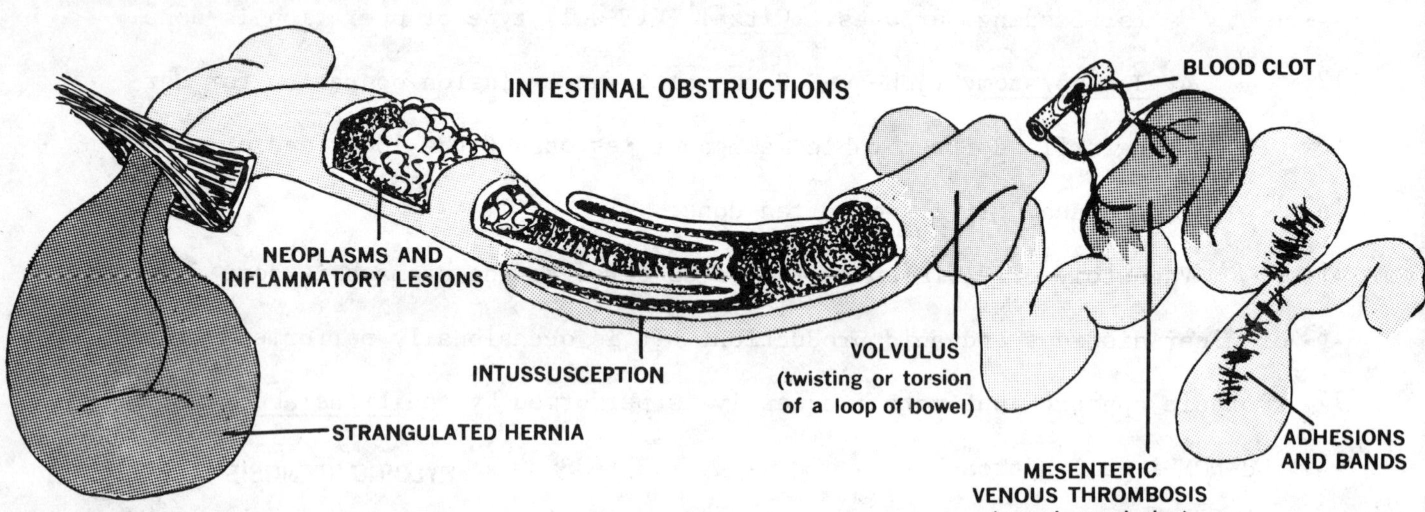

Surgeries performed:

1. hernio/plasty (hernia) (her"nē-ō-PLAS-tē) and intestinal resection and anastomosis for strangulation of intestine;
2. exploration and lysis for adhesions and adhesive bands;
3. reduction of intussusception. In recurrent conditions it is rarely necessary to perform exteriorization and secondary closure of resection. Primary resection and end-to-end anastomosis is usually done.

4. entero/stomy (en-ter-OS-tō-mē) and removal of stone for gallstone obstruction;
5. resection and primary anastomosis of the involved intestine for mesenteric venous thrombosis;
6. resection of gangrenous (GANG-gre-nes) bowel with end-to-end anastomosis.

Hemi/col/ectomy [half colon] (hem"ē-kō-LEK-tō-mē) and ileo-trans/verse [ileum across to turn] (il"ē-ō-trans-VERS) colon anastomosis is performed for carcinoma of the cecum.

INTESTINAL ANASTOMOSIS PROCEDURES

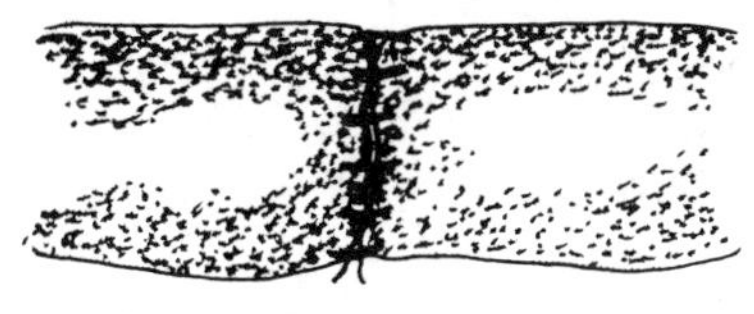
END-TO-END

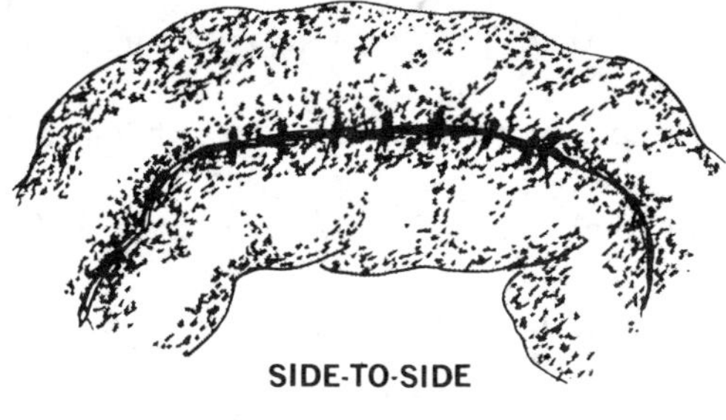
SIDE-TO-SIDE

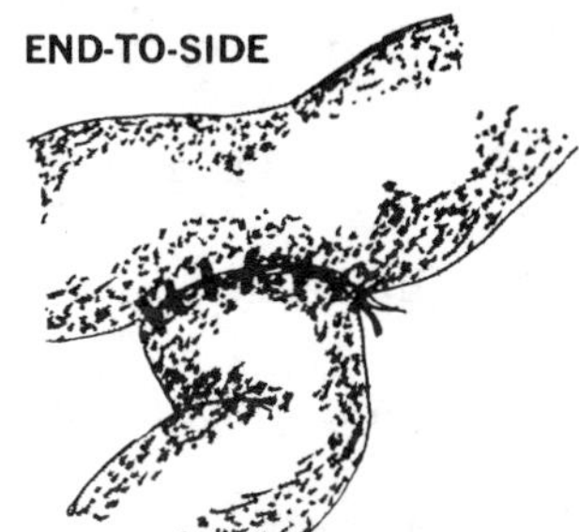
END-TO-SIDE

Indications for ileo/stomy (il-ē-OS-tō-mē) (single-barreled, double-barreled):

1. chronic, non-specific ulcerative colitis (the most common condition);
2. pan-col/ectomy [all colon] (pan-kō-LEK-tō-mē) for polyps of the colon or other conditions;
3. acute, complete obstruction due to cancer in the right colon.

Meckel's diverticulum may be situated anywhere from the ileocecal junction to the ligament of Treitz[1] (trīts) but is most commonly found 25 to 100 centimeters from the cecum. Procedure used is diverticulectomy or resection of the small bowel with end-to-end anastomosis.

Ile/ectomy [ileum] (il-ē-EK-tō-mē) and entero/anastomosis (en"ter-ō-ah-nas-tō-MŌ-sis) are performed for regional ile/itis (il-ē-Ī-tis).

Exposure of the pancreas is obtained through a variety of upper abdominal

1. Wensel Treitz, Austrian physician, 1819-1872

incisions: high transverse, L-shape, reverse-L, inverted-T. Wounds of the pancreas resulting from stab or bullet wounds are closed with interrupted sutures with a soft rubber drain placed to the site of repair.

Operation for pan/creatic [all flesh] (pan-krē-AT-ik) duct lith/iasis [stone] (lith-Ī-ah-sis) and calc/ification [lime to make] (kal"si-fi-KĀ-shun) in the pancreas is excision of calcified areas. Sometimes sympath/ectomy [sympathetic nerve] (sim-pah-THEK-tō-mē) and splanchnic/ectomy [visceral nerve] splank-nē-SEK-tō-mē) are done for relief of the pain due to the calcification in the pancreas.

Transduodenal exploration of the pancreatic duct and transection of the sphincter of Oddi are also performed for calcification.

True cysts of the pancreas are blast/omas [germ,cell] (blas-TŌ-mahs). A small cyst (usually a true blastoma) may be e/nucleated [out kernel][1] (i-NŌŌ-klē-āt-ed). Moderate size cysts may also be excised. Large pseudo/cysts [false sac] (SŪ-do-sists) are marsupialized [pouch] (mar-SŪ-pē-al-īz'd).

Cyst-gastro/anastomosis (sist-gas"trō-ah-nas-tō-MŌ-sis) or enteroanastomosis (internal drainage) consists of evacuation of pancreatic cysts and then anastomosing the cysts with the stomach or a loop of the small bowel in the hope that the contents will be continuously evacuated internally.

Small solid tumors of the pancreas (islet cell adenomas) are resected.

Partial pan/creat/ectomy (pan-krē-ah-TEK-tō-mē) (body and tail) is done for lesions of the pancreas. Total pancreatectomy renders the patient dia/ [through] betic [to go] (dī-ah-BET-ik).

Operations by trans/duodenal (trans-dū-ō-DĒ-nal)[2] exposure are performed upon the ampulla of Vater for small neoplasms or impacted calculi [stonelike mass] (KAL-kū-lī).

Chole/cysto/stomy (kō"le-sis-TOS-tō-mē) (surgical incision into the gall bladder with drainage) is indicated as follows:

1. Where the patient is a very poor operative risk.
2. In the presence of severe inflammation.

1. A more complete definition is "to extract from a sac without cutting." Optional pronunciation ē-NŌŌ-klē-āt-ed
2. Optional pronunciation trans-dū-OD-i-nal

3. Patients with severe symptoms due to gall bladder disease but having some other serious complicating disease and not able to withstand a <u>chole/cyst/ectomy</u> (kō"le-sis-TEK-tō-mē).

Cholecystectomy is indicated for

1. cholelithiasis,
2. tumors which are difficult to diagnose,
3. trauma.

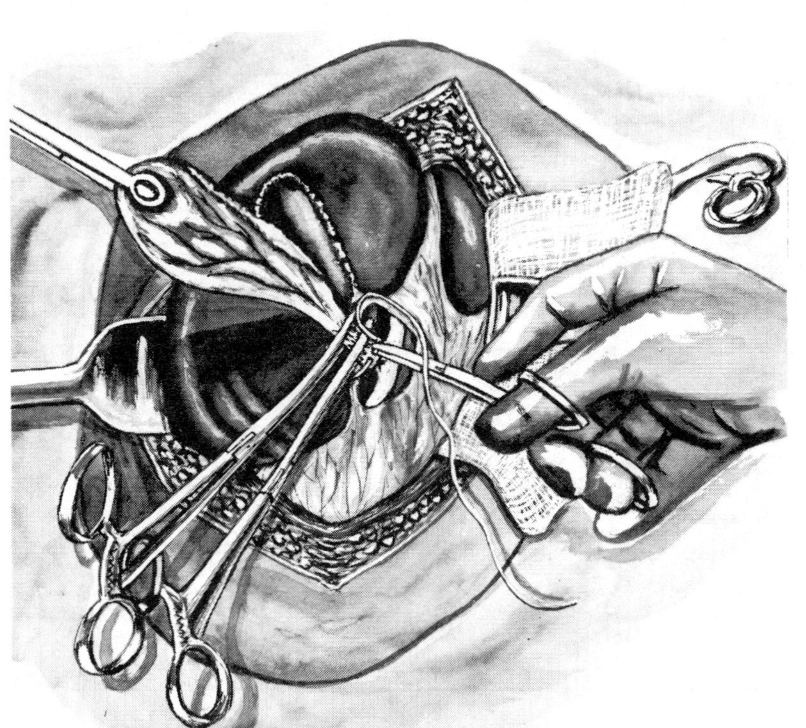

CHOLECYSTECTOMY

This stage of the procedure shows the cystic duct being ligated between clamps. The gall bladder has been dissected by blunt and sharp dissection from the gall bladder bed or fossa. The liver is turned up and to the right. After ligation of the cystic duct is completed the duct will be severed between the ligations and the gall bladder removed.

<u>Chole/docho/tomy</u>[1] (receptacle) (kō"led-ō-KOT-ō-mē) and <u>chole/docho/stomy</u>[2] (kō"led-ō-KOS-tō-mē) (opening of the common bile duct) are indicated:

1. when a stone is palpable in the common duct,
2. dilatation of the duct which indicates obstruction distal to the dilated area,
3. a thickened wall of the common duct which is usually indicative of chronic inflammatory process,
4. the presence of jaundice without pain which usually indicates common duct obstruction from malignancy,
5. miscellaneous indications: suppurative cholangitis, strictures, tumors and obstructions due to lesions in the pancreas.

Transduodenal removal of stones in the common duct is performed when the

1. Optional pronunciation kō"le-dō-KOT-ō-mē
2. Optional pronunciation kō"le-dō-KOS-tō-mē

stone cannot be removed through an opening in the common duct.

Strictures of the common duct are often secondary to operations on the bili/ary [bile] (BIL-ē-ār-ē) system and are produced by trauma. Operative procedures are as follows:

1. resection of stricture with end-to-end anastomosis where possible;
2. anastomosis of the common duct to the duodenum (chole/docho/duodeno/stomy [kō-led"ō-kō-dū-o-den-OS-tō-mē]);
3. anastomosis of the hilar [a small bit or trifle] (HĪ-lar) duct to Roux[1] (ro͞o) Y arm of jejunum;
4. anastomosis of left intra/hepatic [inside] (in"trah-hē-PAT-ik) duct to Roux Y arm of jejunum;
5. chole/cysto/entero/stomy (kō-le-sis"tō-en-ter-OS-tō-mē) (anastomosis between the biliary tract and the intestinal tract);
6. anastomosis of the hilar duct to a loop of the jejunum.

Extra/peri/toneal [outside of] (eks"trah-per-i-tō-NĒ-al) incision and drainage (I & D) is performed for sub/phrenic (sub-FREN-ik) abscess.

Retro/peri/toneal [backward] (re"trō-per-i-tō-NĒ-al) I & D is also performed for subphrenic abscess.

A/spiration[2] [to / to breath] (as"pe-RĀ-shun) of amebic hepatic abscess to evacuate contents.

Transthoracic I & D, extraperitoneal I & D or extra/serous [whey] (eks-trah-SĒ-rus) drainage are performed for pyogenic liver abscess.

Indications and procedures for surgery of the colon:

1. trauma: exteriorization of damaged areas or resection and primary end-to-end anastomosis;
2. intussusception: reduction of the intussusception. If unable to reduce then resection of involved area and anastomosis;
3. volvulus (twisting and looping of the intestine) occurs in the sigmoid colon and cecum: resection of the area of the colon involved with anastomosis and colostomy;

1. César Roux, Swiss surgeon, 1857-1926
2. "to attempt to reach" is another translation for this term.

4. appendicitis: appendectomy;
5. solitary diverticulum of cecum: diverticulectomy;
6. ulcerative colitis: col/ectomy colon (kō-LEK-tō-mē) or ileostomy if the disease involves the whole area of the colon;
7. benign neoplasms:
    a. sub/mucous (sub-MYŌŌ-kus) lip/oma fat (lī-PŌ-mah): excision;
    b. benign polyps: polypectomy if a single polyp;
    c. multiple polyps: radical surgical excision of involved bowel. This sometimes necessitates total colectomy and permanent ileostomy. If polyps are in the rectum and in small numbers they may be fulgurated lightning (FUL-gya-rāt-ed) through a sigmoido/scope sigmoid colon (sig-MOYD-ō-skōp);
8. malignant neoplasms (these are the cause of the majority of operations on the colon): excision of involved area, anastomosis; colo/stomy (kō-LOS-tō-mē) or ceco/stomy cecum (sē-KOS-tō-mē).

Rod colostomy is the permanent type of colostomy. The temporary type, known as transverse colon colostomy, is rarely performed.

The following procedures are used for surgical treatment of malignant lesions of the rectum and lower part of the sigmoid:

1. abdomino/perine/al perineum[1] (ab-dom"i-nō-per-i-NĒ-al) resection of rectum and sigmoid with permanent colostomy;
2. colostomy and lower bowel lesion resections;
3. anterior resection of the upper part of the rectum and lower portion of the sigmoid with preservation of intestinal continuity by colo/recto/stomy rectum (kō"lō-rek-TOS-tō-mē) (anastomosis, usually end-to-end);
4. exteriorization operations with extraperitoneal or intraperitoneal resection;

1. The perineum is the area between the pubis and the anus. It is often called the "floor of the pelvis."

5. modified Mikulicz (MIK-ū-lich) resection;

6. abdominoperineal procto/sigmoid/ectomy [anus,rectum] (prok"tō-sig-moyd-EK-tō-mē) with preservation of the external sphincter (the pull-through or Hochenegg's[1] [HOK-en-egz] operation);

7. posterior proct/ectomy (prok-TEK-tō-mē) and lower excision. Not radical procedure for cancer.

Surgical treatment of abscess and fistula of the ano/rectal [anus rectum] (ā-nō-REK-tal) region includes:

1. incision and drainage for ischio/rectal [ischium] (is"kē-ō-REK-tal) abscess;

2. unroofing of fistula in ano;

3. repair of defect in urethro-vaginal [urethra vagina] (u-rē-thrō-VAJ-i-nal) fistula. Supra/pubic [above pubis] (sū"prah-PYŌŌ-bik) cysto/stomy (sis-TOS-tō-mē) may be performed with repair of fistula;

4. repair of recto/vesical [bladder] (rek-tō-VES-i-kl) fistula.

Other abnormalities of the rectum and anus and the surgical procedures performed to correct them are:

1. prolapse of the rectum: amputation of the rectum or mobilization of the rectum;

2. hemorrhoids, internal, external or combined: excision of (hemo/rrhoid/ectomy [hem-ō-royd-EK-tō-mē]);

INTERNAL
COMBINED
EXTERNAL
BLOOD CLOT
THROMBOSED

HEMORRHOIDS

3. fissure in ano: excision of;

4. pilonid/al [hair+nest] (pī-lo-NĪ-dal) cysts and sinuses: excision of;

5. imperforate anus (infants): sigmoidal (sig-MOYD-al) colostomy and correction of anal defect.

1. Julius von Hochenegg, Vienna surgeon, 1859-1940

Abdominal hernia and repair: operation for hernia has two phases: 1. the treatment (usually the excision) of the sac and 2. the repair of the defect through which the hernia has passed. These may be of varying importance in different types of hernia. Hernio/rrhaphy (her-nē-OR-ah-fē), unilateral or bilateral, is performed for the following:

1. indirect inguinal [groin] (IN-gwin-al) hernia,
2. direct inguinal hernia,
3. combined direct and indirect hernia (also known as "saddlebag" or "pantaloon" hernia),
4. sliding hernia,
5. femoral hernia,
6. umbilical hernia,
7. ventral hernia.

INDEX
CHAPTER VIII

PAGE	LINE	
208	13	suprapubic
204	6	sympathectomy
199	10	thoraco-esophago-gastrostomy
202	4	thrombosis
198	16	tracheo-esophageal
201	17	transabdominal
204	23	transduodenal
200	11	transgastric
199	15	transthoracic
203	23	Treitz
195	8	tuberculosis
195	7	typhoid
195	14	ulcerative
188	23	umbilical
197	2	umbilicus
195	13	uremia
208	12	urethro-vaginal
186	14	uvula
200	16	vagectomy
200	4	vagotomy
195	19	venereum
202	4	venous
190	10	vermiform
190	3	villi
197	10	viscera
197	9	visceroptosis
197	24	volvulus
198	2	Weil's
201	11	Witzel

FEMALE ORGANS OF REPRODUCTION

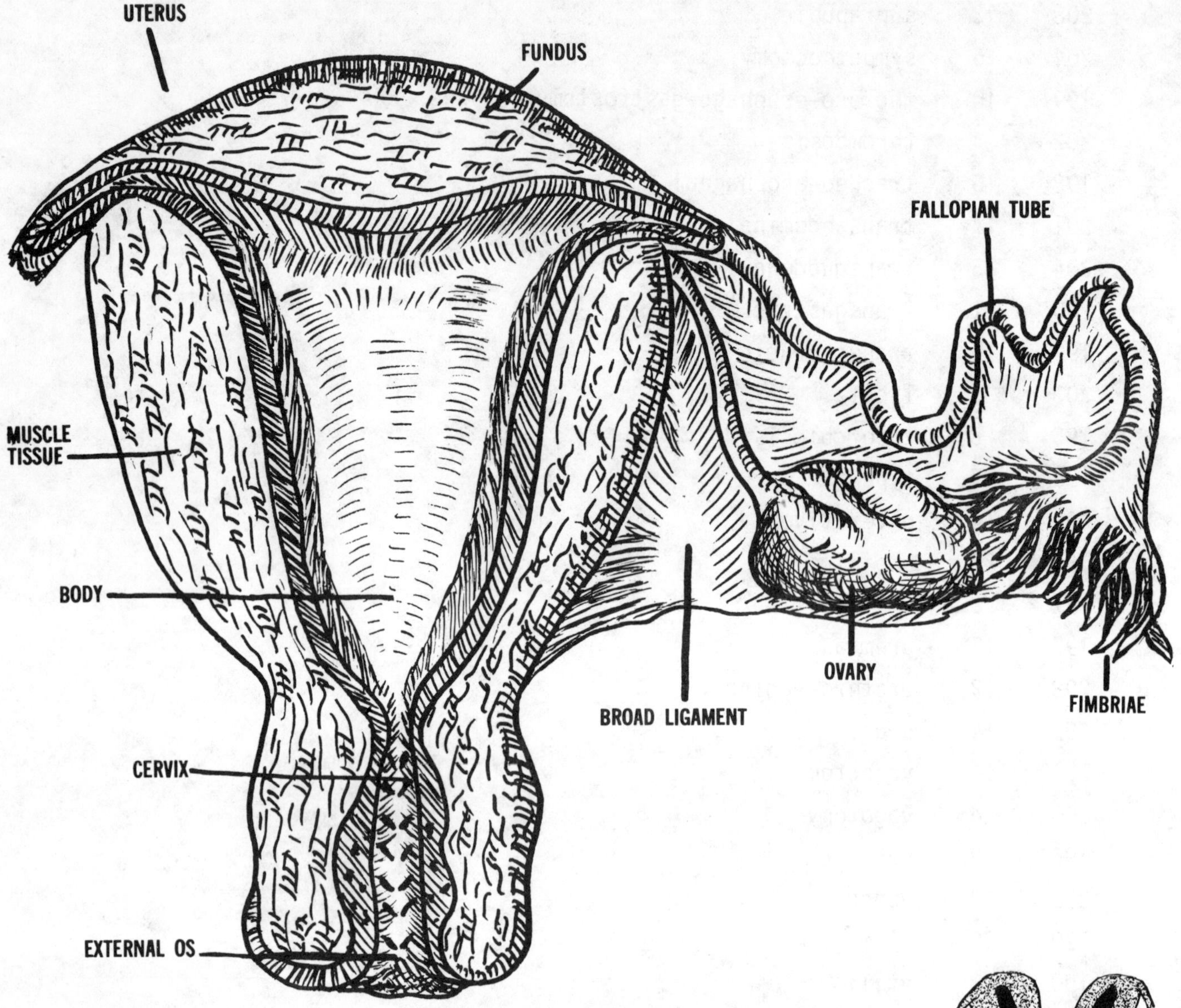

UTERUS
FUNDUS
FALLOPIAN TUBE
MUSCLE TISSUE
BODY
OVARY
FIMBRIAE
BROAD LIGAMENT
CERVIX
EXTERNAL OS

CONGENITAL MALFORMATIONS OF THE UTERUS

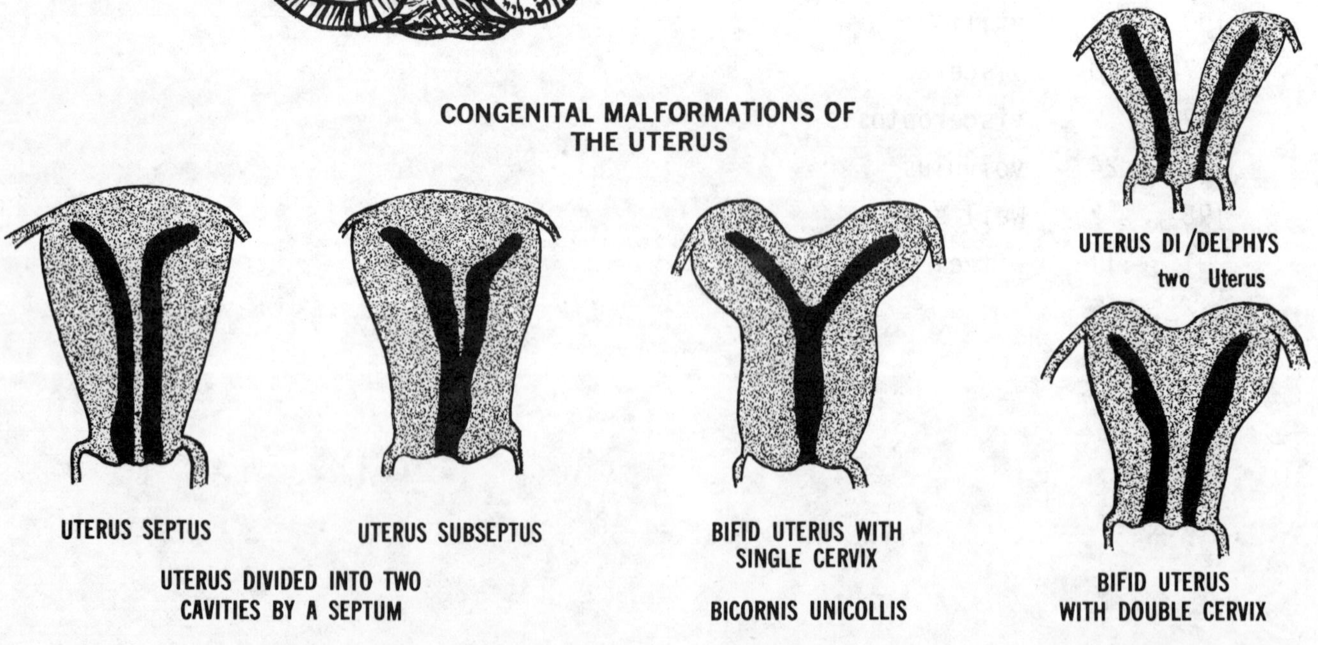

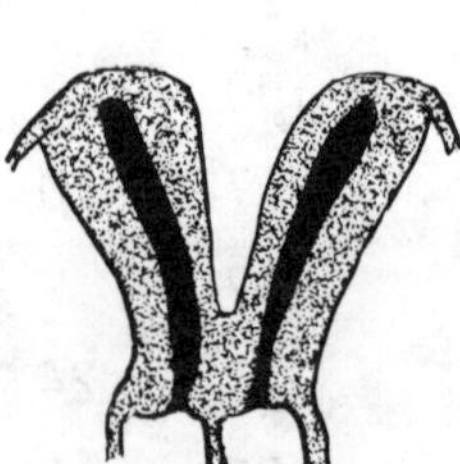

UTERUS DI/DELPHYS
two Uterus

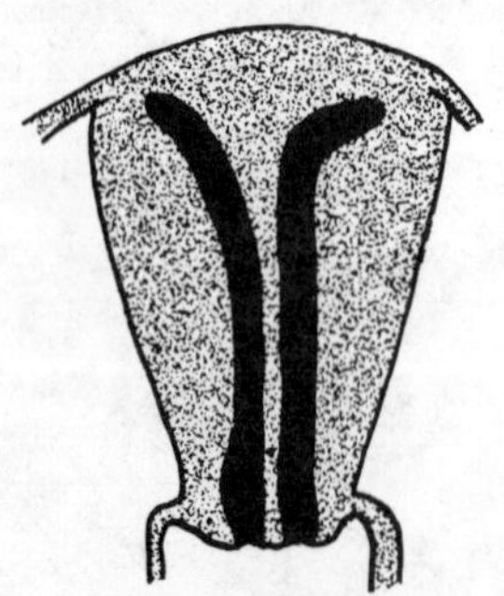

UTERUS SEPTUS

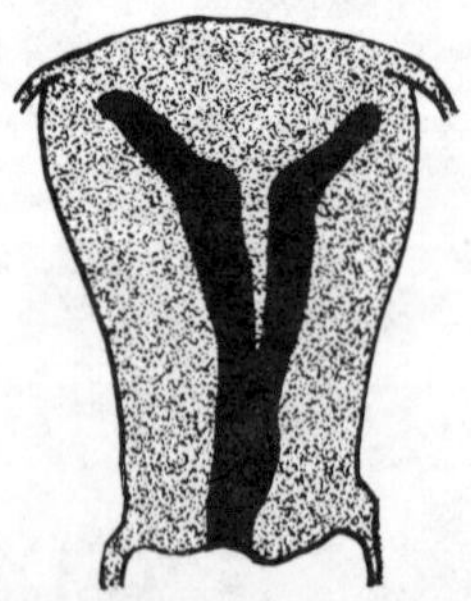

UTERUS SUBSEPTUS

UTERUS DIVIDED INTO TWO CAVITIES BY A SEPTUM

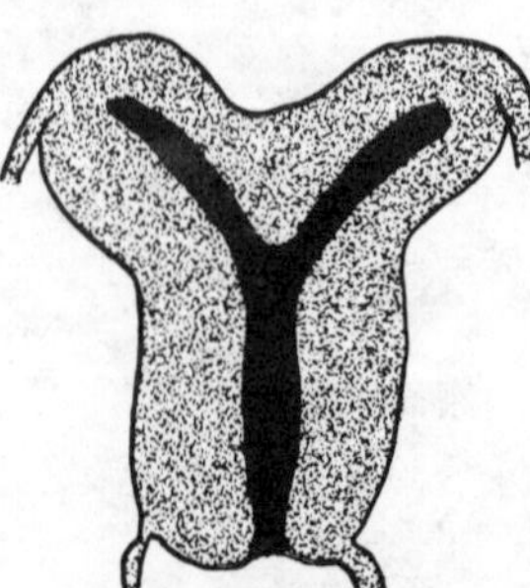

BIFID UTERUS WITH SINGLE CERVIX

BICORNIS UNICOLLIS

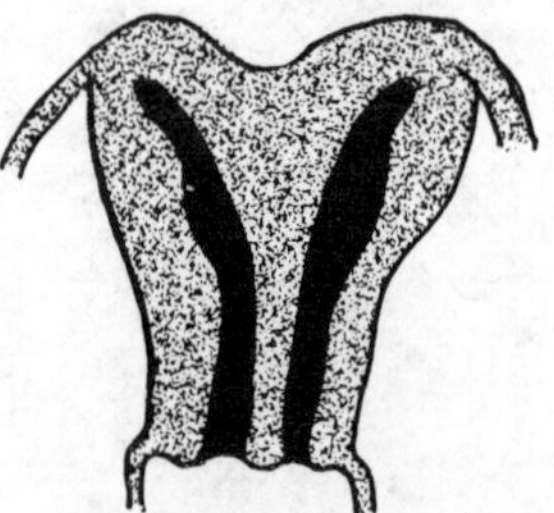

BIFID UTERUS WITH DOUBLE CERVIX

CHAPTER IX
THE GENITO-URINARY SYSTEM

The female reproductive system consists of the two ovaries [egg bearer] (Ō-vah-rēz) which produce the ova [egg] (Ō-vah) and the internal secretions, the two uterine [uterus] (Ū-ter-in)[1] (fallopian[2] [fah-LŌ-pē-an]) tubes, one uterus [womb] (Ū-ter-us), one vagina [hollow] (vah-JĪ-nah), the external genitals [organs of reproduction] (JEN-i-tals), and two breasts.

The ovaries, two almond-shaped, glandular bodies, are attached to the back of the broad ligament behind and below the uterine tubes on each side of the uterus. A short ligament attaches the ovary to the uterus. At the tubal end of the ovary it is attached to the fallopian tube by one of the fringe-like processes of the fimbriated [a fringe] (FIM-brē-āt-ed) extremity of the ovi/duct [egg] (Ō-vi-dukt).

The ovaries produce, develop and mature the ova. They then discharge the ova when they are fully formed. The ovaries also furnish two internal secretions. The Graafian[3] (GRAF-ē-an) (vesicul/ar [bladder] [ve-SIK-ū-lar]) follicles [little bag] (FOL-i-kls) produce one of the internal secretions which is called oestrin [female hormone] (ES-trin). The cells of the corpus [body] (KOR-pus) luteum [yellow] (LŪ-tē-um) produce another secretion known as pro/gestin [in favor gestation] (prō-JES-tin) or pro/gesterone (prō-JES-ter-ōn). The functions of these secretions are given in CHAPTER VI, THE ENDOCRINE SYSTEM.

The uterine tubes, also called fallopian tubes or oviducts, leave the upper angles of the uterus and pass in a somewhat twisted course between the folds and along the upper margin of the broad ligament toward the sides of the pelvis. The oviducts are about four inches long. At their distal end are many fringe-like processes which are called fimbriae (FIM-brē-ē). One of these fimbriae is attached to each ovary. The ova travel from the ovaries to the uterus through the fallopian tubes. When an ovum does not become fertilized it disintegrates and is absorbed in the secretions of the genital tract. Sometimes an im/pregnated [in with child]

1. Optional pronunciation Ū-ter-īn
2. Gabriello Fallopio, Italian anatomist, 1523-1562
3. Reijnier (Regner) de Graaf, Dutch physiologist and histologist, 1641-1673; optional pronunciation GRAH-fē-an

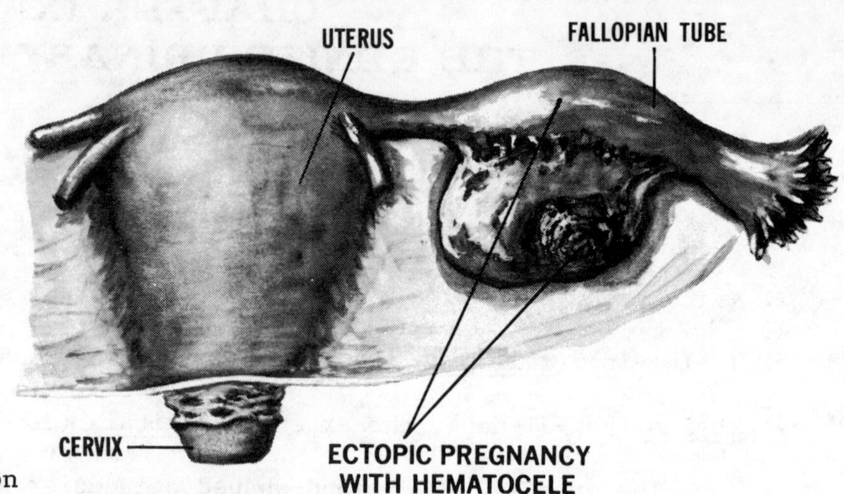

(im-PREG-nā-ted) ovum remains in the tube instead of passing into the uterus. Growth of the impregnated ovum may continue. However, the presence of the impregnated ovum creates an erosive action upon the walls of the tube which usually results in hemorrhage and causes a painful distention of the tube. This condition is known as <u>ec/top/ic</u> [out place] (ek-TOP-ik) <u>pregnancy</u> [with child] (PREG-nen-sē) and usually requires surgical intervention to prevent fatal bleeding.

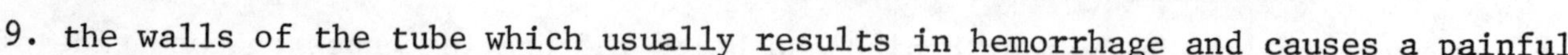

The uterus, a hollow, pear-shaped, muscular organ, is situated in the pelvic cavity between the bladder and the rectum. It is about three inches long, two inches wide at the upper part. It is composed of three parts: the <u>fundus</u> [bottom] (FUN-dus) which is the convex part above the entrance of the oviducts; the body which is the portion between the fundus and the <u>cervix</u> [neck] (SER-viks); and the cervix or neck which is the lower constricted portion extending from the body of the uterus into the vagina. Suspended in the pelvic cavity by ligaments the uterus is not firmly attached or adherent to any part of the skeleton. During <u>gestation</u> [to bear,to carry] (jes-TĀ-shun) it rises into the abdominal cavity. Normally the fundus of the uterus should be inclined forward and the external <u>os</u> [opening] (os) directed downward and backward. When the fundus turns too far forward the condition is known as <u>ante/version</u> [before to turn] (an-te-VER-zhun) and when it inclines backward it is known as <u>retro/version</u> [backward] (ret-rō-VER-zhun). Sometimes a bend may exist where the cervix joins the body. If the body bends forward it is known as <u>ante/flexion</u> [to bend] (an-te-FLEK-shun) and if it bends backward, <u>retro/flexion</u> (ret-rō-FLEK-shun).

Eight ligaments suspend the uterus in the pelvis. Six of these ligaments are arranged in pairs. They are the two broad or lateral ligaments, the anterior ligament, the posterior ligament, the two round ligaments and the two utero-sacral [uterus sacrum] (ū"ter-ō-SĀ-kral) ligaments.

The uterus receives the ovum from the oviducts and, if the ovum is fertilized, retains it during its development. When the ovum has developed into a full-term fetus it is expelled from the uterus aided by the contractions of the uterine walls.

The vagina extends downward and forward from the uterus to the vulva [a covering] (VUL-vah). It is a musculo-membranous canal which is situated in front of the rectum and behind the bladder. The upper portion surrounds the vaginal (VAJ-i-nal) portion of the cervix and forms a deep recess behind the cervix which is called the posterior fornix [arch, vault] (FŌR-niks). The anterior and lateral fornices [(plural)] (FŌR-ni-sēz) are smaller recesses at the front and sides of the cervix.

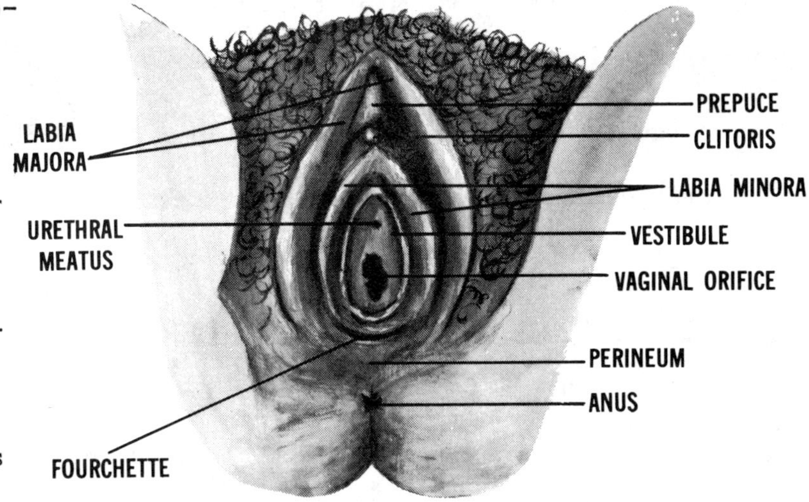

LABIA MAJORA
URETHRAL MEATUS
FOURCHETTE
PREPUCE
CLITORIS
LABIA MINORA
VESTIBULE
VAGINAL ORIFICE
PERINEUM
ANUS

FEMALE GENITALIA

The external genitals are known under the name of vulva or pudendum [to feel ashamed] (pyo͞o-DEN-dum). They include the following: the mons [mountain] pubis [pubic bone] (monz PYO͞O-bis), the labia [lips] (LĀ-bē-ah) majora (mah-JŌ-rah), the labia minora (mi-NŌ-rah), the clitoris (KLIT-or-is),[1] the vestibule [an entrance-court] (VES-ti-būl) of the vagina and the greater vestibular (ves-TIB-ū-lar) glands.

The perineum (per-i-NĒ-um) is the area of the external surface of the floor of the pelvis from the pubic arch to the anus with the underlying muscles and fascia. The vagina perforates the perineum in the female. The perineal

1. Optional pronunciation KLĪ-tor-is. An organ in the female similar to the penis in the male.

(per-i-NĒ-al) body is a wedge-shaped upward extension of the perineum which forms a septum between the vagina and the rectum. Because the perineum is distensible it stretches to a remarkable extent during labor.

The two mamm/ary [breast] (MAM-er-ē) glands or breasts are convex in shape. Near the center of the convexity a papilla [nipple] (pah-PIL-ah) projects called the nipple. The nipple contains the openings of the milk ducts and is surrounded by a small circular area of pink or dark colored skin called the areola [small space] (ah-RĒ-ō-lah). The breasts secrete the milk to nourish the new-born babies.

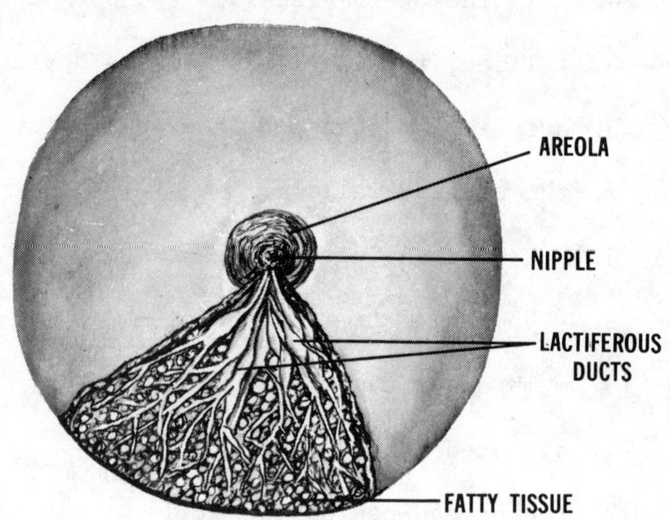

THE BREAST

In the male the urethra[1] (ū-RĒ-thrah) is about eight inches long and passes through the pro/state [before to stand] (PROS-tāt) gland and then through the penis (PĒ-nis). The opening of the urethra is known as the urin/ary [urine] (Ū-ri-nār-ē) meatus [passage] (mē-Ā-tus). In the male the urethra is the terminal portion of both the urinary and reproductive systems.

The testes (TES-tēz) are two glandular organs suspended in the scrotum [bag] (SKRŌ-tum) by the spermat/ic [seed] (sper-MAT-ik) cords. The testes have several coverings: skin, dartos [flayed] (DAR-tōs) tunic [coat] (TŪ-nik) (scrotal [SKRŌ-tal] layers), inter/crur/al [between leg] (in-ter-KRŪ-ral) fascia [band] (FASH-ē-ah), cremaster [to suspend] (krē-MAS-ter), infundibuli/form [funnel] (in-fun-DIB-ū-li-form), tunica [coat] (TŪ-nik-ah) vaginalis (vaj-i-NAL-is). The excretory ducts of the testes are 1. the epi/didymis [on twin] (ep-i-DID-i-mis) which is a tubal structure and lies along the top and side of each testis; 2. the vas [vessel] deferens [to carry down] (vas DEF-er-enz) or seminal [seed] (SEM-i-nal) duct which is a tube leading from the epididymis and passes through the inguinal [groin] (IN-gwin-al)

1. A canal leading from the bladder discharging the urine externally.

The Male Pelvic Organs

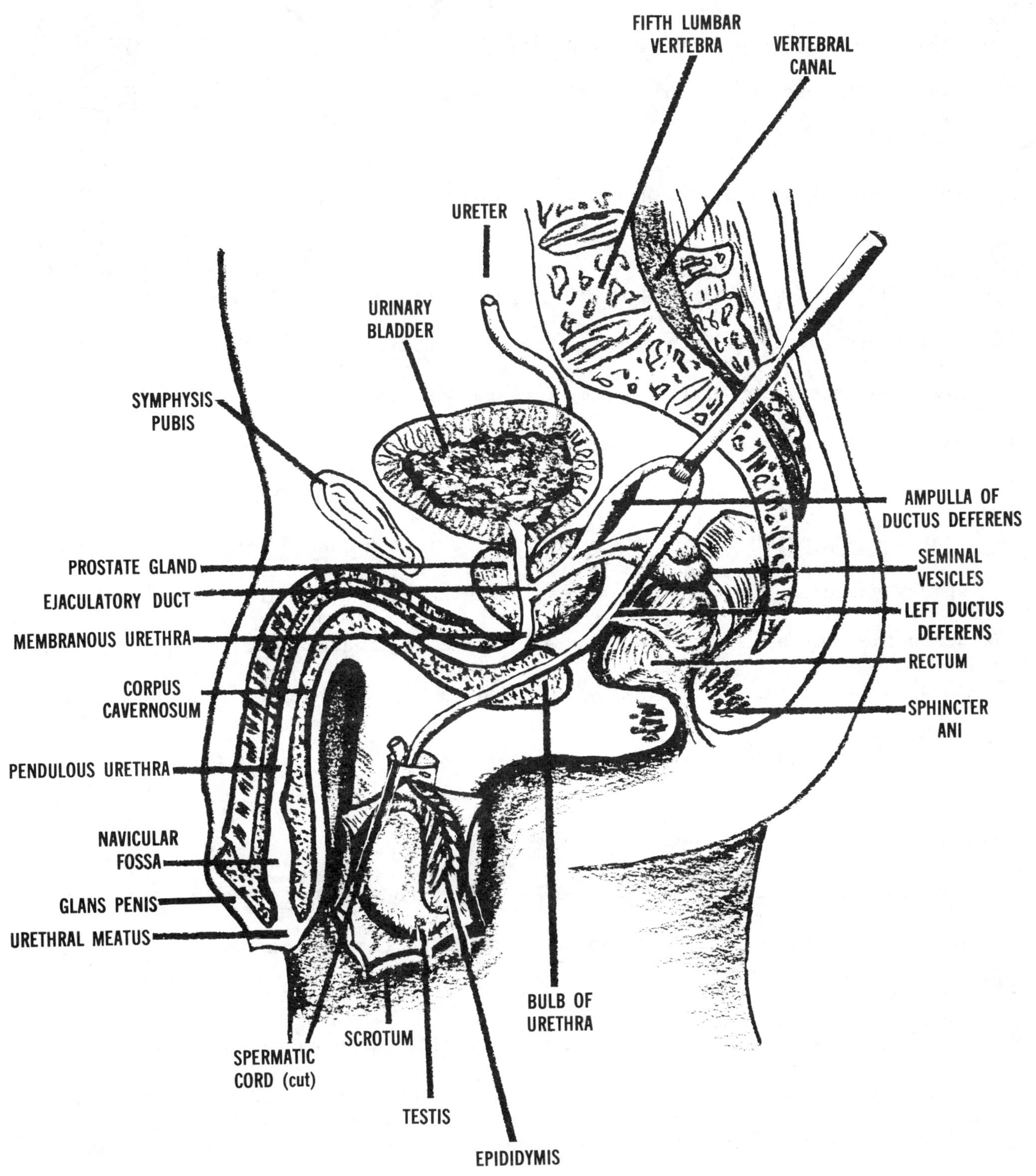

canal into the abdominal cavity. It extends over the posterior surface of the bladder where it is known as the ductus (DUK-tus) deferens and joins with the seminal vesicles [a little bladder] (VES-i-kls) to enter the prostate, emptying into the urethra through the ejaculatory [to throw out] (ē-JAK-ū-lah-tō-rē) ducts; 3. the ejaculatory ducts which are two small tubes passing through the prostate gland to end in the urethra.

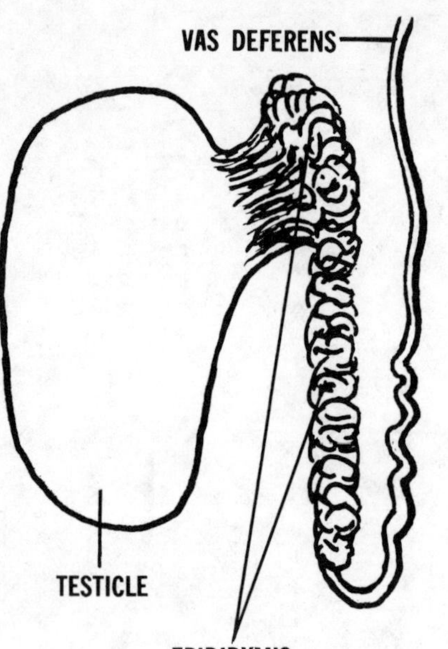

The scrotum is divided into two pouchlike sacs by a septum, each sac containing a testis, epididymis, and lower part of the spermatic cord. It consists of two layers, the in/tegument [in / to cover] (in-TEG-ū-ment) and the dartos tunic.

The penis is suspended from the front and sides of the pubic arch and contains a greater part of the urethra. It is composed of thick fibrous or spongy vascular tissue and is covered with skin. At the distal end of the penis there is a slight thickening of tissue, called the glans [Latin for gland] (glanz) penis. Also at the distal end the skin is folded doubly and is called the pre/puce [before / penis] (PRĒ-pūs) or foreskin [prepuce] (FŌR-skin).

The prostate is a muscular gland through which the urethra courses. Its base lies against the urinary bladder above.

The bulbo/urethral [bulb / urethra] (bul-bō-ū-RĒ-thral) glands (Cowper's[1] [KOW-perz] glands) are small glands situated behind and lateral to the membranous portion of the urethra.

The urinary organs comprise a pair of kidneys which secrete the urine, a pair of ureters [urinary canal] (ŪR-i-ters)[2] or ducts which convey the urine from the kidney to the urinary bladder where it is retained for a time, and a urethra through which the urine is discharged from the body.

The kidneys are situated in the posterior part of the abdomen, on either

1. William Cowper, English surgeon and anatomist, 1666-1709
2. Optional pronunciation ū-RĒ-ters

THE URINARY SYSTEM

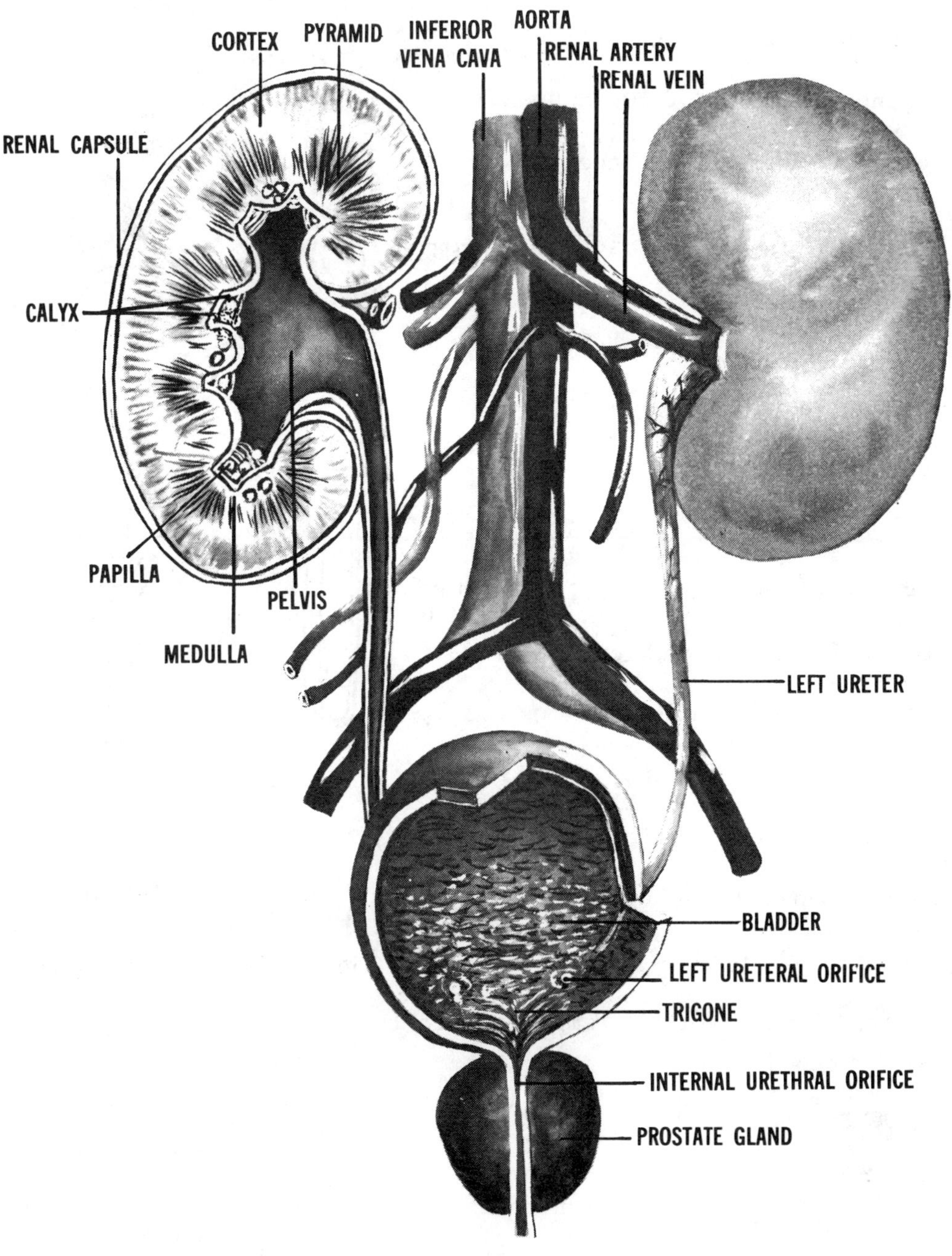
CORTEX
PYRAMID
INFERIOR VENA CAVA
AORTA
RENAL ARTERY
RENAL VEIN
RENAL CAPSULE
CALYX
PAPILLA
PELVIS
MEDULLA
LEFT URETER
BLADDER
LEFT URETERAL ORIFICE
TRIGONE
INTERNAL URETHRAL ORIFICE
PROSTATE GLAND

side of the vertebral column, behind the parietal [wall] (pah-RĪ-i-tal) peri/toneum [around / to stretch] (per-i-tō-NĒ-um), and surrounded by a mass of fat and loose areolar (ah-RĒ-ō-lar) tissue. The external surface of each kidney presents a concave notch called the hilum [a depression] (HĪ-lum). Structures enter the kidney through the hilum. Each kidney is encased in a covering called the tunica fibrosa [fiber] (fī-BRŌ-sah).

The internal structure of each kidney consists of two substances: the outer layer, the cortex, which contains the glomeruli [small ball] (glō-MER-ū-lī) and the functioning tubules [small tubes] (TŪ-būls) and an inner portion, the medulla [middle] (me-DUL-ah) which is arranged in conical masses called renal [kidney] (RĒ-nal) pyramids and which contains the collecting tubules which empty into the minor calices[1] [cup of flower] (KĀ-li-sēz) which, in turn, empty into the major calices. These empty into the pelvis of the kidney which narrows to form the ureter which is about 10 inches long and empties into the bladder.

AFFERENT BLOOD VESSEL
EFFERENT BLOOD VESSEL
PROXIMAL CONVOLUTED TUBE
GLOMERULUS
DISTAL CONVOLUTED TUBE
HENLE'S LOOP
COLLECTING TUBULE

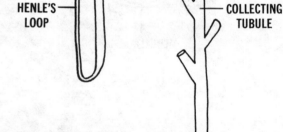

RENAL UNIT (NEPHRON)
OF THE CORTEX OF THE KIDNEY

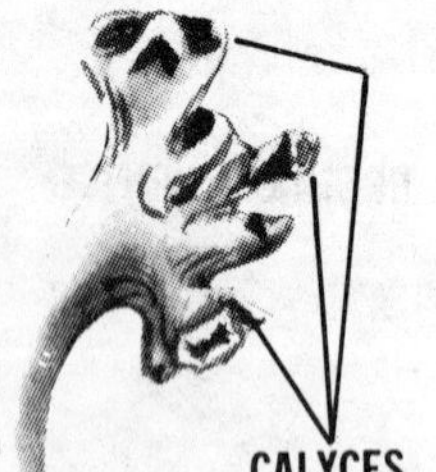

NORMAL LEFT RENAL
PELVIS AND URETER

The urinary bladder is a musculomembranous sac lying in the midline in front of the parietal peritoneum and behind the sym/physis [together / to grow] (SIM-fi-sis) pubis. In the male it lies in front of the rectum above the prostate gland and in the female it lies in front of the uterus and vagina. The fundus of the

1. The older spelling is "calyces." It is still used and will be found as an optional spelling in this text.

bladder is triangular in shape with ureteral (ū-RĒ-ter-al) orifices behind each corner of the base and the urethral (ū-RĒ-thral) orifice at the apex in front. This triangular area is known as the trigone *(triangle)* (TRĪ-gōn).

In the female, the urethra is a tube about one and one-half inches long passing down behind the symphysis, through the peritoneal fascia and opening in front of the vagina, behind the labia minora and clitoris. It is surrounded by a sphincter *(binder)* (SFINK-tur) muscle as it enters the perineum.

DISEASES AND ANOMALIES

Abnormal conditions resulting from glandular disturbances in both the male and female have been discussed in CHAPTER VI on the ENDOCRINE SYSTEM. Many other diseases and conditions are listed in the section which follows on Surgery. There are, however, certain infectious diseases and tumors of the female reproductive system which are included in this section because of the frequent occurrence of some of these conditions.

Infectious diseases of the female genital tract include:

1. tricho/monas *(hair / unit)* (trik-ō-MŌ-nas)[1] vaginalis also called tricho-mon/iasis (trik-ō-mō-NĪ-ah-sis)
2. monilia *(necklace (a fungus))* (mō-NIL-ē-ah) albicans *(to make white)* (AL-bi-kanz)
3. gono/rrhea *(seed)* (gon-ō-RĒ-ah)
4. syphilis

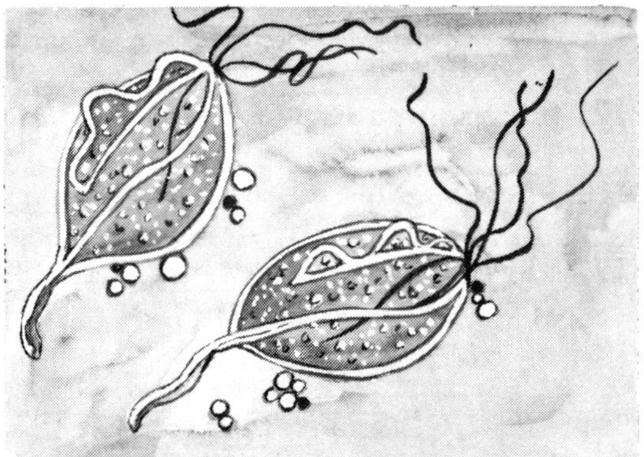

TRICHOMONAS VAGINALIS

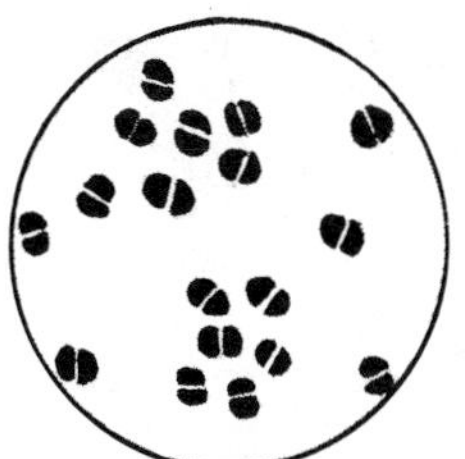

DIPLOCOCCI OF GONORRHEA

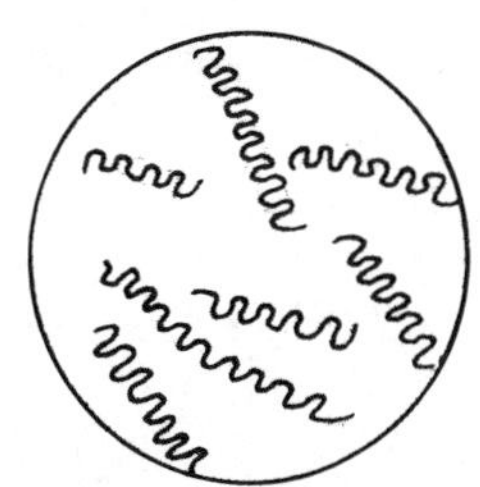

TRIPONEMA PALLIDUM OF SYPHILIS (SPIROCHETES)

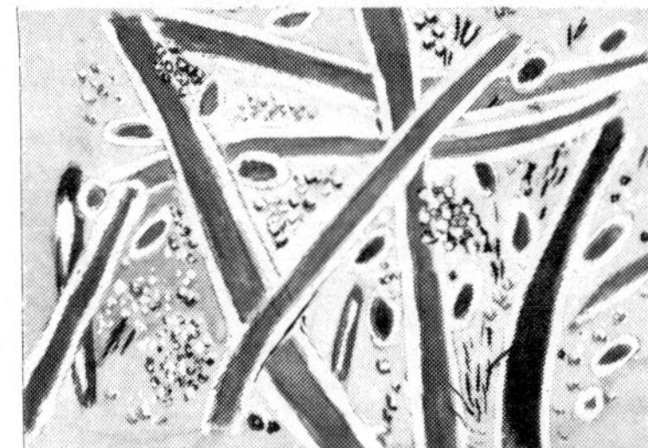

MONILIA ALBICANS

1. Optional pronunciation tri-KOM-ō-nas

5. chancr/oid [cancer] (SHANG-kroyd)
6. lympho/granul/oma [water, grain] (lim"fō-gran-ū-LŌ-mah) venereum [pertaining to Venus, goddess of love] (ve-NĒ-rē-um)
7. granul/oma (gran-ū-LŌ-mah) inguinale [groin] (in-gwin-AL-ē)
8. dia/betic [through, to go] (dī-ah-BET-ik) vulv/itis [vulva] (vul-VĪ-tis)
9. urethr/itis [urethra] (ū-re-THRĪ-tis)
10. skene/itis[1] (skēn-Ī-tis)
11. bartholin/itis[2] (bar-tō-lin-Ī-tis)
12. Bartholin's[2] (BAR-to-linz) abscess

Skin disorders of the vulva include:

1. follicul/itis [follicle] (fō-lik-ū-LĪ-tis)
2. furuncul/osis[3] [furuncle] (fu"rung-kyo͞o-LŌ-sis)
3. herpes [to creep, shingles] (HUR-pēz) genitalis (jen-i-TAL-is)
4. inter/trigo [between, to rub] (in-tur-TRĒ-gō)
5. tinea [moth] (TIN-ē-ah) cruris [leg] (KRO͞O-ris)
6. psor/iasis [itch] (sō-RĪ-ah-sis)

Benign tumors of the vulva include fibroma, fibro/my/oma [fiber, muscle] (fī-brō-mī-Ō-mah), lipoma, papill/oma [nipple] (pap-i-LŌ-mah), condyl/oma [wart] (kon-di-LŌ-mah) acuminatum [to sharpen] (ah-kyo͞o-mi-NĀ-tum), urethral caruncle [small fleshy mass] (KAR-ung-kl), hydr/aden/oma [water, gland] (hī-drad-i-NŌ-mah), angioma, myx/oma [mucus] (mik-SŌ-mah), neuroma, and endo/metrial [within, uterus] (en-dō-MĒ-trē-al) growths.

Malignant tumors of the vulva include carcinoma (primary and, occasionally, secondary) and, infrequently, sarcoma.

Ovarian neoplasms may occur at any age. The majority occur during the reproductive years.

Non-neoplastic cysts of the ovary include

1. follicle cysts
2. hydrops [dropsy] (HĪ-drops) folliculi[4] [follicles] (fo-LIK-u-li)
3. corpus luteum cyst

1. J. C. Skene, Brooklyn gynecologist, This term may also be spelled "skenitis."
2. Casper Bartholin, Jr., Danish anatomist, 1655-1738
3. From the Latin "furunculus" meaning "a petty thief."
4. An unusually large follicle cyst

The most common ovarian neoplasms are cyst/aden/omas *sac* (sis-tad-i-NŌ-mahs). They are of two types: 1. serous and 2. pseudo/ *false* mucinous *mucus* (sū-dō-MYŌŌ-sin-us)

FOLLICLE CYST (BENIGN)

SEROUS CYSTADENOMA MULTILOCULAR (MALIGNANT)

OVARIAN NEOPLASMS

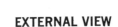

Serous cysts include serous cyst/oma (sis-TŌ-mah) (a simple serous cyst), serous cystadenoma, papillary serous cystadenoma, fibr/omat/ous *tumor* (fī-BRŌ-mah-tus) papillomas, serous adeno/fibr/oma (ad-i-nō-fī-BRŌ-mah), serous cyst/adeno/fibr/oma (sist"ad-i-nō-fī-BRŌ-mah).

Pseudomucinous cysts include pseudomucinous cystadenoma, pseudo/myx/oma (sū"dō-mik-SŌ-mah) peritonei *peritoneum* (per-i-tō-NĒ-ī).

Endometrial cysts (chocolate cysts, endo/metri/osis [en-dō-mē-trē-Ō-sis]) arise from misplaced endometrial implants on the surface of the ovary.

A terat/oma *monster* (ter-ah-TŌ-mah) is composed of body tissues not normal to the part. In the ovary two varieties are found: a benign cystic derm/oid *skin* (DER-moyd) (contents of this type of cyst may be hair, bone, teeth or sebaceous *oily* [se-BĀ-shus] matter), and a malignant, solid teratoma.

Granulosa[1] (gran-ū-LŌ-sah) cell tumors are known as "feminizing" neoplasms and in children may cause the syndrome of precocious puberty.

Theca *case,sheath* (THĒ-kah) cell tumors are benign, unilateral, solid, estro/gen *mad desire to beget* (ES-trō-jen) producing neoplasms. The majority occur during the meno/pausal *month to cease* (MEN-ō-paw-zal) and postmenopausal years.

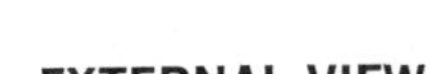

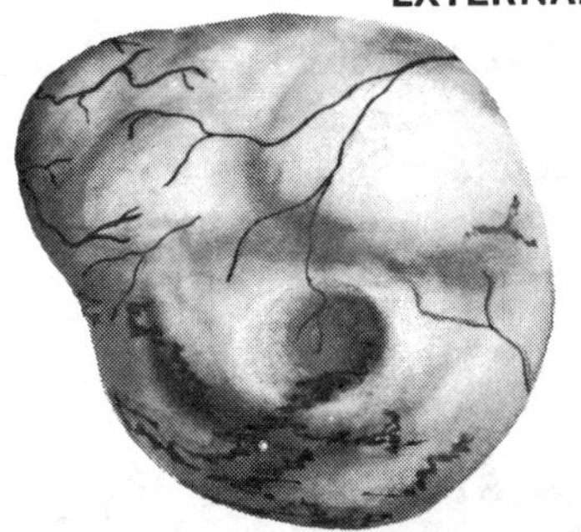

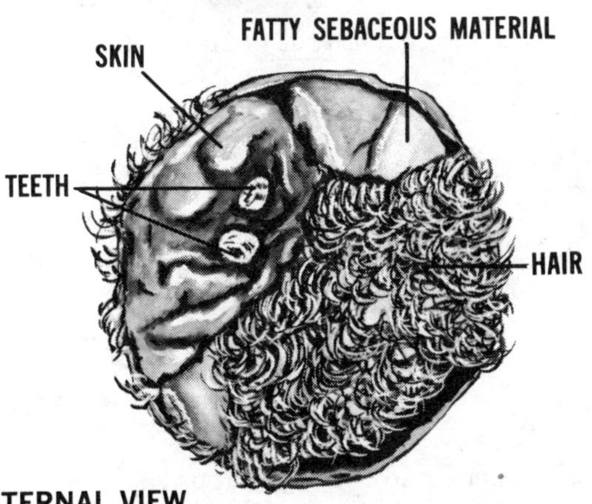

INTERNAL VIEW

BENIGN DERMOID CYST

1. membrana granulosa -- the layer of small cells which form the wall of the Graafian follicle.

Masculinizing tumors of the ovary are divided into three categories: the arrheno/blast/oma *male germ* (ah-rē-nō-blas-TŌ-mah), the adrenal rest tumor, the Leydig[1] (LĪ-dig) cell tumor. These tumors cause defeminization manifested by a/meno/rrhea *without* (ā-men-ō-RĒ-ah),[2] sterility, loss in feminine contour, decrease in the size of the breasts, genital hypo/plasia *below* (hī-pō-PLĀ-zē-ah), and coarse skin texture. Masculinization is evident in hirsut/ism *shaggy,hairy* (HUR-sūt-izm), male escutcheon *a shield* (es-KUCH-an)[3], enlargement of the clitoris, increased muscular development, acne, and hoarseness of the voice.

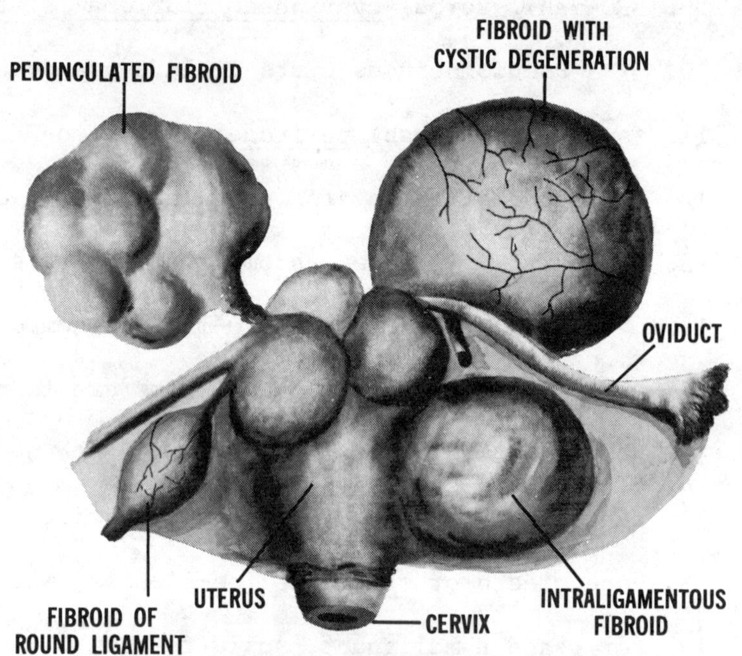

UTERINE FIBROIDS

My/omas (mī-Ō-mahs) (also known as fibroids, fibromyomas or leio/my/omas *smooth* [lī-ō-mī-Ō-mahs]) are benign tumors of the uterus. They are made up of a mixture of smooth muscle and fibrous tissues and are classified according to their relationship to the uterine wall:

1. inter/stitial *between to set* (in-ter-STISH-al) or intra/mural *inside wall* (in-trah-MYŌŌ-ral)
2. subserous
3. submucous

Polyps are growths which arise from the mucosa of the corpus or cervix and may be single or multiple.

Chorion/epitheli/oma[4] *skin epithelium* (kō"rē-on-ep-i-thē-lē-Ō-mah) is a highly malignant tumor of the uterus. One of its main characteristics is its rapid metastasis

1. Franz von Leydig, German anatomist, 1821-1908
2. Optional pronunciation ah-men-ō-RĒ-ah
3. Optional pronunciation i-SKUCH-an; the pattern of distribution of the pubic hair.
4. Also spelled "chorio-epithelioma;" "chorion" means "the membrane enclosing the fetus."

to other areas of the body (the lungs, liver, urinary tract, broad ligaments, tubes and ovaries).

Carcinoma of the cervix of the uterus is more frequent than carcinoma of the corpus. When it does occur in the corpus it is usually an adeno/carcin/oma [cancer] (ad"i-nō-kar-si-NŌ-mah).

Causes of disease of the urinary system: the kidneys may be the seat of inflammation due to infection; organisms may enter them by way of the blood stream, or ascend to them from the bladder by way of the ureters. They are frequently invaded by malignant and benign tumors and may be subjected to trauma and to the deleterious [to injure] (del-i-tē-rē-us) action of chemical agents. The kidneys may also be affected by various congenital anomalies. These include "horseshoe" kidney, bifid renal pelvis (also called reduplication of the renal pelvis) and reduplication of one or both kidneys and/or ureters.

Urinary diseases fall within the scope of the specialist in urology. Among these are all diseases of the urethra, bladder and ureters; stones in the urinary tract, tumors, trauma and infections characterized by pus formation.

In the male the reproductive organs are closely related with the urinary system. Therefore, the various diseases and conditions affecting the male reproductive organs are also treated by the urologist. As many of these fall into the realm of surgery they are included in that section of this chapter.

There are four principal groups of manifestations which appear in cases of Bright's[1] disease. These are 1. the presence of abnormal constituents in the urine; 2. im-

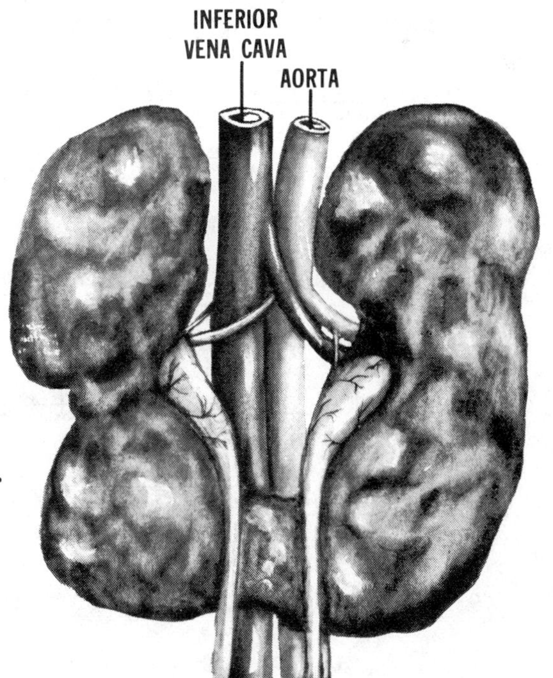

HORSESHOE KIDNEY

1. Richard Bright, English physician, 1789-1858

pairment of the function of the kidneys; 3. hyper/tension [above / to stretch] (hī-per-TEN-shun); and 4. edema [swelling] (ē-DĒ-mah). Nephritic [kidney] (ne-FRIT-ik) edema is due to retention of water and salt in the body because of diminution [to decrease] (dim-i-NŪ-shun) in the output of urine. Nephrotic (ne-FROT-ik) edema is due to diminution of the plasma [shape,form] (PLAZ-mah) proteins. There are three varieties of Bright's disease: the inflammatory type called nephritis (ne-FRĪ-tis); the degenerative type called nephr/osis (ne-FRŌ-sis); and the type secondary to vascular disease called nephro/scler/osis [hard] (nef"rō-skle-RŌ-sis).

Glomerulo/nephr/itis [small ball] (glom-er-ū-lō-ne-FRĪ-tis): this type of Bright's disease is often called diffuse glomerulonephritis, to distinguish it from types of inflammatory disease involving only certain portions of the kidney, and from inflammation accompanied by pus formation.

The term nephrosis refers to the presence of degenerative changes in the kidneys without the occurrence of inflammation. Several varieties of nephrosis are recognized: larval [a mask] (LAR-val) or febrile [fever] (FEB-ril) nephrosis; necrotizing [death] (NEK-ro-tiz-ing) nephrosis (this term applies to extensive death of kidney tubules); amyl/oid [starch] (AM-i-loyd) nephrosis; de/hydration [from / water] (dē-hī-DRĀ-shun) nephrosis; lip/oid [fat] (LĪ-poyd) or true nephrosis.

Nephrosclerosis refers to changes in the kidneys which are due to sclerosis of their vessels.

Floating kidney and nephro/ptosis (nef-rop-TŌ-sis) usually occur in persons who have ptosis (TŌ-sis) of the other abdominal organs as well.

Kidneys may become infected by any of the pus-producing germs: colon bacilli, staphylo/cocci [bunch of grapes] (staf"i-lō-KOK-sī), strepto/cocci [to twist] (strep-tō-KOK-sī), tubercle bacilli, etc.; these organisms may ascend to the kidneys by way of the ureters, or reach them through the blood stream.

Stone in the kidney is known as nephro/lith/iasis [stone] (nef"rō-li-THĪ-ah-sis). Stones damage the kidneys by causing stasis of urine and thus inviting infection or by blocking the passages through which the urine flows and causing hydro/ *water* nephr/osis (hī"drō-ne-FRŌ-sis). Stones usually form in the calices and are often expelled into the ureter; when such an event occurs, the patient experiences renal colic.

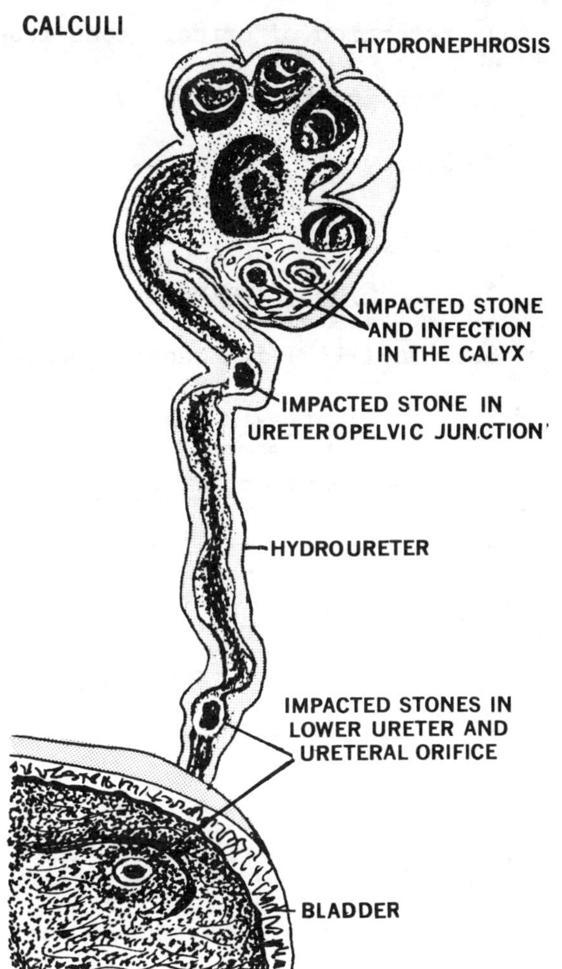

The term hydronephrosis refers to dilatation of the pelvis of the kidney with atrophy (AT-rō-fē) of kidney tissue from pressure, resulting from obstruction in the urinary tract.

Malignant tumors of the kidney occur more frequently than benign ones, and primary tumors more frequently than metastatic ones. The commonest primary tumor of the kidney is the hyper/nephr/oma (hī"per-nē-FRŌ-mah).

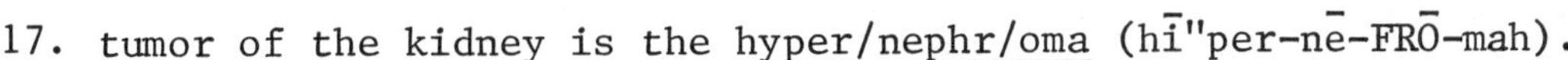

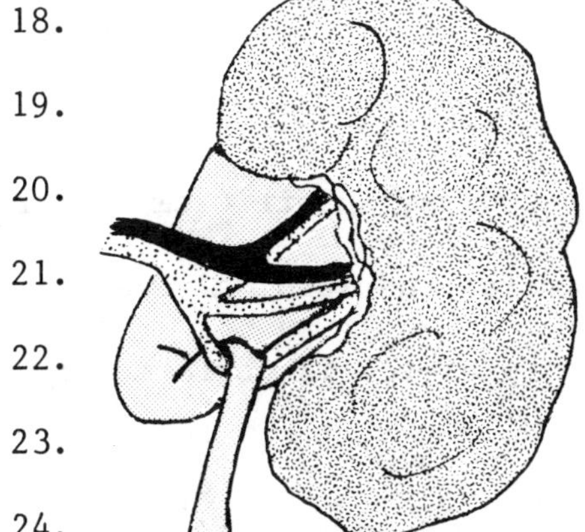

HYDRONEPHROSIS AND URETERAL KINK CAUSED BY ABERRANT BLOOD VESSEL

The kidneys may be involved by two types of cystic disease. One is the solitary cyst, which is due, presumably, to blockage of the collecting tubes in a portion of the kidney; urine collects and forms a tumor of variable size. The other type, called congenital poly/cyst/ic *many* (pol-i-SIS-tik) kidneys, is a disease in which multiple cysts gradually destroy the tissue of both kidneys.

PELVIS OF KIDNEY

CONGENITAL BILATERAL POLYCYSTIC DISEASE

Ur/emia *urine* (ū-RĒ-mē-ah) is the symptom complex due to the retention of urinary constituents within the body. It may occur in any condition in which there is widespread destruction of the functioning tissue of both kidneys.

SURGERY

Gyneco/logical [woman,wife] (gī"ne-kō-LOJ-i-kl)[1] surgery of the external genitalia (jen-i-TĀ-lē-ah) includes: *(Diagnosis is listed first, then the surgical procedure.)*

1. atresia [without opening] (ah-TRĒ-zē-ah) of the hymen [membrane] (HĪ-men): hymeno/tomy (hī-men-OT-ō-mē) or hymen/ectomy (hī-men-EK-tō-mē)
2. congenital hyper/trophy (hī-PER-trō-fē) of clitoris: partial clitorid [clitoris]/ectomy (kli"tō-rid-EK-tō-mē) (amputation of clitoris), female circumcision (removal of foreskin)
3. abscess of Bartholin's gland: I & D
4. chronic bartholinitis and cysts of Bartholin's gland: excision of Bartholin's gland, marsupialization [pouch] (mar-sū"pē-al-i-ZĀ-shun) of Bartholin's cyst or abscess
5. kraurosis [dry] (kraw-RŌ-sis) vulvae (VUL-vē) and leuko/plakia [white plate] (lū-kō-PLĀ-kē-ah): vulv/ectomy (vul-VEK-tō-mē)
6. vulvar carcinoma, epi/derm/oid [skin] (ep-i-DER-moyd) type: Basset operation (vulvectomy and lymph/aden/ectomy [lim"fad-i-NEK-tō-mē]). This is a radical procedure consisting of excision of vulva, superficial inguinal lymph nodes and wide dissection of deep femoral and inguinal glands.
7. episio/perineo/plasty [vulva perineum] (ē-piz"ē-ō-per-i-NĒ-ō-plas-tē) is performed for injury to vulva and perineum
8. episio/tomy (ē-piz-ē-OT-ō-mē), mediolateral, is performed for tense perineum in second stage labor, and perineo/rrhaphy (per"i-nē-OR-ah-fē) is done for obstetrical [midwife][2] (ob-STET-re-kal) laceration of the perineum
9. colpo/rrhaphy [vagina] (kōl-PŌR-ah-fē) (repair of the vagina) is performed for relaxation of vaginal musculature [muscle] (MUS-kyōō-le-chur)

1. Optional pronunciation jin"i-kō-LOJ-i-kl
2. Actually translates as "to stand before" which denotes the position formerly taken by the midwife.

Obstetrical conditions amenable to surgery include conditions resulting from pregnancy and some of the conditions which occur during parturition [delivery] (par-tu-RISH-un) (childbirth).

1. dilatation and curettage [a scraping] (ky o͞o -re-TAHZH) (D & C) is performed for early incomplete abortion (AB);
2. suction curettage is the removal of products of conception utilizing a plastic curette to which suction is applied;
3. cesarean[1] [to cut] (si-ZAR-ē-an) section is indicated for many reasons including dys/tocia [difficult] (dis-TŌ-sē-ah), cervical stenosis, carcinoma of the cervix in pregnancy, inlet contraction of pelvis, total placenta [flat cake] (plah-SEN-tah) previa[2] [leading the way] (PRĒ-vē-ah) and intra/partum [within childbirth] (in"trah-PAR-tum) hemorrhage;
4. unilateral salping/ectomy (sal-pin-JEK-tō-mē) is performed for ruptured ectopic pregnancy;
5. salpingo/stomy [oviducts] (sal-pin-JOS-tō-mē) is performed for removal of ectopic pregnancy and repair of the fallopian tube;
6. for obstetrical laceration of the cervix trachelo/rrhaphy [neck] (trā-ke-LOR-ah-fē) is done.

The part of the body of the fetus which is in advance at birth is called a presentation. Some of the more common fetal presentations, which may occur as either right or left, include:

1. sacro/anterior [sacrum / in front] (sā"krō-an-TĒ-rē-or) breech
2. sacro/posterior [in back] (sā"krō-pos-TĒ-rē-or) breech
3. mento/anterior [chin] (men"tō-an-TĒ-rē-or) face
4. mento/posterior (men"tō-pos-TĒ-rē-or) face
5. occipito/anterior [back of head] (ok-sip"i-tō-an-TĒ-rē-or) vertex [crown of head] (VUR-teks)
6. occipito/posterior (ok-sip"i-tō-pos-TĒ-rē-or) vertex
7. transverse (shoulder) or scapulo/anterior [scapula] (skap"ū-lō-an-TĒ-rē-or)
8. transverse (shoulder) or scapulo/posterior (skap"ū-lō-pos-TĒ-rē-or)

1. This is the surgery reported to have been performed at the birth of Julius Caesar. The Latin words are "sectio cesarea" coming from "caesus" which is the past participle of "caedere" meaning "to cut."

2. The condition in which the placenta is implanted in the lower segment of the uterus, extending to the margin of the internal os of the cervix or partially or completely obstructing the os. Various types (depending on the coverage) are called complete, total or central, incomplete, lateral or marginal.

Different obstetrical methods for delivery of the fetus include forceps, vacuum extractor and breech extraction.

Ballottement [to toss up (French)] (bal-ot-MON) is a maneuver used particularly as a method of diagnosis of pregnancy. It is also used for determining the size of an organ, particularly when there is ascites [a bag] (ah-SĪ-tēz) and to determine the mobility of a kidney.

Vers/ion [to turn] (VER-zhun) is a change of position of the fetus in the womb. It may occur spontaneously or it may be performed manually. Types of version are abdominal, ano/pelvic [anus pelvis] (ā"nō-PEL-vik), bimanual or bipolar, Braxton-Hicks,[1] cephalic [head] (se-FAL-ik), combined, external, forced, internal, pelvic, podalic [foot] (pō-DAL-ik), postural [position] (POS-tū-ral), Potter's, spontaneous, and Wright's.

Amnio/centesis [lamb puncture] (am"nē-ō-sen-TĒ-sis) is removal of amniotic fluid by inserting a needle transabdominally into the amniotic (am-nē-OT-ik) cavity.

Intrauterine transfusions are performed for aiding the fetus.

Surgical procedures performed on the female reproductive organs because of functional disturbances include the following:

1. dilatation and curettage (D & C) is performed for treatment of dys/meno/rrhea [difficult month] (dis"men-ō-RĒ-ah), for stenosis of the cervical canal which may result from senile atresia or damage to the mucosa [mucus] (myōō-KŌ-sah) by radium. A pyo/metrium [pus uterus] (pī-ō-MĒ-trē-um) may follow and dilatation is necessary to provide drainage of the uterine cavity. D & C is also performed for dia/gnostic [through to know] (dī-ag-NOS-tik) exploration of the uterine cavity for malignant disease, for obtaining an endometrial biopsy in patients with functional menstrual [month] (MEN-strōō-al) difficulties, and for the introduction of a radium applicator in malignant disease.
2. perineorrhaphy (repair of the perineum) is indicated when anatomical reconstruction is necessary following damage from delivery; in all reconstruction operations such as the Donald, Fothergill, or Manchester

1. John Braxton-Hicks, English gynecologist, 1825-1897

operations; for tightening of the muscles of the perineum;

3. trachelorrhaphy or repair of the cervix is performed wherever laceration of the cervix has occurred which results in exposure of the cervical mucosa; in many instances of severe erosion or chronic infection. In less severe erosion of the cervix cauterization [to burn] (kaw"ter-i-ZĀ-shun) or conization [cone] (kō-ni-ZĀ-shun)[1] may be performed;
4. uterine suspension (hystero/pexy [uterus] [HIS-ter-ō-pek-sē]) is performed for a uterus that prolapses to the intro/itus [into / to go] (in-TRŌ-ī-tus) if childbearing is still a factor; for acquired or congenital retroversion of the uterus. Other types of procedures are the Olshausen[2] (OLS-how-zen) operation and the Coffey suspension;
5. cysto/cele [sac] (SIS-tō-sēl) (hernial protrusion of the urinary bladder) is repaired when various urinary symptoms develop. The surgical procedure is known as anterior colporrhaphy or colpo/plasty (KOL-pō-plas-tē);
6. repair of a recto/cele [rectum] (REK-tō-sēl) (hernial protrusion of part of the rectum) is known as posterior colporrhaphy or colpo/perineo/plasty (kol"pō-per-i-NĒ-ō-plas-tē). When both cystocele and rectocele are repaired together the surgery is known as anterior-posterior colporrhaphy or A & P repair;
7. vaginal hyster/ectomy (his-ter-EK-tō-mē) (removal of the uterus through the vagina) is performed for small tumors, cancer in situ [in / position] (in SĪ-tyōō) and for relaxation of the pelvic floor with varying degrees of prolapse even to the extreme prolapse of procidentia [to fall forward] (prō-si-DEN-shē-ah). For patients who cannot withstand the rigors of more common surgical methods of curing a procidentia, the LeFort operation (partial colp/ectomy [kōl-PEK-tō-mē]) or obliteration of the vagina are performed;
8. fibr/oids (FĪ-broyds), abnormal uterine bleeding in the meno/pause (MEN-ō-pawz) group, prolapse, fibrosis uteri, as a necessary part of

1. Excision of a cone of tissue such as of the mucosa of the cervix. Optional pronunciation kon-i-ZĀ-shun
2. Robert von Olshausen, Berlin obstetrician, 1835-1915

an operation for certain diseases of the adnexae (ad-NEK-sē), and carcinoma are all indications for hysterectomy. Besides vaginal hysterectomy other types of hysterectomy are
(adnexae: appendages)

A. total hysterectomy or pan/hyster/ectomy (pan"his-ter-EK-tō-mē) is removal of the corpus (body) and cervix (neck) of the uterus. This is the operation of choice for uterine my/omata (mī-Ō-mah-tah), adeno/my/osis (ad"i-nō-mī-Ō-sis) and uterine cancer. It may be used in prolapse when combined with A & P repair. A frequently used incision is the Pfannenstiel[1] incision called by some surgeons the "bikini" incision for obvious reasons.
(pan: all; my/omata: muscle tumors)

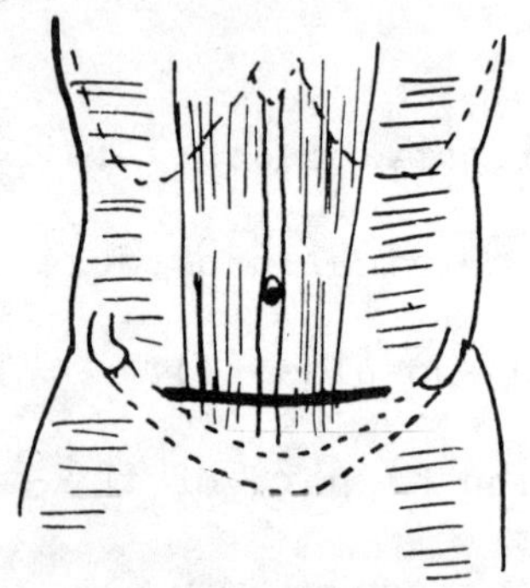

SKIN INCISION

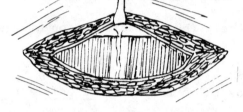

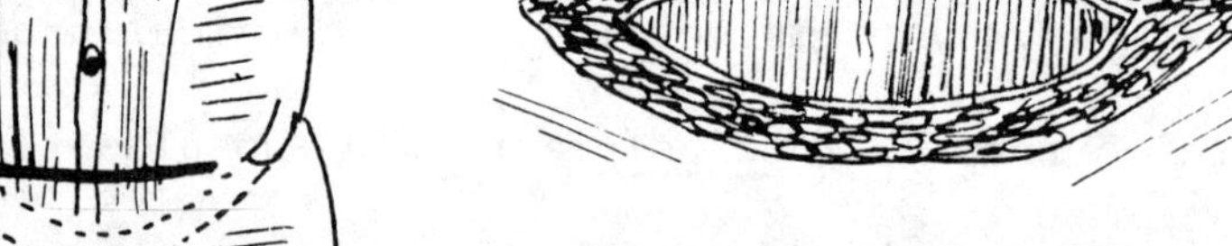

Anterior rectus sheath incised transversely and reflected upward by sharp dissection.

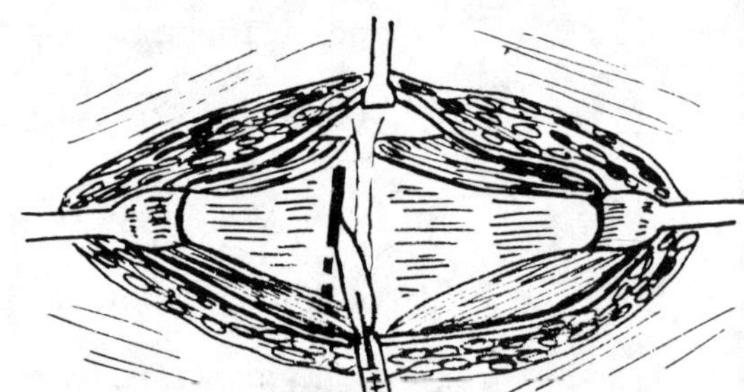

Rectus muscles freed, retracted laterally. Incision completed by incising remaining layers vertically.

PFANNENSTIEL INCISION

B. Wertheim[2] (VER-tīm) or radical hysterectomy with bilateral pelvic lymph node dissection is performed for cancer of the cervix and uterus with extension of cancer to lateral structures.

9. for submucous myomas in the corpus uteri a my/om/ectomy (mī-ō-MEK-tō-mē) is performed;
(om: tumor)

10. repair or closure of vesico/vaginal (ves"i-kō-VAJ-i-nal) fistula may be performed through three approaches: the vaginal, the supra/pubic (sū"prah-PYŌŌ-bik) route and the trans/peritoneal (trans"per-i-tō-NĒ-al) attack;
(vesico: bladder; vaginal: vagina; supra: above; pubic: pubic bone; trans: across)

11. a hernio/rrhaphy (her"nē-ŌR-ah-fē) type of surgery is performed for entero/cele (EN-ter-ō-sēl) (herniation of the bowel into the cul-de-sac
(hernio: hernia; entero: intestine; cul-de-sac: bottom of bag)

1. Pronounced FAN-en-stēl or PFAN-en-stēl; Johann Pfannenstiel, German gynecologist, 1862-1909
2. Ernest Wertheim, Vienna gynecologist, 1864-1920

[KUL-de-sak] or pouch of Douglas);

12. salpingo-oophor/ectomy (sal-ping"gō-ō"oo-fōr-EK-tō-mē) or adnex/ectomy (ad-nek-SEK-tō-mē) is the removal of the oviducts and ovaries and may be unilateral or bilateral. It is performed for disease of the adnexae secondary to salping/itis (sal-pin-JĪ-tis), oophor/itis (ō-of-ōr-Ī-tis), endometriosis, or ovarian cyst. Where a bilateral condition exists hysterectomy may also be performed;
    tube ovary adnexae

13. oophoro/cyst/ectomy (ō-of-ōr-ō-sis-TEK-tō-mē) is the excision of an ovarian cyst. Oophoro/plasty (ō-of-ŌR-ō-plas-tē) is plastic surgery on the ovary for ovarian cyst;

14. adnexo/pexy (ad-NEK-sō-pek-sē) is the operation of elevating and fixing the fallopian tube and ovary to the broad ligament for obstructed tubes;

15. oophor/ectomy (ō-of-ō-REK-tō-mē) (removal of the ovary) is performed for torsion of ovarian pedicle, malignant growths, cystic condition and endometriosis;

16. tubo/plasty (TŪ-bō-plas-tē) is plastic repair of a scarred fallopian tube;
    oviducts

17. tubal ligation is a sterilization procedure performed by tying and cutting the fallopian tubes.

Surgeries of the breast may be performed by gynecologists or plastic surgeons. Types of procedures performed include:

1. incision and drainage (I & D, masto/tomy [mas-TOT-ō-mē] with drainage) is done for infections;
    breast

2. benign tumors and cysts are excised;

3. simple mast/ectomy (mas-TEK-tō-mē) is performed for diffuse benign disease of the female breast. It is also performed in the male for chronic mast/itis (mas-TĪ-tis) or for gyneco/mastia (gī-ne-kō-MAS-tē-ah);
    woman

4. radical mastectomy is done for carcinoma of the breast;

5. mammilli/plasty [nipple] (mam-IL-i-plas-tē) is performed for umbilicated [navel] (um-BIL-i-kā-ted) or depressed nipple.

Genito/urinary (jen"i-tō-YŌŌR-i-nār-ē) or urological surgery not only is performed on the organs which comprise the urinary system but also upon the male reproductive organs because of the close relationship of these two systems in the male.

Surgery upon the kidneys is performed through oblique kidney, flank, anterior and anterior transperitoneal incisions. The hockey stick incision is rarely used today.

Nephr/ectomy (ne-FREK-tō-mē) is performed for tumors of the kidney, stag horn calculus [stone] (KAL-kū-lus), pyo/nephr/osis [pus] (pī"ō-ne-FRŌ-sis), pyelo/nephr/itis [renal pelvis] (pī"el-ō-ne-FRĪ-tis) and trauma [wound] (TRAW-mah).

Nephro/pexy (NEF-rō-pek-sē) is occasionally done when nephroptosis (floating kidney) causes an interference in the flow of urine because of the formation of a ureteral kink.

Incision and drainage (I & D) and excision of infected areas of the kidney is done for carbuncle [a little coal] (KAR-bung-kal) of the kidney and peri/nephritic [around] (per-ē-ne-FRIT-ik) abscess. In some cases nephrectomy is necessary.

Calyc/ectomy [cup of flower] (kā-li-SEK-tō-mē)[1] is performed when a calyx (KĀ-liks) is markedly dilated and scarred and its infundibulum [funnel] (in-fun-DIB-ū-lum) scarred and, therefore, incapable of draining the calyx into the pelvis.

Hemi/nephr/ectomy [half] (hem"ē-ne-FREK-tō-mē) is done when the upper or lower half of the kidney is destroyed by stone, tuberculosis (TBC), pyel/ectasis (pī-el-EK-tah-sis) and infection; for kidney preferably with bifid[2] (BĪ-fid) pelvis.

Nephro/rrhaphy (nef-RŌR-ah-fē) (suture of the kidney) is performed for traumatic (traw-MAT-ik) injuries.

Renal calculi [(plural)] (KAL-kū-lī) are sometimes removed by nephro/litho/tomy (nef-rō-lith-OT-ō-mē) or hemi/nephro/tomy (hem"ē-ne-FROT-ō-mē).

1. Optional pronunciation kal-i-SEK-tō-mē

2. Means "cleft in two parts"

In cases of hypernephroma, pelvic carcinoma, ureteral carcinoma and Wilm's[1] (vilms) tumor (malignant renal tumor of young children), total nephrectomy with ureter/ectomy (ū"rē-ter-EK-tō-mē) and sometimes partial cyst/ectomy [bladder] (sis-TEK-tō-mē) is performed.

For calculi in the renal pelvis pyelo/litho/tomy (pī"el-ō-lith-OT-ō-mē) is indicated and uretero/litho/tomy (ū-rē"ter-ō-lith-OT-ō-mē) is done for a stone in the ureter which cannot be extracted endo/scopically [within / to look] (en-dō-SKOP-ik-ah-lē).

Uretero/plasty (ū-RĒ-ter-ō-plas-tē) and pyelo/plasty (PĪ-el-ō-plas-tē) are performed for stricture of the ureter, ureteral injury or retroperitoneal fibrosis (R.P.F.).

Hypo/plastic [below / formation] (hī-pō-PLAS-tik) kidneys or kidneys with deficient blood supply or chronic infection, sclerotic [hard] (skle-ROT-ik) or not, are removed in persons with hypertension and occasionally for the relief of infection or pain.

Ectopic kidneys usually are not removed. However, if they cause pressure or pain and are associated with stone or chronic infection they are removed.

Bladder surgery may be either open or closed. Open surgery is necessary for infiltrating and some large ped/unculated [foot / small] (pe-DUNG-kyo͞o-lā-ted) tumors; for very large or hard stones; malformations, congenital or acquired; and often, although not always, for the effects of trauma, either blast, puncture by missile from without, or by pelvic bone from within. Some of the open procedures are diverticul/ectomy [to turn aside] (dī"ver-tik-ū-LEK-tō-mē) (for bladder diverticula [dī-ver-TIK-ū-lah]), partial cystectomy, cystectomy with uretero-intestinal (ū-rē"ter-ō-in-TES-ti-nal) anastomosis [to make an opening] (ah-nas-tō-MŌ-sis) or uretero/cutaneous [skin] (ū-rē-ter-ō-kyo͞o-TĀ-nē-us) anastomosis, uretero/neo/cysto/stomy [new] (ū-rē-ter-ō-nē"ō-sis-TOS-tō-mē), cysto/tomy (sis-TOT-ō-mē) and cystostomy (sis-TOS-tō-mē) (usually for the purpose of introducing a tube or catheter into the bladder for elimination of urine).

1. Marx Wilms, German surgeon, 1867-1918

Closed surgery of the bladder consists of two methods:

1. electricity: dessicating *to dry up* (DES-i-kāt-ing), coagulating *to curdle* (kō-AG-ū-lāt-ing) and cutting currents using active Bugbee electr/odes *amber way* (ē-LEK-trōds), cutting loops with re/secto/scope *back to cut* (rē-SEK-tō-skōp), and the ureteral orifice incisor of Neil Moore or the Collins' knife
2. nonelectric instruments: scissors, crushing instruments, curets, rongeur *to gnaw* (rawn-ZHER) cysto/scopes (SIS-tō-skōps) and forceps, litho/trites *stone to rub* (LITH-ō-trīts), and the Johnson basket.

Hunner's[1] (HUN-erz) ulcer or elusive ulcer (interstitial cyst/itis [sis-TĪ-tis]) is often relieved with silver nitrate dilatations of the bladder. Sometimes cystoscopic electrocoagulation gives relief.

There are two types of bladder stones: primary (formed entirely within the bladder) and secondary (stone having passed from the kidney, increases in size after entering the bladder). Litho/lapaxy *removal* (lith-ŌL-ah-pak-sē) is done with the visual or blind lithotrite for bladder stones.

Bladder tumors are papillary, sessile *low-growing* (SES-il), pedunculated or invasive. Operations are performed trans/urethrally (trans-ū-RĒ-thrah-lē). Biopsy of tumor is obtained with the Stern-McCarthy resectoscope or biopsy punch. Many tumors can be destroyed by electrocoagulation. When the grade of malignancy is sufficient to warrant it, radon *radium* (RĀ-don) seeds may be implanted through an operating cystoscope.

Ex/trophy *out* (EKS-trō-fē) of the bladder, a congenital malformation, may be divided into complete and incomplete bladder extrophy. Corrective surgery consists of uretero/sigmoido/stomy *sigmoid colon* (ū-rē-ter-ō-sig-moyd-OS-tō-mē) and ileal *ileum* (IL-ē-al) bladder for diverting the urinary stream. Later the abdominal defect is closed.

Pro/static (pros-TAT-ik) obstruction may be caused by benign prostatic hypertrophy (BPH) found in the older group, by carcinoma of the prostate, or

1. Guy LeRoy Hunner, Baltimore surgeon, born 1868

by the small scarred prostate usually associated with median bar found in the younger group. Sometimes the two types are mixed. Surgical procedures performed are:

1. suprapubic <u>pro/stat/ectomy</u> (pros-tah-TEK-tō-mē), one-stage or two-stage. With the latter, a cystostomy is performed, and five to 10 days later prostatic enucleation.
2. perineal prostatectomy
3. transurethral prostatectomy (transurethral resection of the prostate)(TURP)
4. retropubic prostatectomy

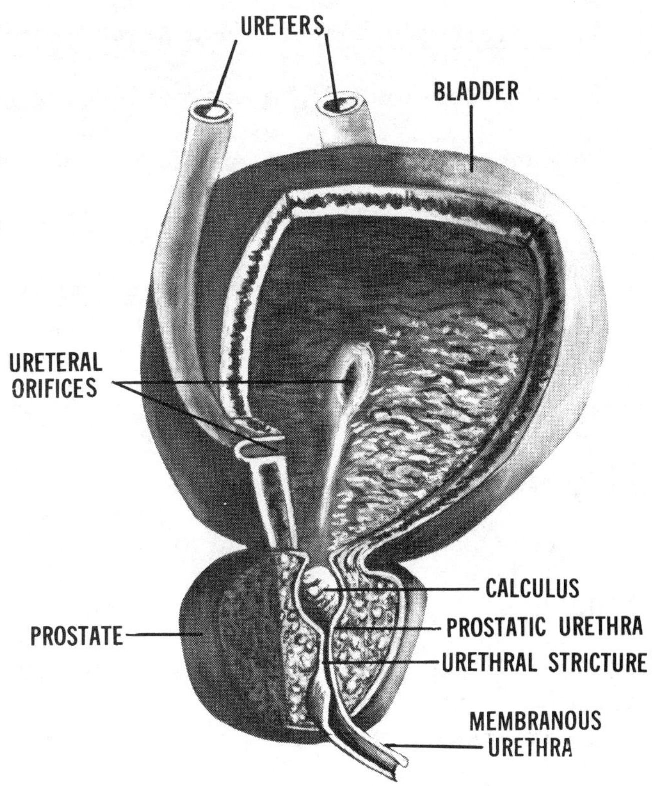

CALCULUS IN URETHRAL STRICTURE CAUSED BY PROSTATISM

This type of stricture of the prostatic urethra is rare. Stricture of the membranous urethra is more common.

Carcinoma of the prostate: if fixation or metastasis has not occurred a radical prostatectomy is performed either retropubically or perineally. Partial or complete <u>orchi/ectomy</u>[1] *testicle* (or-kē-EK-tō-mē) or <u>castration</u>[2] (kas-TRĀ-shun) may also be performed.

<u>Epi/didym/ectomy</u> (ep"i-did-i-MEK-tō-mē) is performed for chronic recurrent <u>epi/didym/itis</u> (ep"i-did-i-MĪ-tis).

<u>Varico/cel/ectomy</u> *swollen vein hernia* (var"i-kō-se-LEK-tō-mē) is performed for <u>varico/cele</u> (VAR-i-kō-sēl).

<u>Spermato/cele</u> *seed* (SPUR-ma-tō-sēl) is usually a primary <u>hydro/cele</u> *water* (HĪ-drō-sēl) that has established an opening with the vas or epididymis. <u>Spermato/cel/ectomy</u> (spur-mat"ō-se-LEK-tō-mē) is done.

Hydrocele in the young is frequently associated with hernia in which case

1. Is also spelled "orchidectomy"
2. To deprive a male or female of generative power. The removal of the gonads (ovaries or testes).

hydro/cel/ectomy (hī"drō-se-LEK-tō-mē) and herniorrhaphy are performed.

Torsion of the spermatic cord complicated by testicul/ar *testicle* (tes-TIK-ū-lar) gangrene *an eating sore* (GANG-grēn) is corrected by orchiectomy or detorsion; also scrotal fixation of the opposite testis is performed.

Tumors of the testicle: semin/oma *seed* (sem-i-NŌ-mah)[1], em/bryonal *in to be full of life* (EM-brē-on-al)[2] carcinoma, terato/carcinoma *monster cancer* (ter"ah-tō-kar-si-NŌ-mah), teratoma, and chorio-epithelioma are all highly malignant. Unilateral orchid/ectomy *testicle* (or-ki-DEK-tō-mē) with removal of the tunica vaginalis and the fascial layers of the spermatic cord and scrotum is performed. Sometimes retroperitoneal node dissection is done.

Castration or bilateral orchidectomy is also performed for andro/gen *man to produce* (AN-drō-jen) control of prostatic carcinoma.

The Torek[3] (TŌ-rek) operation, orchio/plasty (OR-kē-ō-plas-tē), orchio/pexy (or-kē-ō-PEK-sē) are procedures performed for undescended testicle (crypt/orch/ism *to hide* [krip-TOR-kizm]).

Radical removal of the affected organ is necessary in cancer of the penis. Removal of the urethra because of cancer is rarely done.

Urethral strictures are treated by dilatation. Urethral meato/tomy *passage* (mē-ah-TOT-ō-mē) is performed for urethral meatal (mē-Ā-tal) stenosis, male or female.

Epi/spadias *a rent or tear* (ep-i-SPĀ-dē-as) and hypo/spadias (hī-pō-SPĀ-dē-as) are congenital abnormalities of the penis and surgical correction is done in a two-stage procedure.

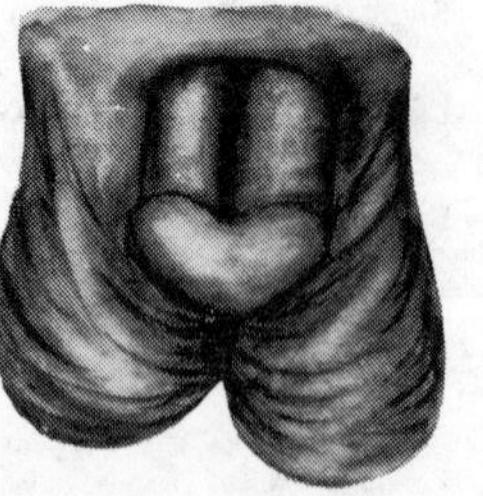

EPISPADIAS

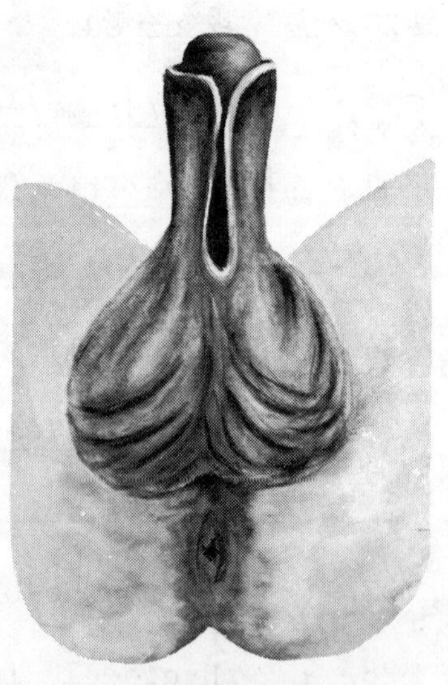

HYPOSPADIAS

Circum/cision *around to cut* (ser-kum-SIZH-un) of the penis is performed for redundant prepuce, phimosis *to muzzle* (fī-MŌ-sis) or balano/posth/itis *glans penis prepuce* (bal"ah-nō-pos-THĪ-tis).

1. Optional pronunciation se-mi-NŌ-mah
2. Optional pronunciation EM-brē-ō-nal
3. Franz J. A. Torek, New York surgeon, 1861-1938

INDEX
CHAPTER IX

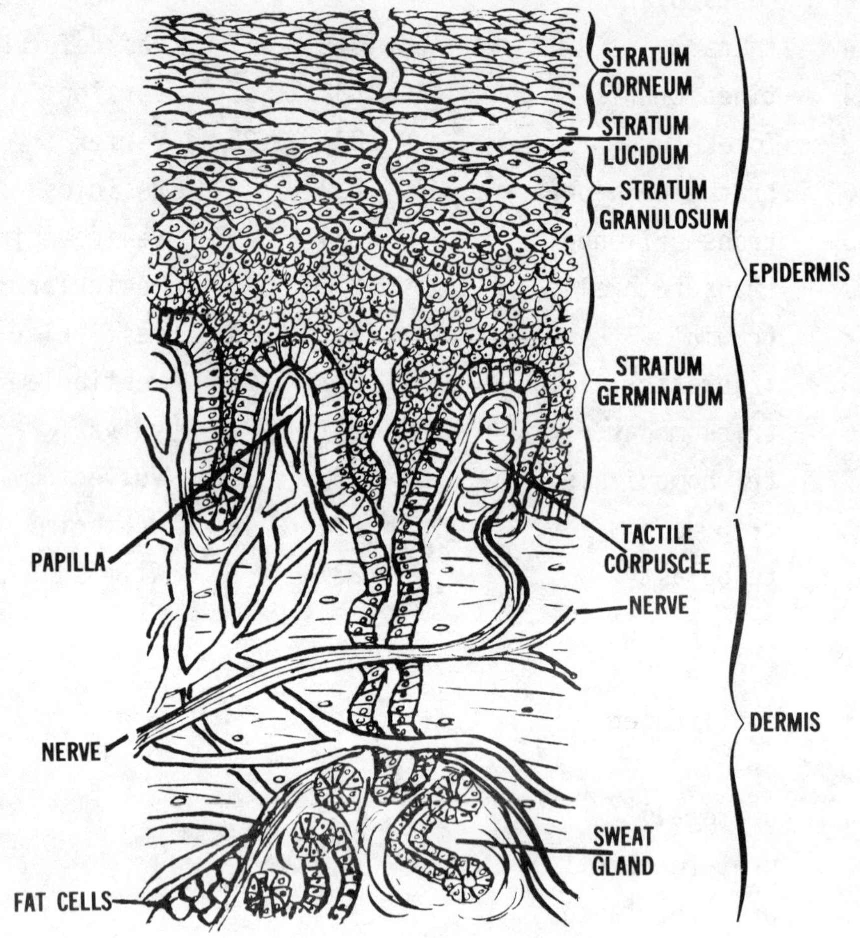

STRUCTURE OF THE SKIN (Touch)

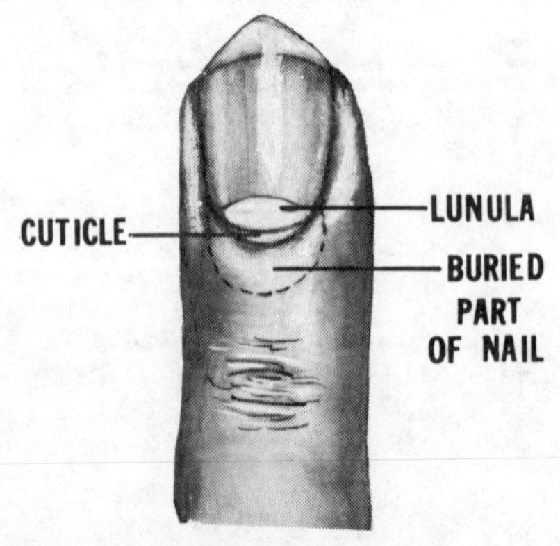

THE FINGERNAIL

CHAPTER X
THE SENSES
Touch, Taste, Smell, Hearing, Sight

ANATOMY OF TOUCH (The Skin and Appendages)

The functions of the skin are 1. to cover the body; 2. to protect the deeper tissues from drying, from injury, and from invasion by foreign organisms; 3. as an important factor in heat regulation; 4. as a limited excretory and absorbing power because the skin contains the end organs of many of the sensory nerves.

The skin consists of two distinct layers:

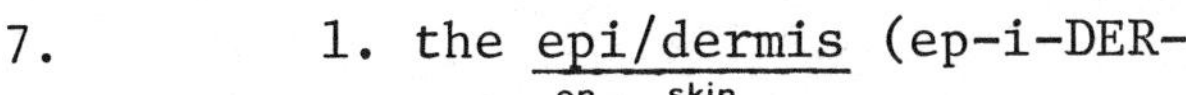

1. the epi/dermis *(on skin)* (ep-i-DER-mis), cut/icle *(skin small)* (KYŌŌ-te-kl) or scarf skin;
2. the corium *(skin,hide)* (KŌ-rē-um), cutis *(skin)* (KYŌŌ-tis) vera *(true)* (VĒ-rah), or derma *(skin)* (DER-mah).

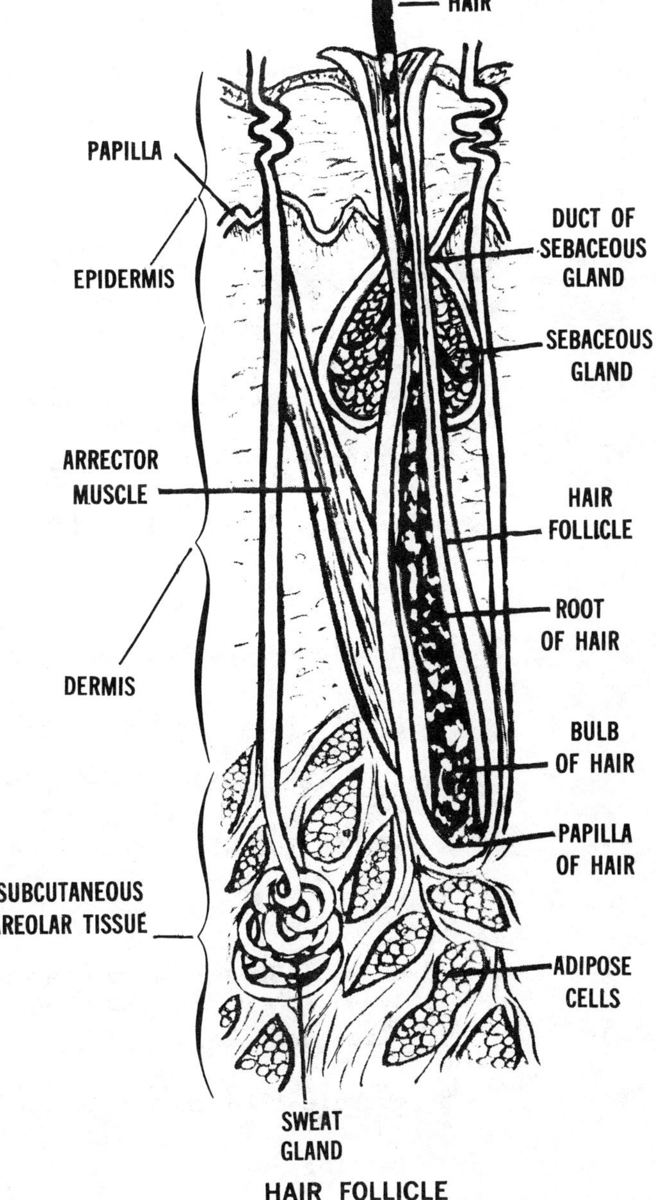

HAIR FOLLICLE

The epidermis is a stratified epi/thelium *(on nipple)* (ep-i-THĒ-lē-um) consisting of layers of cells. It consists of four layers: the stratum *(layer)* (STRĀ-tum) corneum *(horny)* (KŌR-nē-um), the stratum lucidum *(clear)* (LŪ-sid-um), the stratum granulosum *(granules)* (gran-ū-LŌ-sum) and the stratum mucosum *(mucus)* (myōō-KŌ-sum). The corium is a highly sensitive, vascular layer and consists of two layers: the papill/ary *(papilla)* (PAP-i-lār-ē) or superficial layer and the reticul/ar [a little net] (re-TIK-ū-lar) layer.

The appendages of the skin are the nails, the hairs, the sebace/ous [oily] (se-BĀ-shus) glands, the sudori/ferous [sweat to bear] (sū-do-RIF-er-es) or sweat glands and their ducts. The skin lining the external audit/ory [to hear] (AW-de-tō-rē) canal contains modified sweat glands called cerumin/ous [wax] (se-RŪ-min-us) glands. They secrete a yellow, pasty substance resembling wax which is called cerumen (se-RŪ-men).

DISEASES OF THE SKIN

There are two classes of skin lesions:

1. primary lesions (the type which appear initially or into which the lesions soon evolve);
2. secondary lesions (these result from development of primary lesions, either naturally or from effects of topical applications, scratching, rubbing, etc.).

Primary lesions include the following:

1. macule [a spot] (MAK-yo͞ol) -- small (up to fingernail size) discoloration which is level with the surface,
2. patch -- an oversized macule,
3. papule [pimple] (PAP-yo͞ol) -- firm, small (up to buck-shot size) elevated lesion,
4. nodule -- similar to a papule but larger,
5. tumor -- a firm elevation which is larger than a half-marble,
6. vesicle [a blister] (VES-i-kl) -- an elevated lesion within the size range of a papule containing clear fluid,
7. bulla [bubble] (BŪL-ah) or bleb [small blister] (bleb) -- an oversized vesicle,
8. pustule [blister] (PUS-cho͞ol) -- vesicle or bleb containing pus,

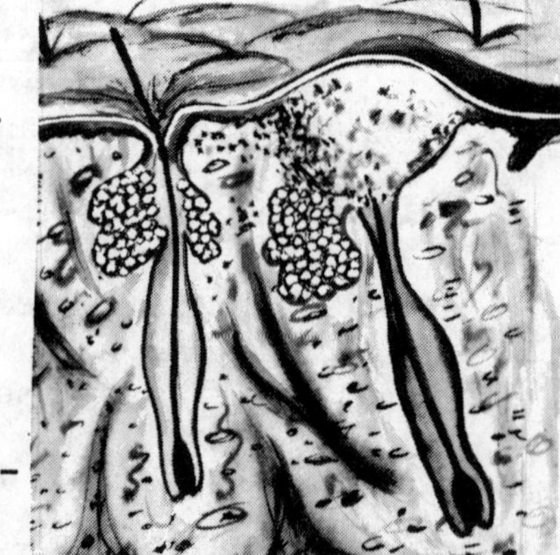
PUSTULE

9. wheal [hive] (hwēl) -- elevated, usually transient lesion of irregular shape from whose borders narrow processes commonly extend.

Secondary lesions consist of:

1. ex/cori/ation [out skin] (eks-kō-rē-Ā-shun) -- an area denuded of the horny layer, exposing the moist pink cellular layer of the epidermis,
2. scale -- a particle of denuded horny layer,
3. crust -- mass or plate of dried ex/udate [out sweat] (EKS-yōō-dāt),
4. fissure -- a "crack" extending through the epidermis,
5. ulcer -- an excavation; an area uncovered by skin.

When pink or red lesions blanch (turn white) on pressure they are said to be erythemat/ous [redness] (er-i-THEM-ah-tus). This is caused by dilatation of small blood vessels in the skin and is known as erythema [redness] (er-i-THĒ-mah). If these discolorations are macular in size they are called purpuric [purple] (pur-PŪ-rik) spots; if they are larger in size they are called ec/chymoses [out to pour] (ek-ē-MŌ-sēz). Minute hemorrhagic spots of pinpoint to pinhead size which also occur in the skin are called petechiae (pe-TĒ-kē-ē).[1]

Dermat/itis (der-mah-TĪ-tis) or inflammation of the skin may be acute or chronic. It is characterized by hyper/emia [excessive blood] (hī-per-Ē-mē-ah) of and exudation into the layers of the skin. The following are a few of the diseases which come under the heading of dermatitis:

1. erythema inter/trigo [between to rub] (in-ter-TRĒ-go),
2. miliaria[2] [millet] (mil-ē-Ā-rē-ah) or prickly heat,
3. pompholyx [bubble] (POM-fo-liks),
4. pityr/iasis [bran] (pit-ē-RĪ-ah-sis) rosea [rosy] (RŌ-sē-ah),
5. eczema [to boil over] (EK-se-mah),
6. pemphigus [blister] (PEM-fe-gus),
7. psor/iasis [itch] (sō-RĪ-ah-sis),
8. acne vulgaris [common] (vul-GĀ-ris),

1. Optional pronunciation pē-TĒ-kē-ī
2. So named because the vesicles resemble the seeds of millet, a grass once raised as a grain.

9. ex/foliative (eks-FŌ-lē-ah-tiv) dermatitis.
out leaf

Comedo (KOM-i-dō) (more commonly known as "black-
to eat up
head") is a blackish plug of dried, fatty (sebaceous) matter excreted by a skin follicle. The skin of the face is often subject to blackheads.

BLACKHEAD

Discoloration of the skin (either patchy or diffuse) may occur in association with or following inflammatory conditions and neoplasms, as a manifestation of metabolic and endocrine disorders, or without any detectable cause. Some of these abnormalities are:

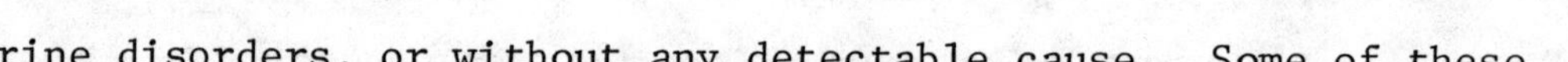

1. lentigo (len-TĪ-gō) also known as lentigines (len-TIJ-i-nēz) or
   freckle / freckles(plural)
   freckles,
2. chloasma (klō-AZ-mah) or "liver spots" refers to patches which other-
   to be green
   wise are identical to freckles. However, they have nothing to do with the liver.
3. albin/ism (AL-bin-izm) which is a congenital absence of pigment in
   white
   skin that is otherwise normal. Persons affected with this condition are known as albinos (al-BĪ-nōs).
4. vitiligo (vit-i-LĪ-gō) or leuko/derma (lū-kō-DER-mah) which is an
   blemish / white
   acquired disorder of unknown cause and which is characterized by patches of depigmentation (loss of color), the skin otherwise remaining normal.

Benign tumors of the skin are common and numerous. They may arise from the cells of the epidermis or the fibrous tissue, blood vessels, or the nerves of the deeper layer. Primary malignant tumors, which usually arise from cells of the epidermis, are also common, but metastatic cancers are rare.

Kel/oids (KĒ-loyds) are benign tumors due to overgrowth of fibrous tissue
scar
in scars which result from trauma, burns, inflammation or ulceration.

Angi/omas [vessel] (an-jē-Ō-mahs) are benign tumors which are caused by overgrowth of blood vessels in the skin.

Pigmented nevi [birthmarks] (NĒ-vī) or moles are round or oval in shape, vary in color from light brown to black, are slightly elevated flat tumors of variable size or number. They are usually benign but occasionally one becomes malignant (malignant melan/oma [black] [mel-ah-NŌ-mah]) and meta/stasizes [beyond to stand] (me-tas-tah-SĪ-sez) to distant organs, often without apparent change in the primary mole itself.

Neuro/fibr/omas [nerve fiber] (nū"rō-fī-BRŌ-mahs) are multiple rounded, elevated, often ped/unculated [foot small] (pe-DUNG-kyōō-lāt-ed) tumors of varying size which arise from the connective tissue sheaths of nerves.

Carcin/omas [cancer] (kar-si-NŌ-mahs) are malignant tumors arising in the cells of the epidermis.

The sebaceous (oil) glands or the sweat glands may secrete excessive or subnormal amounts. This gives rise to oiliness, or dryness, or moistness of the skin. Each of these conditions, in turn, may result in other abnormal states. Some of these conditions are:

Sebo/rrhea [suet] (seb-ō-RĒ-ah) refers to excessive secretion of the sebaceous glands. These glands are most abundant in the scalp and upon the face and neck. The condition is responsible for "oily skin," "dandruff," and is responsible for a susceptibility toward the formation of blackheads, "pimples" and ezcema-like lesions.

A sebaceous cyst results when a sebaceous gland whose duct is blocked continues to secrete until the accumulated secretion forms a tumor of considerable size. The size of the tumor may range from that of a marble to as large as a hen's egg.

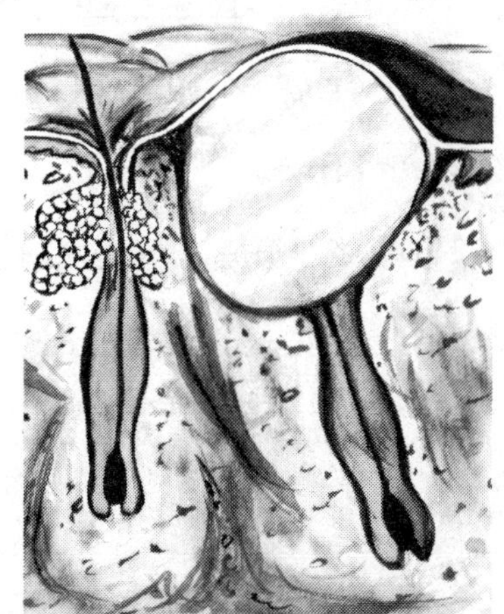
SEBACEOUS CYST

Hyper/hidr/osis [excessive sweat] (hī"per-hi-DRŌ-sis) applies to excessive sweating which may cause prickly heat or small non-inflamed vesicles called sudamina [to sweat] (sū-DAM-i-nah). This condition may also bring about inflammation and excoriation of the skin at the sites of pressure or friction.

Disease of the skin of the scalp may involve the roots of the hair which may cause the hair to fall out or break off. This results in thinning of the hair or patches of baldness. Loss of hair may also occur in the absence of detectable disease of the scalp.

Baldness is known as alopecia[1] [fox] (al-ō-PĒ-shē-ah). In its familiar form in the male it is a hereditary condition which begins in early adult life or adolescence and is known as alopecia prematura [early ripe] (prē-mah-TŪR-ah). This progresses gradually. At middle age only a fringe of hair may remain about the sides and back of the head. This condition is known as alopecia senilis [old age] (se-NIL-is).

Baldness occurring in patches and not due to any detectable disease of the scalp is known as alopecia areata [patches] (ar-ē-Ā-tah). It occurs for the most part in children and young adults. It affects both sexes.

Hyper/trich/osis [hair] (hī"per-trik-Ō-sis) is the excessive, abnormal or premature growth of hair in any region or regions of the body.

Hypo/trich/osis (hī"pō-trik-Ō-sis) is a condition in which there is decreased growth, scantiness or absence of hair in regions where hair should grow.

The fingernails and toenails have a number of abnormalities which include changes in color, contour and thickness, loss of a nail or nails, and inflammation of the nail beds and the tissues about their borders and which may be caused by other conditions of the body.

Hypertrophy refers to an overgrowth of the nails in size or thickness. Atrophy refers to thinning or decrease of size. Either hypertrophy or atrophy

1. A disease like fox mange.

may be associated with roughness or brittleness. Ingrowing is present if growth of the nails presses in upon the soft tissues at the sides of the nails. Onych/ia *nail* (ō-NIK-ē-ah) indicates inflammation of the nail bed. Par/onych/ia *beside* (par-ō-NIK-e-ah) refers to inflammation of tissues adjacent to the nail. Onycho/lysis (on-i-KOL-i-sis) is loosening of the nail.

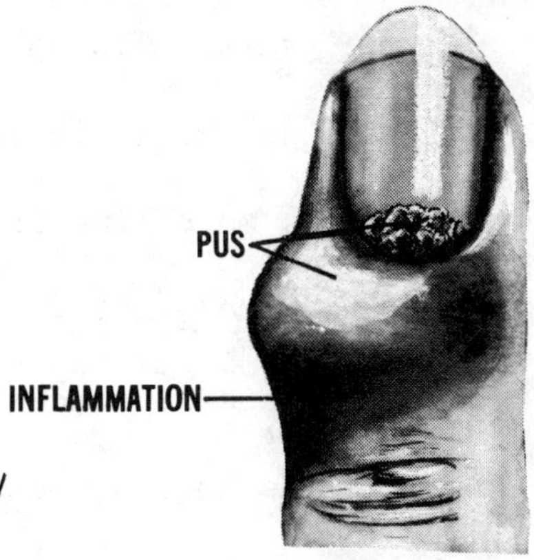

PUS

INFLAMMATION

PARONYCHIA

PLASTIC SURGERY, SURGERY OF SKIN AND SUBCUTANEOUS TISSUES

Skin grafts can be made to grow successfully in practically any viable area that is free of major infection. Generally, the thinner the graft, the greater will be the chance of growing. The thicker the graft, the more difficult it will be to obtain complete growing but the maximum degree of function and cosmesis *an adorning* (koz-MĒ-sis) will be obtained.

Skin grafts are classified as

1. free grafts
   a. split-thickness
   b. free full-thickness
2. pedicle grafts, "flaps"
   a. open (direct)
   b. tubed

Intermediate split-thickness grafts may be called thick Thiersch[1] (teersh) grafts. They can be cut from 25 to 85% of the total skin thickness.

Full thickness grafts give the maximum degree of cosmetic and functional result but are the most difficult in which to obtain growth.

Pedicle flaps may be open or tubed. They are utilized in extensive reconstruction about the face, particularly about the mouth and tip of the nose. They are also used when it is doubtful whether the viability of the graft can be maintained, and when it is necessary to transfer a subcutaneous fat pad with

1. Karl Thiersch, German surgeon, 1822-1895; optional pronunciation TĒR-shez

the graft. The open flap is quicker but is subject to contamination of its open pedicle. The tubed pedicle flap is a closed mechanism throughout but requires more time in its construction and transfer.

Homo/grafts *same* (HŌ-mō-grafts) (skin grafts taken from other individuals) are considered unsuccessful except in identical twins.

Methods of cutting skin grafts:

1. with scalpel
   a. small pinch grafts
   b. free full-thickness grafts
2. with free hand knife (often aided by a Blair-Brown suction box or vacuum retractor)
   a. split-thickness skin grafts
3. with derma/tome *cutting instrument* (DER-mah-tōm)
   a. split-thickness skin grafts

Preservation of unused auto/genous *self to produce* (aw-TOJ-i-nus) split-thickness grafts: these may be transferred successfully, after freezing or refrigeration for at least three to four weeks.

Z-plasty consists of sliding flaps of skin after a "Z" incision has been made and the triangular flaps undermined.

Transplantation of tissues other than skin:

1. A dermal or "cutis" graft consists of full-thickness skin from which the epidermal layer has been removed.
2. Free fat grafts often prove unsuccessful because of nearly complete absorption.
3. Free fascia lata grafts when rolled up to build out a depression are usually replaced by fibrous tissue. This causes scar contracture in the area of the graft.
4. Costal cartilage is frequently used for correction of surface de-

pressions. This may be either autogenous (removed from the same patient) or preserved. It may be used in large pieces or diced into small bits and molded into shape. Sometimes the cartilage is grated very finely and injected into the prepared cavity with a coarse syringe.

5. Bone grafts may be used in massive pieces or molded in a mass from small chips. Because of its relatively simple accessibility and because it is a soft cancellous bone that vascularizes[1] *vessel* (VAS-kū-lar-ī-zez) rapidly, the iliac crest of the hip bone is the most frequent source of bone grafts for use in plastic surgery.

The following are some of the indications for plastic surgery:

1. granulating defects following burns and avulsions
2. healed defects: scar contractures of the neck, extremity contractures, ec/tropion *out to turn* (ek-TRŌ-pē-on) of the eyelid, nasal tip and ala defect, intraoral scarring, scar contractures of hands
3. syn/dactyl/ism *together digit* (sin-DAK-til-izm)
4. poly/dactyl/ism *many* (pol-ē-DAK-til-izm)
5. reconstruction of the thumb
6. electrical burns
7. plantar *sole of foot* (PLAN-tar) warts
8. scars and keloids
9. chronic leg ulcers
10. tattoos
11. congenital absence of the vagina
12. penile (PĒ-nīl) hypo/spadias *a rent,tear* (hī-pō-SPĀ-dē-as)
13. anal stenosis (often occurs following operations for imperforate anus)

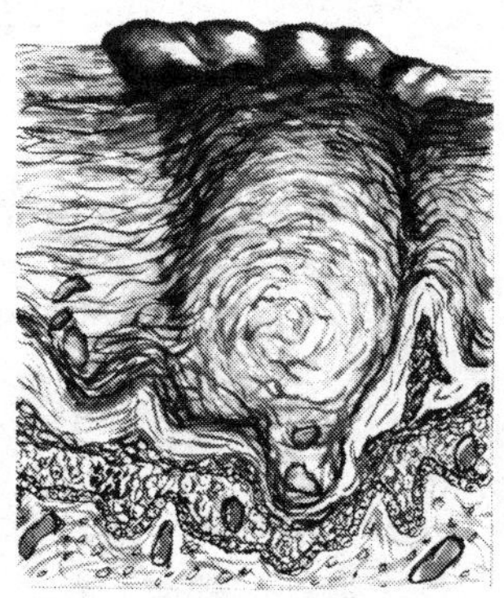

PLANTAR WART

1. To supply with vessels.

14. nasal deformities: developmental deformities, fracture deformities, saddle deformities, fracture dislocations of the nasal septum
15. protruding ear
16. cleft lips (surgical procedure: cheilo/plasty *lip* [KĪ-lō-plas-tē])
17. cleft palate (surgical procedures: staphylo/rrhaphy *palate* [staf-i-LŌR-ah-fē] and palato/plasty *palate* [pal"ah-tō-PLAS-tē])
18. partially cleft palate

Surgery of the skin and subcutaneous tissues is done for the following conditions:

Infections:

1. furuncle *a petty thief* (FYO͞OR-ung-kl) or boil: incision of the area to promote free drainage of pus and necrotic matter (I & D);
2. carbuncle *a little coal* (KAR-bung-kl) while like a furuncle, is much more virulent and extensive and requires excision;
3. tuberculosis of the skin (lupus *wolf* [LŪ-pus] vulgaris): excision of all infected skin and subcutaneous tissue;
4. actino/myc/osis *ray fungus* (ak"tin-ō-mī-KŌ-sis) gives rise to a granul/oma *grains* (gran-ū-LŌ-mah) that forms a sinus or fistula *pipe* (FIS-tū-lah) and discharges a thin pus which contains yellow sulphur-like granules. There are three types: cervico/facial *neck face* (ser-vi-kō-FĀ-shē-al), abdominal and thoracic. Treatment consists of chemo/therapy *chemical treatment* (kē"mō-THER-ah-pē) (the use of antibiotics), the excision of all sinus tracts and granul/omat/ous (gran-ū-LŌ-mah-tus) tissue;
5. granuloma pyo/genica *pus to produce* (pī-ō-JEN-i-kah) is caused by infection or implantation of a foreign body: excision of granuloma pyogenica and irritation focus;
6. decubitus *lying down* (dē-KYO͞O-be-tus) ulcer (bedsore): excison of ulcer and

grafting if necessary;

7. epi/dermo/phytosis (plant) (ep"i-der-mō-fī-TŌ-sis) (athlete's foot) is caused by fungi. Treated by chemotherapy and I & D of encapsulated pus;

8. perforating ulcer occurs over the plantar aspect of the foot at the metatarso/phalangeal (metatarsus, phalanges) (met-ah-tar"sō-fah-LAN-jē-al) joint in patients suffering from chronic diseases such as arteriosclerosis, diabetes, syphilis and the degenerative diseases of the nervous system. If conservative treatment is not satisfactory the simple excision of the ulcer and skin grafting may be done. Pedicle grafts are often used.

Benign tumors of the skin and subcutaneous tissues:

hemangioma, neurofibroma, lipoma, fibro/lip/oma (fī"brō-lī-PŌ-mah), angioma, lymphangioma, hemo/lymph/angi/oma (blood, water) (hē"mō-lim-fan-jē-Ō-mah), endo/theli/oma (en"dō-thē-lē-Ō-mah), keloid

Epithelial tumors:

plantar wart, xanth/omata (yellow) (zan-THŌ-mah-tah), callus (KAL-us), sub/ungual (below, nail) (sub-UNG-gwal) corn or callus (onych/oma (nail) [on-i-KŌ-mah]) glomus (a ball) (GLŌ-mus) tumor

Malignant epithelial tumors:

squamous cell epi/theli/oma (ep"i-thē-lē-Ō-mah), basal cell epithelioma (Rodent ulcer), columnar epithelioma and gland cell carcinoma, melanoma (malignant pigmented nevus (birthmark) [NĒ-vus] or melano/sarc/oma (black, flesh) [mel"ah-nō-sar-KŌ-mah] [the most malignant of all tumors]). Two of the most malignant melanosarcomas are melanotic (mel-ah-NOT-ik) whitlow (a felon) (HWIT-lō) and subungual melanoma.

Surgery of tumors consists of excision of the tumor, grafting where necessary, and, in the case of malignant tumors, radical excision of infected area.

Sebaceous cysts and dermoid cysts are excised.

Paronychia is an infection caused by a torn hang-nail or some injury to the cuticle. Partial excision of the nail is performed.

Three common plastic procedures are:

1. rhytid/ectomy [wrinkle] (rit-i-DEK-tō-mē) (face lifting) which is performed for ptosis [prolapse] (TŌ-sis) senilis [old age] (se-NIL-is) of the face;
2. blepharo/plasty [eyelid] (BLEF-ah-rō-plas-tē) for aging eyelids;
3. mamma/plasty [breast] (MAM-ah-plas-tē) for pendulent or large breasts.

ANATOMY OF TASTE (The Mouth)

The tongue, a freely movable muscular organ, consists of two halves united in the center. The root of the tongue is attached to the hyoid ["U"shaped] (hī-OYD) bone by several muscles. Four varieties of papillae [nipple] (pah-PIL-ē) cover the tongue: the vallate [to wall] (VAL-āt) or circum/vallate [around] (ser-kum-VAL-āt), the fungi/form [fungus] (FUN-je-form), the fili/form [thread] (FIL-i-form), and simple papillae. These papillae contain capillaries and nerves.

The taste-buds occur chiefly on the surface of the tongue. However, some are scattered over the soft palate [roof of mouth] (PAL-at), fauces [throat] (FAW-sēz), epi/glottis [on, mouth of windpipe] (epi-i-GLOT-is) and even the vocal cords.

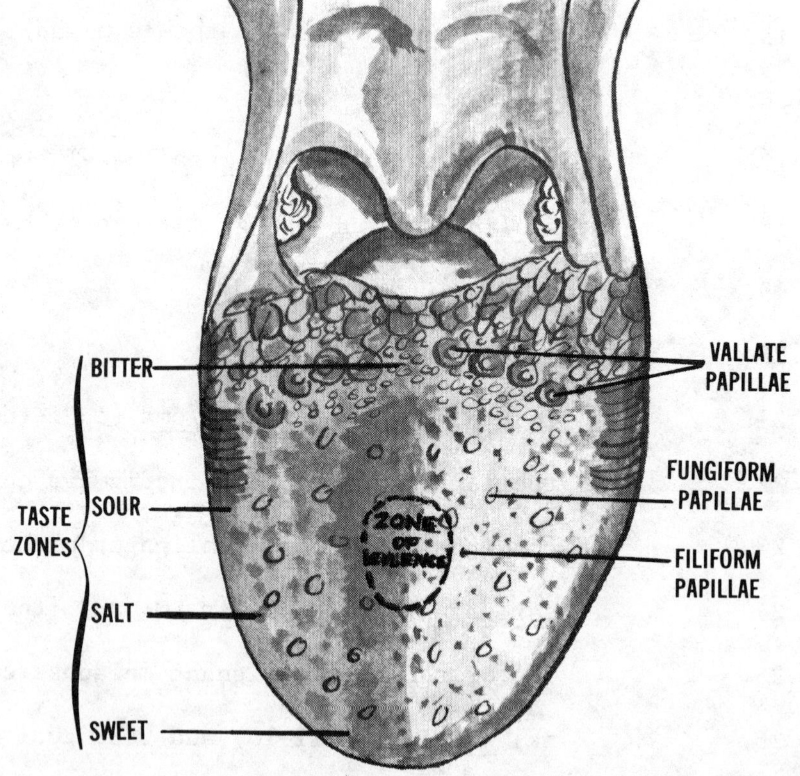

THE TONGUE (Taste)

ANATOMY OF SMELL (The Nose)

The olfact/ory (to smell) (ōl-FAK-tō-rē) nerves spread out in a fine network over the surface of the superior nasal conchae (shell (plural)) (KONG-kē) and the upper third of the septum. These nerves are the special nerves of the sense of smell. The tact/ile (touch) (TAK-til) sense which enables nasal perception of the sensations of cold, heat, pain, tickling and tension or pressure is furnished by the tri/geminal (three twin) (trī-JEM-i-nal) or fifth cranial nerve.

BRANCHES FROM OLFACTORY NERVE
BRANCHES FROM NERVE OF PTERYGOID CANAL
ANTERIOR ETHMOIDAL NERVE
NASOPALATINE NERVE

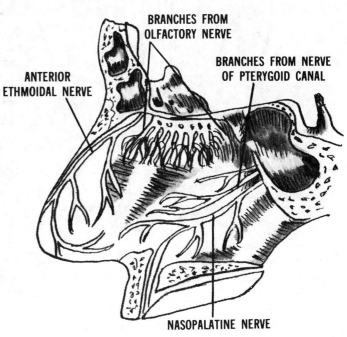

THE NOSE (Smell)

Diseases and Surgeries of the Nose and Mouth have been included in CHAPTER VII and CHAPTER VIII on the RESPIRATORY and GASTRO-INTESTINAL SYSTEMS respectively.

ANATOMY OF HEARING (The Ear)

The external ear, the middle ear or tympanic (a drum) (tim-PAN-ik) cavity, the internal ear or labyrinth (a maze) (LAB-i-rinth), and the acoustic (ah-KOOS-tik) center and acoustic nerve comprise the auditory apparatus.

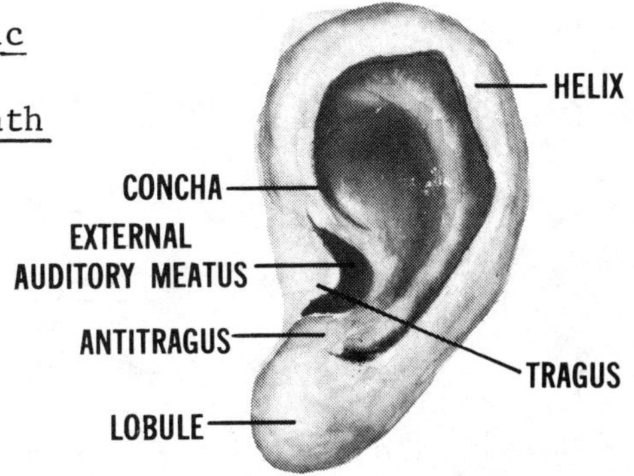

AURICLE (PINNA) OF EXTERNAL EAR

The external ear is composed of the aur/icle (ear little) (AW-re-kl) or pinna (wing) (PIN-nah), and the external auditory canal.

The membrana (membrane) (MEM-brah-nah)[1] tympani (drum) (TIM-pah-nī) or tympanic membrane (ear drum) separates the external auditory canal

1. Optional pronunciation mem-BRĀ-nah

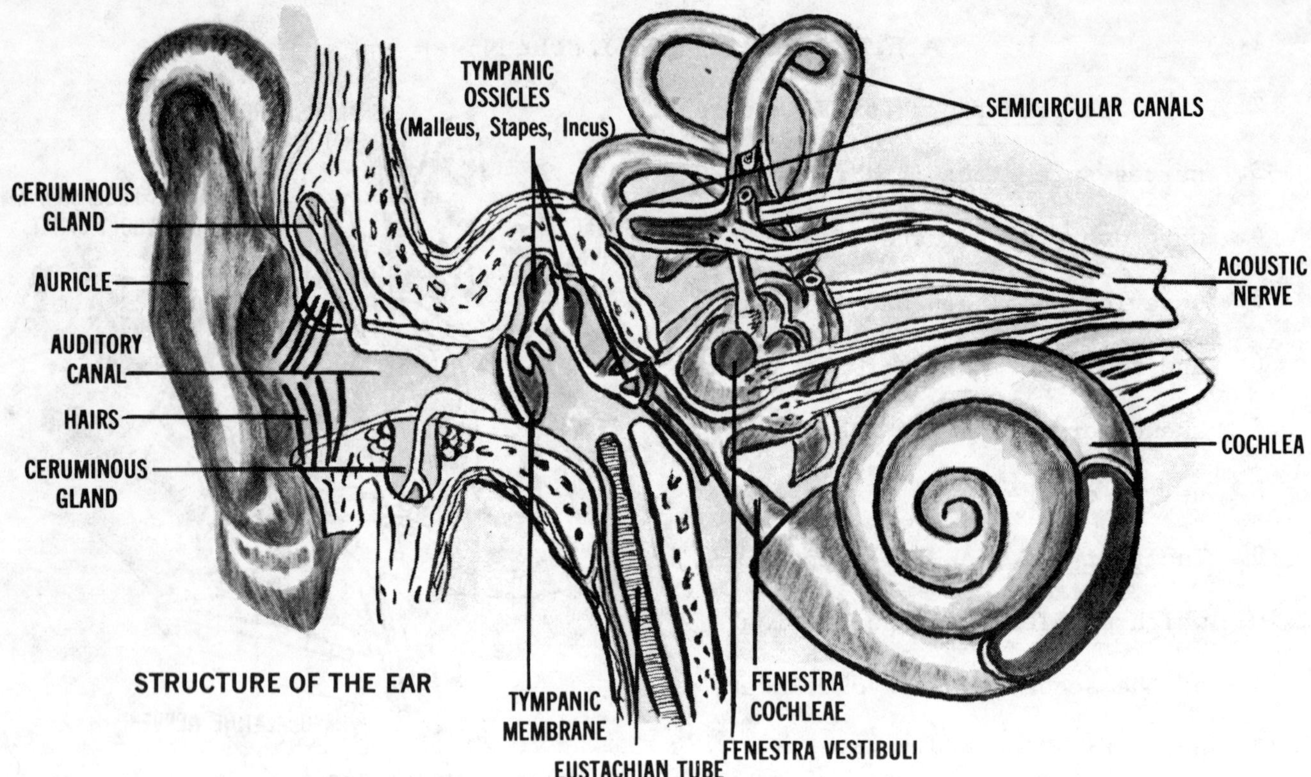

STRUCTURE OF THE EAR

from the tympanic cavity. This cavity, more commonly called the middle ear, is a small, irregular bony cavity located in the petrous *a rock* (PET-rus) portion of the temporal bone. The middle ear is separated from the internal ear by a very thin bony wall. In this wall are two small openings: the fenestra *window* (fe-NES-trah) vestibuli *vestibule* (ves-TIB-ū-lī), also known as the ovalis *oval* (ō-VĀ-lis), and and the fenestra cochleae *snail shell(plural)* (KŌK-lē-ē), also known as the rotunda *rotund, round* (rō-TUN-dah). In the cavity of the middle ear, which occurs from the tympanic membrane to the fenestra vestibuli, are three tiny, movable bones which have been named because of their shapes: the malleus (MAL-ē-us) or hammer, the incus (ING-kus) or anvil, and the stapes (STĀ-pēz) or stirrup.

The eustachian (ū-STĀ-kē-an)[1] (auditory) tube connects the cavity of the middle ear with the pharynx. Then, through the pharynx to the exterior. It is the eustachian tube which equalizes the pressure of the air on both sides of the tympanic membrane.

The terminations of the auditory nerve occur in the internal ear or the labyrinth. The internal ear is, therefore, an essential part of the organ of

1. Optional pronunciation ū-STĀ-shē-on; named after Bartolommeo Eustachio, Italian anatomist, 1520-1574.

hearing. It contains the osseous [bone] (OS-ē-us) labyrinth which is made up of a series of oddly shaped cavities. These cavities have been hollowed out of the petrous portion of the temporal bone and are named for their shape: the vestibule, the cochlea (KŌK-lē-ah) and the semi/circular [half] (sem-i-SER-kyōō-lar) canals.

The acoustic nerve is composed of two sets of fibers. One set is known as the cochlear (KŌK-lē-ar) division and the other set as the vestibular (ves-TIB-ū-lar) division. These divisions differ in function, origin and destination. The acoustic nerve is a sensory nerve.

DISEASES AND ANOMALIES OF THE EAR

Congenital malformations of the ear include poly/otia [many ear] (pol-ē-Ō-shē-ah) (the presence of more than one ear on one or both sides of the head), micr/otia [small] (mī-KRŌ-shē-ah) (undersize of the external ear), macr/otia [large] (mak-RŌ-shē-ah) (excessive size of the ears) and atresia [without opening] (ah-TRĒ-zē-ah) of the external canal.

The middle ear is subject to many types of infection due to its close relationship with the upper respiratory tract. Some of the more common middle ear infections are acute, subacute and chronic catarrhal [to flow down] (kah-TAHR-al) ot/itis [ear] (o-TĪ-tis) media [middle] (MĒ-dē-ah), acute and chronic otitis media, sup/purative [under pus] (SUP-ū-rah-tiv) otitis media.

Tumors of the middle and inner ear may be benign or malignant. True tumors occurring are ex/ostoses [out bone] (ek-sos-TŌ-sēz), chondr/oma [cartilage] (kon-DRŌ-mah) or en/chondr/oma (en-kon-DRŌ-mah), derm/oid (DER-moyd) cyst, nevus or hem/angi/oma [blood vessel] (hē-man-jē-Ō-mah), and fibr/oma [fiber] (fī-BRŌ-mah). Malignant tumors include carcin/oma [cancer] (kar-si-NŌ-mah), sarc/oma [flesh] (sar-KŌ-mah) and endothelioma.

Mast/oid/itis [breast] (mas-toyd-Ī-tis) is an inflammation of the lining of the mastoid cells. Because the relationship of these cells is so closely allied with the middle ear the resulting inflammation can involve the middle ear, the mastoid antrum and the mastoid cells. Mastoiditis may be acute or chronic.

The use of antibiotics has greatly lessened the dangers of this infection to a point where surgery is rarely necessary.

Chole/steat/oma *bile fat* (kō"les-tē-ah-TŌ-mah) and pseudo/chole/steat/oma *false* (sū"dō-kō"les-tē-ah-TŌ-mah) are pathologic changes associated with middle ear disease. They almost always require surgical intervention.

Oto/genic *ear to produce* (ō-tō-JEN-ik) mening/itis *membrane* (men-in-JĪ-tis) is a complication which may occur in both acute and chronic otitis media and is most frequent in children.

There are two types of labyrinth/itis (lab"i-rin-THĪ-tis): the etio/logic *cause study of* (ē-tē-ō-LOJ-ik) type which occurs in the course of a middle ear infection, as a result of trauma, or as a postoperative condition; the pathologic type which may be circum/scribed *around to write* (SER-kum-skrī-bd), dif/fuse *apart to pour* (de-FŪZ), or which may occur as a postoperative condition after radical operations of the middle ear.

The internal ear may be affected primarily by conditions usually of a non/sup/purative *not* (non-SUP-ū-rah-tiv) character such as from skull injuries, infections and general diseases of the bones and circulatory diseases or secondarily which is commonly due to some disease of the surroundings of the internal and middle ear.

Conduction hearing loss can be caused by impacted wax, infection of the middle ear, mastoiditis, and oto/scler/osis *hard* (ō"tō-skle-RŌ-sis). Infections of the middle ear and mastoiditis, if given prompt medical attention with antibiotic treatment, are no longer the threat they once were.

Otosclerosis is a progressive disease. It begins as a spongy growth near the base of the stapes -- one of the three small bones in the middle ear -- and, in time, the growth turns to bone, freezing the stapes into immobility. Stapedial *stapes* (stā-PĒ-dē-al) surgery has become virtually routine in the treatment of otosclerosis.

Diseases of the inner ear which can also produce a hearing loss are

Ménierè's[1] (man-YAIRZ) disease which also causes sudden attacks of vertigo [dizziness] (VUR-ti-gō)[2] and tinnitus [a tinkling] (tin-Ī-tus)[3], boilermaker's deafness, and presby/cusis [old hearing][4] (pres-bē-KŪ-sis). Drugs have helped in Ménierè's disease but the others are essentially uncurable at this time.

SURGERY OF THE EAR

Surgical correction of conditions of the ear is aimed at the improvement and preservation of hearing.

Oto/plasty [ear] (Ō-tō-plas-tē) is used for plastic repair of the ear following removal of malignant growths which may also necessitate amputation of the ear.

Oto/scopy (ō-TOS-kō-pē) is used for diagnostic purposes. It is also used for removal of foreign bodies or lesions in the external auditory canal.

Surgical treatment of otitis media is determined by the type of inflammation present. In cases of acute otitis media and acute chronic purulent otitis media (O.M.P.A.) either of these procedures may be performed:

1. myringo/tomy [drum] (mir-in-GOT-ō-mē) (incision of the ear drum and drainage of the middle ear),
2. paracentesis (puncture of the ear drum) and evacuation of fluid from the middle ear,
3. simple mastoid/ectomy (mas-toyd-EK-tō-mē) (the scooping out and obliterating of infected air cells) if the infection extends into the mastoid area.

Perforation (or hole) of the ear drum (tympanic membrane) is repaired by myringo/plasty (mi-RING-gō-plas-tē) which is a graft applied over the perforation.

The surgical treatment of chronic suppurative otitis media consists of various procedures whose use is determined by the extent of the infection. Some of these procedures are radical mastoidectomy, modified radical mastoidectomy and end/aural (end-AWR-al) mastoidectomy and, in certain cases,

1. Prosper Ménierè, French physician, 1799-1862
2. Optional pronunciation vur-TĪ-gō
3. Optional pronunciation TIN-i-tus
4. Optional spelling is presby/acusis (pres-bē-ah-KŪ-sis); it means "that lessening of the acuteness of hearing which characterizes old age."

ossic/ul/ectomy (bone, small) (os"i-kyo͞o-LEK-tō-mē).

Otosclerosis is the formation of spongy bone in the capsule of the labyrinth usually associated with conductive deafness with fixation of the stapes. Two of the surgical procedures used are stapes mobilization and the Lempert endaural fenestration operation.

Various types of mastoidectomy are performed for many conditions besides mastoiditis. Cases of mastoiditis which require surgery have decreased considerably with the advent of antibiotics. There are three common types of mastoidectomy procedures performed and the nature of the condition determines which will be used.

1. Simple mastoidectomy which does not extend beyond the mastoid process of the temporal bone. It consists of the removal of all cellular structure of the mastoid process without invasion of the middle ear or external auditory canal.
2. Modified radical mastoidectomy in which the posterior canal wall is removed but the oss/icles (bone, small) (OS-i-kls) and tympanic membrane are not disturbed.
3. Radical mastoidectomy which is performed only when the middle ear is so diseased that its tympanic membrane and ossicles have to be removed.

A more recent surgical procedure performed for old, chronic cases of mastoiditis is tympano/plasty (drum) (TIM-pah-nō-plas-tē) which consists of radical mastoidectomy and reconstruction of the middle ear.

Tumors of the external auditory canal include carcinoma, xanth/omat/osis (yellow, tumor) (zan-thō-mah-TŌ-sis), fibro/tuberc/ul/oma (node, small) (fī-brō-tū"ber-kyo͞o-LŌ-mah), granulo-tubercul/oma (grains) (gran"ū-lō-tū"ber-kyo͞o-LŌ-mah), cholesteatoma, benign aur/al (ear) (AWR-al) polyps. Treatment for malignant neoplasms consists of radical mastoidectomy with postoperative irradiation. Benign tumors are excised unless their growth and size involves important structures of the ear, in which case more radical procedures are performed.

Tumors of the middle ear are benign and malignant. Surgery consists of excision of benign tumors and radical dissection for malignant growths. The latter is usually done by radical mastoidectomy with postoperative irradiation.

Types of labyrinthitis include diffuse, diffuse serous, purulent, diffuse purulent latent and postoperative labyrinthitis. Surgical procedures may be simple or radical mastoidectomy with or without labyrinth/ectomy [a maze] (lab"i-rin-THEK-tō-mē).

ANATOMY OF SIGHT (The Eye)

The essential organs of the eye are the bulb of the eye or the eyeball, the optic nerve, and the visual center in the brain. The accessory organs of the visual apparatus are the eyebrows, eyelids, con/junctiva [together to join] (kon-junk-TĪ-vah), lacrimal [tear] (LAK-re-mal) apparatus, muscles of the eyeball, and the fascia [band] (FASH-ē-ah) bulbi [bulb] (BUL-bī).

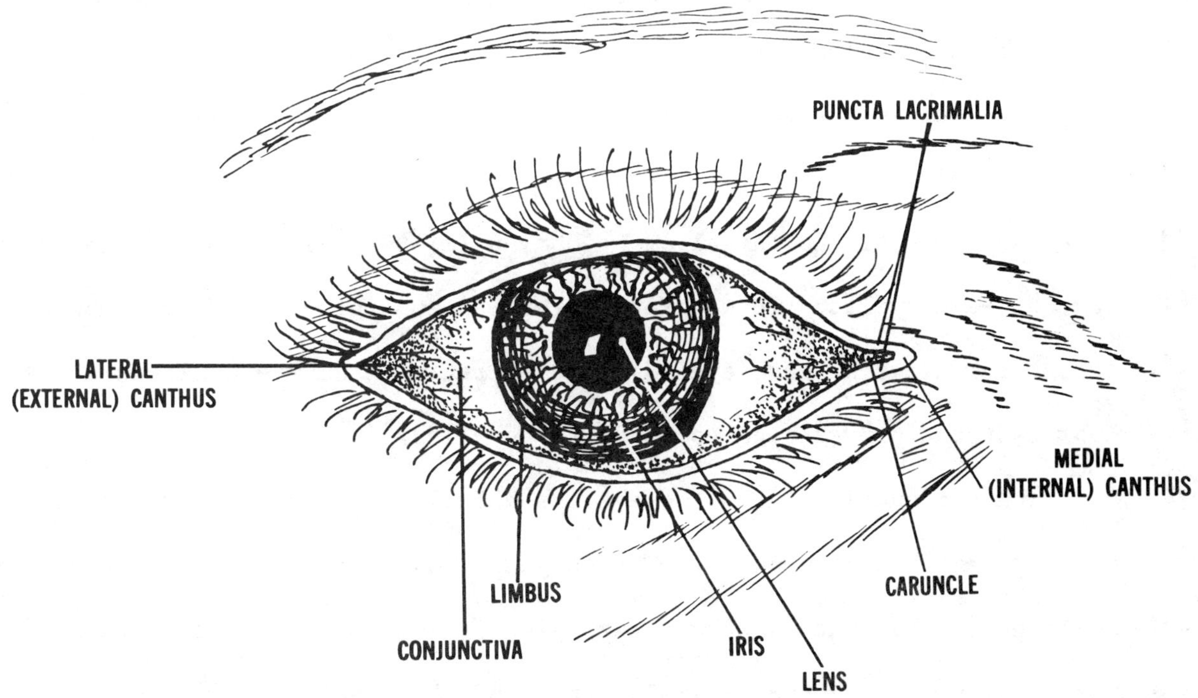

Front View of Right Eye

On the upper ridge of each of the orbits (also called the supraorbital margins) is a thick ridge of skin covered with short hairs. These two areas are known as the eyebrows. They protect the eyes to a certain degree from excessive brightness, dust, perspiration, etc.

The two movable folds of skin placed in front of each eye are known as eyelids or palpebrae [eyelid(plural)] (PAL-pe-brē). They are lined by a mucous membrane (the conjunctiva) which continues over the bulb of the eye. The dense and fibrous connective tissue, which forms the eyelids with the muscle fibers, is called tarsal [a broad flat surface] (TAHR-sal) plates. The levator [lifter] (le-VĀ-tor) palpebrae superioris [above] (sū-PĒ-rē-or-is), the "eye-opening" muscle, is a small muscle attached to the upper lid. The "eye-closing" muscle is called the orbicul/aris [a small disk] (or"bik-ū-LĀ-ris) oculi [eye] (OK-ū-lī). It is a sphincter muscle around both lids and its function is to close the eyelids.

The palpebral (PAL-pe-bral) fissure is the slit between the edges of the upper and lower lids. At each end of this fissure are angles which are called the lateral palpebral com/missure [together to join] (KOM-i-sūr) or the external canthus [corner of eye] (KAN-thus) and the medial palpebral commissure or the internal canthus.

The eyelashes are a row of short, thick hairs projecting from the margin of each eyelid.

The ducts of the tarsal or Meibomian[1] (mī-BŌ-mē-an) glands open on the edge of each eyelid. These glands are sebaceous glands and are embedded in the tarsal cartilage of each eyelid. The secretion from these glands serves as a lubricant and prevents adhesion of the eyelids.

The conjunctiva lines the eyelids and also continues from them to cover the forepart of the eyeball. The conjunctiva is continuous with the lining membrane of the ducts of the tarsal glands, the lacrimal ducts, lacrimal sac, naso/lacrimal [nose] (nā-zō-LAK-ri-mal) duct, and the nose.

The lacrimal gland, lacrimal ducts, lacrimal sac and nasolacrimal duct all

1. Heinrich Meibom, German anatomist, 1638-1700;"Meibomian" is usually capitalized, "meibomitis" is not.

comprise the lacrimal complex. Situated at the medial commissure is a small reddish body, the caruncula [small flesh] (kar-UNG-kyo͞o-lah) lacrim/alis (lak-ri-MĀ-lis) or caruncle (KAR-ung-kl). The whitish secretion which collects in this area is secreted by the caruncula as it contains sebaceous and sudoriferous glands. The tears are secreted by the lacrimal glands.

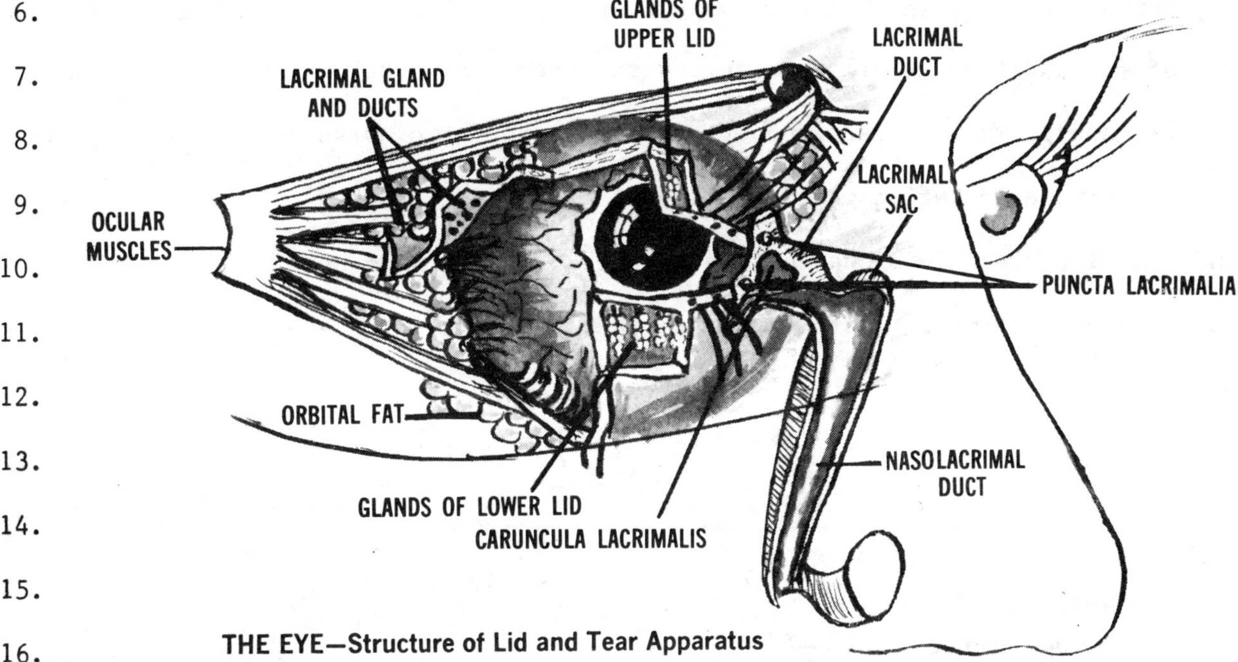

THE EYE—Structure of Lid and Tear Apparatus

There are two groups of eye muscles: the intrinsic muscles which are the ciliary [eyelash] (SIL-ē-ār-ē) muscle and the muscles of the iris; and the extrinsic muscles which hold the eyeball in place and control its movements. The extrinsic muscles include the four straight or recti [straight] (REK-tī) and the two oblique muscles. Squint or strabismus [a squinting] (strah-BIZ-mus) (cross-eye) results when these muscles, particularly the medial and lateral recti muscles, are unequal in length or strength. The equilibrium of the opposing muscles is upset and the eye turns in the direction of the stronger muscle.

The optic, oculo/motor [eye mover] (ok"ū-lō-MŌ-tor), trochlear [pulley] (TRŌ-klē-ar), ab/ducent [away from to draw] (ab-DŪ-sent), and ophthalmic [eye] (of-THAL-mik) cranial nerves all furnish in/nerv/ation [into nerve] (in-er-VĀ-shun) to the eye.

The orbits, the bony cavities in which the eyeballs are contained, are formed by seven bones: the frontal, malar [cheek] (MĀ-lar), maxilla [jawbone] (mak-SIL-ah), palatine [palate] (PAL-ah-tīn), ethm/oid [sieve] (ETH-moyd), sphen/oid [wedge] (SFĒ-noyd), and lacrimal. The funnel-shaped orbit contains the eyeball, muscles, nerves, vessels, lacrimal glands, fat, the fascia bulbi, and the fascia that holds these structures in place. The inner part of the orbit is lined with fibrous tissue and contains a fat pad which serves as a cushion for the eyeball. Between this pad of fat and the eyeball is a serous sac, the fascia bulbi (capsule of Tenon[1] [TĒ-non]), which covers the eyeball from the optic nerve to the ciliary region. It forms a socket in which the eyeball rotates.

The eyeball is shaped like a sphere. It is made up of three coats (tunics). From the outside inward they are 1. the fibrous, which forms the

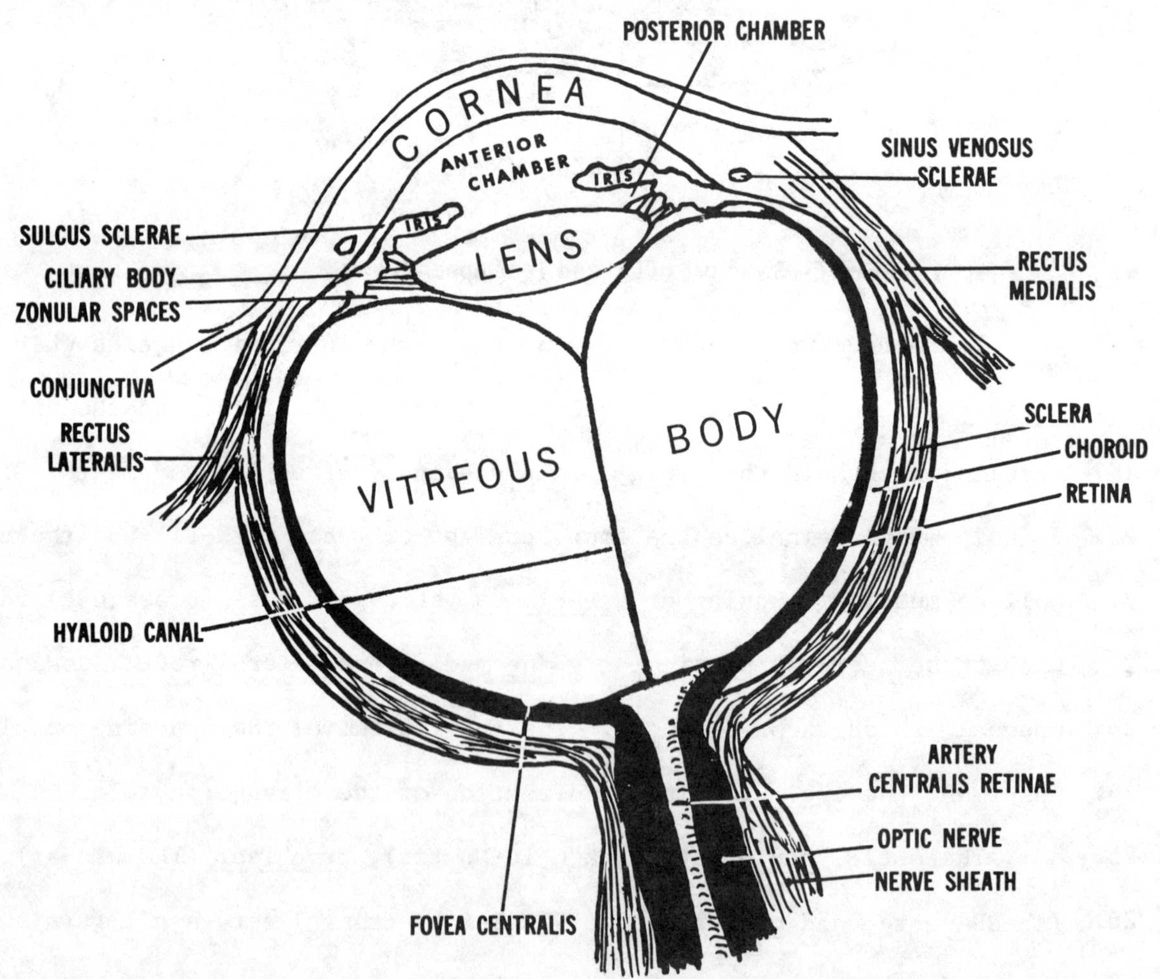

Schematic Cross Section of the Eye

1. Jacques René Tenon, French surgeon, 1724-1816

sclera [hard] (SKLĒ-rah) and cornea [horny] (KŌR-nē-ah); 2. the vascular, which forms the choroid [skinlike] (KŌ-royd), the ciliary body and the iris; and 3. the nervous, which makes up the retina [a net] (RET-i-nah). The eyeball contains three refracting media: 1. the aqueous [water] (Ā-kwē-us) humor, 2. the crystalline [crystal] (KRIS-tal-in) lens and capsule, and 3. the vitreous [glassy] (VIT-rē-us) body.

The posterior five-sixths of the eyeball is covered by the sclera, or white of the eye. The anterior sixth of the eyeball is covered by the cornea. Although the cornea is directly continuous with the sclera, it has no color. The cornea is perfectly transparent and has been called the "window of the eye."

The orbicularis cili/aris [eyelash,eyelid] (sil-ē-ĀR-is), the ciliary processes and the ciliaris muscle make up the ciliary body.

Suspended in the aqueous humor in front of the lens and behind the cornea is the iris, a circular, colored disc. In its middle is a circular hole, the pupil, through which light is admitted into the eye chamber. The number and size of the pigment bearing cells in the iris determine the color of the eye. The iris has two sets of muscles: the sphincter pupillae [girl] (PŪ-pil-ē), the contractor of the pupil; the dilator pupillae, the dilator of the pupil. These muscles are antagonistic in action.

The uvea [grape] (Ū-vē-ah) is the pigmentary layer of the eye and consists of the choroid, the ciliary body and the iris.

The iris regulates the amount of light which enters the eye. This function enables the eye to obtain clear images.

The retina is the inner, nervous coat of the eyeball. It is the perceptive structure of the eye formed by the expansion of the optic nerve. It covers the back part of the eye as far as the ora [margin,edge] (Ō-rah) serrata[1] [notched] (ser-RĀ-tah). The retina receives the images observed and transfers the impressions produced by them to the center of sight in the cortex of the cerebrum. In the center of the posterior part of the retina is the macula [spot] (MAK-ŭ-lah) lutea [yellow] (LŪ-tē-ah),

1. "ora serrata" is Latin for "zigzag border." The plural of "os" (the mouth) is "ora." However, the "ora" as shown here is the Latin singular of "an edge or margin." The plural is "orae."

the most sensitive portion of the retina. In the center of the macula lutea is a depression, the fovea [pit] (FŌ-vē-ah) centr/alis [center] (sen-TRĀ-lis) which is the center of direct vision. This is the part of the retina which is always turned toward the object looked at. About 1/10th inch inside the fovea is the point of entrance of the optic nerve and its central artery. At this point the retina is incomplete and forms the blind spot as this spot is insensitive to light.

The aqueous chamber is the space bounded by the cornea in the front and by the lens, suspensory ligament and ciliary body behind. It is filled with aqueous humor. The iris partially divides this space into an anterior and posterior chamber.

The transparent crystalline lens is the principal refracting medium of the eye. It has convex anterior and posterior surfaces and is enclosed in a capsule. It lies between the iris and the vitreous body.

Four-fifths of the bulb of the eye is filled by the vitreous body, a semi-fluid albuminous [white] (al-BYŌŌ-min-us) tissue, which is enclosed in a thin membrane, the hyal/oid [glass] (HĪ-ah-loyd) membrane. The spher/oidal [sphere] (sfē-ROYD-al) shape of the eyeball is maintained by the vitreous body. It also distends the greater part of the sclera, and supports the retina which lies upon its surface.

DISEASES AND ANOMALIES OF THE EYE

The normal eye is one in which at a distance of about twenty feet parallel rays of light focus on the retina when the eye is at rest. This is known as em/metr/opia [in measure eye] (em-i-TRŌ-pē-ah). A/metr/opia [lack] (am-i-TRŌ-pē-ah) is a condition in which any abnormality in the refractive surfaces or the shape of the eyeball prevents this focusing of parallel rays. Hyper/metr/opia [above] (hī"per-me-TRŌ-pē-ah) or farsightedness, myopia[1] [to shut,to wink] (mī-Ō-pē-ah) or nearsightedness, presby/opia [old] (pres-bē-Ō-pē-ah) (a defective condition of accomodation in which distant objects are seen distinctly, but near objects are indistinct) and a/stigmat/ism [without point] (ah-STIG-

1. The root is "myo" meaning "muscle." This in turn is what shuts the eye, hence the translation "to shut, to wink."

mah-tizm) (in which the curvature of the refracting surfaces is unequal) are the most common refractive troubles of the eye. The commonest form of astigmatism is that in which the vertical curvature is greater than the horizontal and is described as regular astigmatism "according to rule."

Glaucoma[1] (glaw-KŌ-mah), acute or chronic, is a disease characterized by increased tension or pressure within the eye. This increased intra/ocular (inside eye) (in-trah-OK-ū-lar) tension may be noted with the fingers but more accurately by means of a tono/meter (tone to measure) (tō-NOM-i-ter).

Cataract (to rush down) (KAT-ah-rakt) is the term applied to an opacity of the crystalline lens or of its capsule. The most common type occurs in adults past middle age, but it may occur in younger individuals as a result of trauma or disease. Occasionally it occurs at birth (congenital cataract).

Strabismus or squint is a condition in which one eye deviates from the object at which the person is looking (lay term is "cross-eyed"). It may result from paralysis of the nerves supplying the extra-ocular (outside) (eks-trah-OK-ū-lar) muscles, due to injury or disease. Double vision or dipl/opia (double) (dip-LŌ-pē-ah) may result from this condition. Con/vergent (together to incline) (kon-VER-jent) strabismus where the eyes turn inward is known as eso/tropia (inward to turn) (es-ō-TRŌ-pē-ah)[2] and di/vergent (apart) (dī-VER-jent) strabismus where the eyes turn outward is known as exo/tropia (out) (ek-sō-TRŌ-pē-ah).

Congenital anomalies (irregular) (ah-NOM-ah-lēz) of the eyelids include:

1. Coloboma (to mutilate) (kōl-ō-BŌ-mah) of the lid is a triangular notching of the lid margin with absence of the lashes and glands in the affected area.
2. Epi/canthus (ep-i-KAN-thus) is sometimes associated with ptosis and is usually bilateral. A perpendicular fold of the skin extends from the root of the nose to the inner end of the brow,

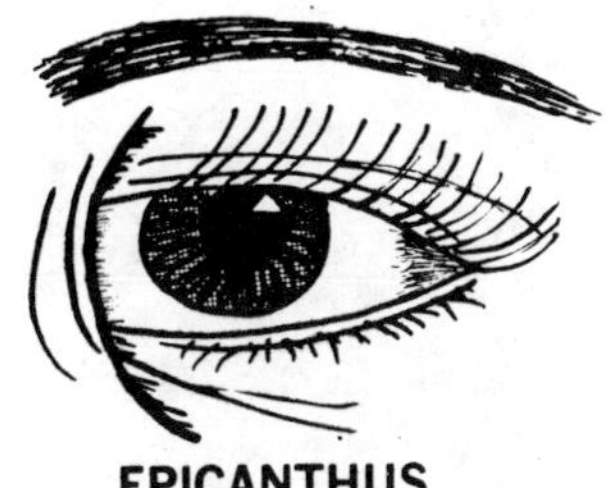
EPICANTHUS

1. Translates to "opacity of the crystalline lens" because of the "dull gray gleam" of the infected eye.
2. Optional pronunciation ē-sō-TRŌ-pē-ah

concealing the inner canthus and caruncle. In Mongolians it is a racial characteristic.

3. Dis/tich/iasis *apart row* (dis-te-KĪ-ah-sis) is a rare condition in which the Meibomian glands are replaced by a second row of lashes.

4. Ptosis is a drooping of the upper lid due to weakness or absence of the levator muscle. It is usually bilateral.

Common affections of the eyelids are:

1. Blephar/itis *eyelid* (blef-ah-RĪ-tis) ciliaris is a very common, chronic inflammation of the margin of the lids, in which reddening and thickening are usually associated with the formation of scales and crusts; it occurs under two forms: non-ulcerative or squamous *scale* (SKWĀ-mus) blepharitis and ulcerative blepharitis.

2. Hordeolum *barleycorn* (hor-DĒ-ō-lum) or stye (stī) is a circumscribed, acute inflammation at the edge of the lid, resulting from a staphylo/ *bunch of grapes* coccus (staf"i-lō-KOK-kus) infection of the glands of Zeiss[1] (tzīs) or of Moll[2], usually ending in sup/pur/ation *under pus* (sup-ū-RĀ-shun).

ACUTE HORDEOLUM

3. Chalazion *small lump or stye* (kah-LĀ-zē-on) is a quiet or inflammatory enlargement of one of the Meibomian glands resulting from stoppage of its duct and accompanied by involvement of surrounding tissues.

4. Meibom/itis (mī-bō-MĪ-tis) is a fairly common, chronic infection of some of the Meibomian glands. It causes red and swollen lid margins, sometimes with foamy secretion upon the conjunctiva. Pressure upon the Meibomian ducts expels glairy, yellowish fluid.

5. Trich/iasis *hair* (tri-KĪ-ah-sis) is an inversion of a varying number of lashes, so that they rub against the cornea. The margin of the lid has a normal position. The displacement affects only the lashes.

1. May also be spelled Zeis. Named for Edward Zeis, Dresden ophthalmologist, 1807-1868.
2. Jacob Antonius Moll, Dutch oculist, 1832-1914

6. En/tropion [in / to turn] (en-TRŌ-pē-on) is a rolling in of the margin of the lid and with it the lashes. Cicatricial [scar] (sik-ah-TRISH-al) entropion is due to cicatricial changes in the conjunctiva and tarsus, most commonly affecting the upper lid. Spastic [to draw] (SPAS-tik) entropion is due to spasm of the palpebral portion of the orbicularis muscle, almost always occurring in the lower lid.

7. Ectropion is an eversion of the lid with exposure of more or less con/junctival (kon-junk-TĪ-val) surface. It may affect the upper or lower lid, or both.

Benign tumors of the eyelids include xanth/elasma [yellow / plate] (zan-thel-AZ-mah), molluscum [soft] (mol-LUS-kum), papill/oma (pap-i-LŌ-mah), milium [millet seed] (MIL-ē-um), cyst and others.

Malignant tumors are commonly carcinoma, rarely sarcoma.

Injuries to the eyelids are ec/chym/osis [out / to pour] (ek-ē-MŌ-sis) ("black-eye"), insect bites, incised wounds, lacerated and contused wounds, burns and em/physema [in / to inflate] (em-fi-SĒ-mah).

Ankylo/blepharon [adhesion] (ang-kil-ō-BLEF-ah-ron) is the adhesion of the margins of the two lids.

Blepharo/phimosis [narrowing] (blef"ah-rō-fī-MŌ-sis) is an apparent contraction of the palpebral fissure at its outer canthus due to this angle being covered and hidden by a vertical fold of skin.

Blepharo/chalasis [relaxation] (blef"ah-rō-kah-LĀ-sis)[1], occasionally occurring in elderly persons, is a redundancy of the skin of the upper lid, causing a fold to hang down over the lid margin.

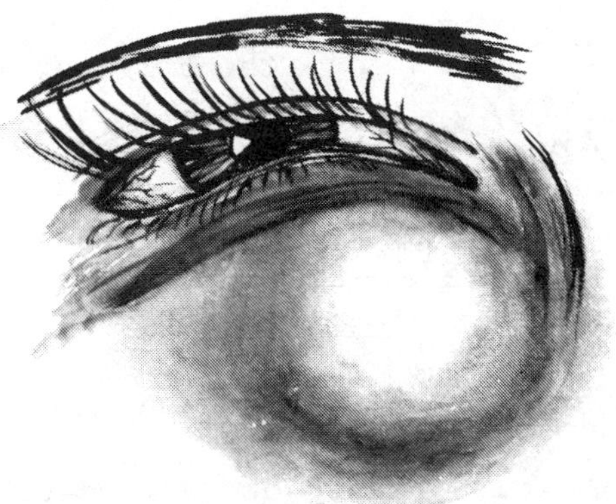
DACRYOCYSTITIS

Sym/blepharon [together] (sim-BLEF-ah-ron) is a cicatricial attachment between the conjunctiva

1. Optional pronunciation blef"ah-rō-KAL-as-is

of the lid and the eyeball.

Inflammation of the lacrimal sac results in a condition known as dacryo/ *tear* cyst/itis *sac* (dak"rē-ō-sis-TĪ-tis).

SURGERY OF THE EYE AND EYELIDS

Strabismus, also known as crossed or wandering eyes, is caused by an extra-ocular muscle or muscles being too strong or too weak. There are three types of strabismus: 1. para/lytic *beyond loosening* (par-ah-LIT-ik), 2. kinetic *motion* (ki-NET-ik) and 3. con/comit-ant *together companion* (kon-KOM-i-tant) or comitant. Either type may be convergent (esotropia) or divergent (exotropia). If the muscle is too strong either of three procedures may be employed.

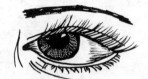

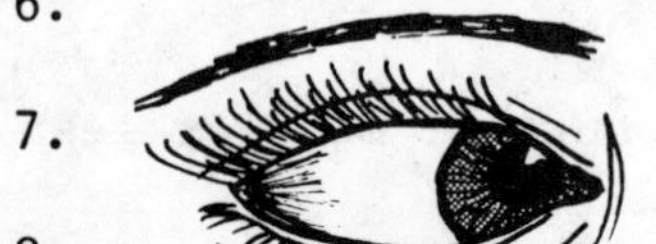

CONVERGENT STRABISMUS

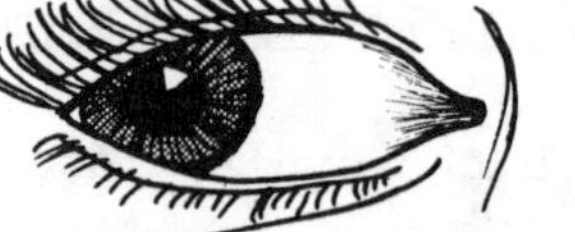

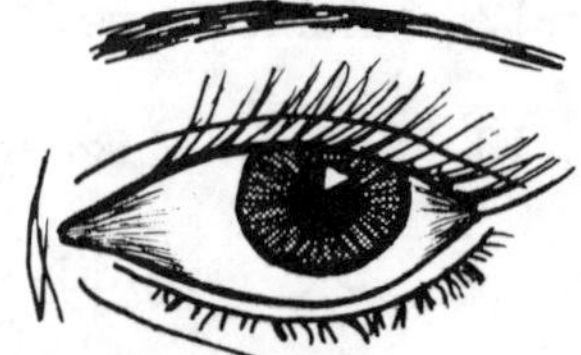

DIVERGENT STRABISMUS

1. teno/tomy *tight stretched band* (ten-OT-ō-mē) (cutting the tendon attachment partially or completely),
2. recession (moving the muscle attachment back on the eyeball),
3. my/ectomy *muscle* (mī-EK-tō-mē) (cutting the muscle partially or completely).

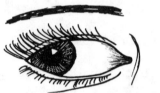

If the muscle is too weak there are two procedures which may be performed to strengthen it.

1. resection (removal of a piece of the muscle and reattachment to the original insertion which draws it tighter and thus makes it stronger),
2. advancement (moving the muscle attachment forward on the eyeball).

Pterygium *wing* (te-RIJ-ē-um) is a fan-shaped growth of conjunctiva and blood vessels with the apex of the fan progressing slowly toward the cornea. It is scraped or excised from the corneal surface. Sometimes a corneal transplant is necessary.

Corneal grafting or kerato/plasty *cornea* (KER-ah-tō-plas-tē), either partial or full thickness, is performed to restore sight in eyes whose impaired vision is caused by opacity of the cornea when the rest of the eye and optic nerve are normal. Keratoplasty is also performed for kerato/conus *cone* (ker"ah-tō-KŌ-nus) and corneal scars.

PTERYGIUM

Para/centesis *beyond puncture* (par"ah-sen-TĒ-sis) of the cornea (kerato/centesis [ker"ah-tō-sen-TĒ-sis]) or removal of aqueous fluid is employed for diagnostic and treatment purposes. In diagnosis it is used to obtain specimens of secretion for smear culture for sensitivity of the infection and for biopsy for microscopic study for tumor. As a treatment it is done to relieve pus infection and relieve the pressure of glaucoma.

Glaucoma is a symptomatic condition characterized by increased intraocular pressure. Surgical procedures performed depend on the type and degree of glaucoma encountered. Several procedures are employed to provide an exit channel for the escape of the internal ocular fluid.

1. irid/ectomy *iris* (i-rid-EK-tō-mē) (excision of the iris) which opens more area for the release of the fluid;
2. irid/en/cleisis *in to lock,to close* (ir"i-den-KLĪ-sis) in which a tunnel of iris is enclosed under the conjunctiva;
3. cyclo/dia/lysis *circle through* (sī"klō-dī-AL-i-sis) in which a channel is opened by a cleavage at the base of the iris to permit the escape of the fluid;
4. trephin/ation *a boring* (tref-i-NĀ-shun) in which a round hole is made in the sclera for the release of the fluid. Other procedures in which openings are made in the sclera are scler/ectomy *hard* (skle-REK-tō-mē) and sclero/tomy (skle-ROT-ō-mē).

Cyclo/dia/thermy *heat* (sī-klō-DĪ-ah-ther-mē) is a procedure which cuts down the aqueous production by inducing atrophy of the ciliary body (the source of the fluid) through the use of <u>dia/thermy</u> (DĪ-ah-ther-mē).

A cataract is an opacity of the crystalline lens or of its capsule. Senile cataracts are the most common type. Surgical procedures consist of:

1. <u>dis/cission</u> *apart to cut* (dis-SIZH-un), or needling, to rupture the lens contents and allow its absorption by the eye fluids;
2. linear extraction which is the removal of all the lens except its capsule. Another similar procedure is extracapsular extraction.
3. intracapsular extraction which is the removal of the entire lens in its capsule. It is performed with the aid of an enzyme <u>alpha</u> *Greek "A"* <u>chymo/trypsin</u> *juice a rubbing*[1] (AL-fah kī"mō-TRIP-sin) and is performed on adults.

Discission and linear extraction are used on patients from 6 months of age to adulthood.

The vitreous humor which lies between the retina and the lens is a semi-liquid, transparent gel. It may become cloudy from old infections, inflammation or hemorrhage in which case it is possible to transplant the vitreous from a donor eye. As yet this procedure is rarely done.

Diathermy or <u>cryo</u> *cold* (KRĪ-ō) application is performed on the retina as follows:

1. for detachment (to close tears or holes or to tack the retina in place),
2. to destroy abnormal blood vessel formations or neoplasms such as angiomas,
3. <u>photo/coagulation</u> *light clotting* (fō-tō-kō-ag-ū-LĀ-shun) (use of the <u>laser</u>[2] [LĀ-ser] beam) is another procedure used on the retina.

<u>E/nucle/ation</u> *out kernel* (ē-nū-klē-Ā-shun) (removal of the eyeball) is indicated for the following conditions: malignant tumors of the eyeball, blind painful glaucoma and hopeless infections.

1. Translation "a rubbing" refers to the process used in the preparation of this drug.
2. "laser" has been coined from the first letters of light amplification by stimulated emission of radiation.

Ex/enter/ation *out intestine* (eks-en-ter-Ā-shun) of the orbit (removal of all of the contents of the orbit) is performed for advanced tumors, usually malignant.

E/viscer/ation *out organ* (ē-vis-er-Ā-shun) is the removal of the contents of the eyeball but leaving the sclera. It is performed only in eyes which have been lost by infection such as from pan/ophthalm/itis *all eye* (pan"of-thal-MĪ-tis).

Trichiasis (an eversion of a various number of eyelashes) is surgically treated by e/pil/ation *out hair* (ep-i-LĀ-shun) (removal) of the misdirected eyelashes or electrocoagulation (diathermy).

Entropion (rolling in of the lid) occurs in two forms: spastic and cicatricial. Cantho/plasty *corner of eye* (KAN-thō-plas-tē), permanent or temporary, is performed for the spastic type and Burow's[1] (BŌŌ-rovz) operation and the Jaesche-Arlt[1] (jāsh-arlt) operation are performed for the cicatricial type.

Ectropion (rolling out of the lid) occurs in several forms: the chief ones are spastic, cicatricial, senile and paralytic. Various types of surgical procedures are used including lateral tarso/rrhaphy *a broad flat surface* (tahr-SŌR-ah-fē), the V-Y operation and blepharoplasty.

Symblepharon is the condition of adhesion of the lid to the globe. Surgical procedure consists of lysis *loosening* (LĪ-sis) of adhesions and sometimes mucous membrane grafting.

Ankyloblepharon is adhesion of the margins of the two lids. It is corrected by blepharoplasty with mucous membrane transplant.

Blepharophimosis is the condition in which the palpebral fissure appears to be contracted at the outer canthus. Canthoplasty is performed.

Ptosis is the drooping of the upper lid usually due to paralysis or defective development of the levator palpebrae superioris muscle. Surgeries consist of various methods of either recession of the levator muscles or the use of other muscles to lift the lid. Blepharoplasty may be required in some cases.

1. Oculists from Vienna, Austria of the early eighteen hundreds.

Dacryo/cyst/ectomy [tear, sac] (dak"rē-ō-sis-TEK-tō-mē) (the removal of the lacrimal sac) and dacryo/cysto/rhino/stomy [nose] (dak"rē-ō-sis-tō-rī-NOS-tō-mē) (creation of a new opening between the tear sac and the nose) are performed for chronic dacryocystitis (an inflammation of the lacrimal sac usually due to an obstruction of the nasal duct). Incision and drainage (I & D) is performed in cases of acute dacryocystitis.

The majority of orbital tumors require surgical treatment. Three procedures may be performed depending on the type, size and location of the tumors: 1. anterior orbito/tomy [track] (or-bi-TOT-ō-mē), 2. lateral orbitotomy or 3. exenteration of the orbit.

INDEX
CHAPTER X

PAGE	LINE	
253	21	Thiersch
263	2	tinnitus
271	8	tonometer
275	24	trephination
272	26	trichiasis
259	14	trigeminal
267	25	trochlear
259	19	tympanic
264	22	tympanoplasty
269	19	uvea
258	13	vallate
255	8	vascularizes
263	1	vertigo
248	22	vesicle
261	7	vestibular
260	17	vestibuli
250	19	vitiligo
269	5	vitreous
249	28	vulgaris
249	1	wheal
273	10	xanthelasma
257	17	xanthomata
264	24	xanthomatosis
272	17	Zeiss

APPENDIX

CASE HISTORY AND INVENTORY BY SYSTEMS

Case histories are written on every patient. The extent of the history is dependent upon the illness, the required treatment and whether admittance to a hospital for surgery or medical treatment will be required.

The fundamentals of case histories are similar. However, each medical specialty has specific symptoms and examination procedures. The following material in no way attempts to cover all symptoms encountered or the examinations performed.

The first section is the basic case history and is concerned with material which must be elicited from the patient.

The second section is known by various titles: "Review of Systems (ROS)," "Inventory by Systems" or "Physical Examination." This section concerns the patient's physical condition which includes subjective symptoms (the patient's description of the complaint, for example, "I've had a sore throat for the past three days.") and the objective symptoms (what the doctor sees or observes, for example, that the patient's throat is red and inflamed). It is the compilation of the material in this second section which helps the doctor arrive at a diagnosis or diagnoses in order to prescribe treatment.

Abbreviations used appear beside all words which are routinely abbreviated.

The medical term for Case History is <u>anamnesis</u> (an-am-NĒ-sis) which means "the information obtained concerning the patient, his family, his previous experiences, and sensations." The translation of the term is "a recalling."

FUNDAMENTALS OF A CASE HISTORY

Chief Complaint (CC)

Present Illness (PI) (elaboration of chief complaint)

Past History (PH)
- Infectious diseases:
  - exanthems (eruptive diseases): measles (rubella, rubeola), chickenpox (varicella), smallpox (variola), meningitis, scarlet fever (scarlatina)
  - non-exanthems: mumps, whooping cough, typhoid fever, malaria, pneumonia, pleurisy
- Operations:
  - tonsillectomy and adenoidectomy (T&A), appendectomy, cholecystectomy, hysterectomy, prostatectomy, etc.
- Onset of menses or menarche (in examination of the female) and the last menstrual period (LMP)
- Injuries:

Family History (FH)
- mother and father living and well (M & F l & w)
- siblings (brothers and sisters)

Marital History (MH)
para 3 - 1 - 2 (3 pregnancies, 1 abortion, 2 children living and well)

Social History (SH)
occupation, habits, diet, alcohol, drugs, etc.

REVIEW OF SYSTEMS (ROS), INVENTORY BY SYSTEMS, PHYSICAL EXAMINATION (PE or PX)

HEAD
exostosis (a bony growth projecting outward)

EYES
amblyopia (dimness of vision)
scotoma (blind or partially blind area in visual field)
diplopia (double vision)
exophthalmos (bulging of eyes)
enophthalmos (eyes set back in head)
ptosis (drooping of eyelids)
extraocular movements (EOM)
pupils round, regular and equal; react to light and accommodation
(pupils r.r.e.; react to l & a)
ophthalmic examination
disc A/V (arteriovenous ratio)
papilledema (edema of optic papilla [checked disc])

EAR
tinnitus (ringing in the ears)
otorrhea (discharge from the ear)
otalgia (pain in the ear)
otitis media (middle ear infection)
mastoiditis (inflammation of the mastoid cells)
otoscopic (inspection of the ear by an instrument)

NOSE
epistaxis (nose bleed)
coryza (cold in the head)
rhinitis (inflammation of the mucous membrane of the nose)

MOUTH (some of these symptoms relate to disturbances in other areas of the body)
dysphonia (difficulty in speaking)
dysarthria (imperfect utterance due to a disorder in the nervous system)
polydipsia (excessive thirst)
polyphagia (excessive eating)
dysphagia (difficulty in swallowing)
herpes (fever blisters on the lips)
gingivitis (inflammation of the gums)
pyorrhea alveolaris (purulent inflammation of dental periosteum)

NECK
swelling as in goiter or of the glands
masses
tenderness
rigidity
trachea -- should be in the midline
tracheal tug -- tug against hand during examination

CARDIORESPIRATORY (C-R) (Heart and Lungs)(Cardiac and Chest Examination)

CHEST

clear to P & A (percussion and auscultation)
sputum -- bloody (blood thoroughly mixed with sputum in type III pneumonia)
prune juice (in pneumonia)
frothy (with pulmonary edema in heart failure)
rusty (stained with blood or blood pigments)
hemoptysis (spitting up blood)
night sweats (primarily in tuberculosis)
eupnea (normal breathing)
dyspnea (difficult breathing)
tachypnea (rapid breathing)
bradypnea (abnormal slowness of breathing)
orthopnea (inability to breath except in upright position)
Cheyne-Stokes (periodic breathing)
apnea (transient cessation of breathing)
breath sounds:
vesicular - normal
tubular - high pitched sounds
bronchovesicular - between tubular and vesicular răles - abnormal - a popping sound when air sacs of lung pop open
rhonchi - dry coarse răle due to partial obstruction
vocal fremitus - a thrill caused by speaking which can be heard in auscultation of the chest
supraclavicular (above the clavicle)
infraclavicular (below the clavicle)
point of maximum impulse (P.M.I.)
palpation (act of feeling with the hand)
percussion (thumping on chest with finger to determine size and position of heart and lungs by the vibrations of normal resonance -- over a solid organ there is no resonance)
auscultation (listening for sounds within the body usually with a stethoscope)
thrill (feels like purring of a cat sounds)
tactile fremitus (the vibrations which can be felt while the patient is speaking)

HEART

embolism (embolus) (a clot breaks off and travels to another organ)
infarction (infarct) (embolus produces an infarct - an area of dead and scarred tissue)
A-2 (aortic second sound)
P-2 (pulmonic second sound)
murmurs (a gentle blowing auscultatory sound present with leakage of a heart valve from stenosis or from the narrowing or stricture of a duct or canal)
insufficiency (valves open when they should be closed)
midclavicular line (MCL)
left border cardiac dullness (LBCD)(should be inside MCL)
valves of the heart: tricuspid, pulmonic, mitral, aortic
systole (interval of heart's contraction)
diastole (interval of heart's relaxation)
rhythm (the beat of the heart)

GASTRO-INTESTINAL (G-I)

icterus or jaundice (yellow discoloration of skin and mucous membrane)
anoxeria (lack or loss of appetite)
nausea or vomiting
flatus (gas or air in the G-I tract)
borborygmus (noise made by flatus in the bowels)
flatulence (distension of stomach or intestines with air or gas)
hematemesis (vomiting of blood)
coffee grounds vomitus (dark partially digested blood)
tarry stools (result of pathology in G-I tract)
clay colored stools (result of pathology in bile ducts)

ABDOMEN

scaphoid (shaped like a boat)
round
obese
palpate for liver, kidneys and spleen (LKS)
palpate for masses, tenderness, rigidity
rebound (outbreak of fresh reflex activity following withdrawal of stimulus)
ascites (accumulation of a clear yellow fluid in the peritoneal cavity)
surgical scars
peristalsis (the worm-like movement of the intestines)
suprapubic tenderness
costovertebral angle (CVA)(the angle where the ribs join the vertebrae. An important area for kidney symptoms.)
hernia: inguinal, femoral, umbilical, diaphragmatic (located by x-ray)

NEUROMUSCULAR (NM) (A neurological history is not taken in full unless the patient has a neurological complaint, symptom or history of a neurological condition.)

vertigo (dizziness)
convulsions
syncope (fainting)
pain in back or limbs
neurological (reflexes) (a reflex test is the striking of a tendon to determine if the nerves are intact with the spinal cord)
biceps (muscles in upper arm)
triceps (muscles in back of upper arm)
knee jerk (KJ)
ankle jerk (AJ)
superficial abdominal wall
Hoffman's sign (digital)
Babinski's sign (Achilles tendon)
Kernig's sign (lower extremities) (if positive a sign of meningitis)
Romberg's sign (swaying of body when standing with feet close together and the eyes closed - a sign of locomotor ataxia)
ankle clonus (a series of convulsive movements of the ankle induced by a sudden pushing up of the foot while the leg is extended)
reflexes are given as + or 1+, ++ or 2+ (the above reflexes are a very small portion of those which are present in the body)
reaction (whether a patient is cooperative, stuporous, has disturbances in speech [sing-song or explosive, slurring due to disturbance of the brain])

extremities

anesthesia (loss of feeling or sensation)
analgesia (absence of sensibility to pain)
paresthesia (abnormal sensation as burning, prickling, etc.)

EXTREMITIES

- varix (varices) (dilated [varicose] veins)
- edema (abnormally large amounts of fluid in the intercellular tissue spaces)
- tremor (an involuntary trembling or quivering)

GENITO-URINARY (G-U)

- dysuria (difficult, painful urination or micturition, terminal dysuria, strangury)
- nocturia (excessive urination at night)
- hematuria (the passage of blood in the urine)
- pyuria (presence of pus in the urine)
- oliguria (deficient secretion of urine)
- polyuria (excessive secretion and discharge of urine)
- enuresis (involuntary discharge of urine)
- nocturnal enuresis (that which occurs at night and during sleep)
- incontinence (inability to control the discharge of urine)
- stress incontinence (involuntary discharge of urine caused by sneezing, coughing, etc.)
- venereal disease (gonorrhea [gc], syphilis [lues], lymphogranuloma venereum, granuloma inguinale)

SKIN

- moist, warm or dry
- jaundiced
- cyanosis (blueness of skin, nails, etc.)

GLANDULAR

- cervical (neck)
- epitrochlear (bend of elbow)
- axillary (arm pit)
- inguinal (groin)

SKELETAL

- spine
  - scoliosis (lateral curvature)
  - kyphosis (increase in dorsal curvature [humpback])
  - lordosis (increase in lumbosacral arch anterior curvature [sway back])

ROUTINE PHYSICAL EXAMINATION:

- temperature (T)
- pulse (P)
- respiration (R)
- blood pressure (BP)
- general appearance (GA)
- well developed (wd)
- well nourished (wn)

ROUTINE LABORATORY REPORTS

An important part in the care of a patient is the analysis of the patient's blood and urine. Both of these liquid media are capable of indicating the presence or absence of certain diseases and conditions. As a means of eliminating probable diseases or of ascertaining their presence these laboratory tests have become a routine procedure for every patient from office visit to hospital admission.

There are many other laboratory tests performed in addition to those listed in the following pages. However, these are specific tests to determine specific conditions and are not used routinely. Only the routine tests are given here to follow the format of this book which deals with the basics only.

Normal values have not been included in the tests because these values depend on the type of test performed in each laboratory. The method of measurement is, however, listed beside each item in addition to the abbreviation for that particular test. These abbreviations are also included in the "Abbreviations for Patient Care."

BLOOD CHEMISTRY

	Method of Measurement
Glucose WB. S.P. (Fasting/Non-Fasting/ 2 hrs. after eating) (also called Glucose Tolerance)	mg%
Carbon Dioxide (CO_2)	mEq/L
Chloride (Cl)	mEq/L
Sodium (Na)	mEq/L
Potassium (K)	mEq/L
Calcium (Ca)	mg%
Phosphorus (P)	mg%
Bilirubin (bili)	Direct/Total
Blood Urea Nitrogen (BUN)	mg%
Creatinine	mg%
Total Protein A/G Ratio (albumin/globulin)	gms%
Protein Bound Iodine (PBI)	mcg%
Uric Acid	mg%
Thyroxine (T_4 or T4)	mcg%
Thymol Turbidity	units
Prothrombin	seconds/% of activity
Transaminase	
SGOT (Serum Glutamic Oxalacetic Transaminase)	units
SGPT (Serum Glutamic Pyruvic Transaminase)	units
CPK (Creatine Phosphokinase)	units
L.D.H. or LDH (Lactic Dehydrogenase)	units
Amylase	units
Lipase	units
Alkaline Phosphatase (alk.p'tase)	Bod. units*
Acid Phosphatase (acid p'tase)	Bod. units
Cholesterol (chol.)	mg%

*Bodansky units

HEMATOLOGY

	Method of Measurement
Complete Blood Count (CBC)	
Red Blood Cells (RBC)	mil/cmm or /cu.mm
Hemoglobin (Hb or Hgb)	gms or gms%
Hematocrit	Vol.%
Mean Corpuscular Hemoglobin Count (MCHC)	%
White Blood Cells (WBC)	/cmm or /cu.mm
Polymorphonuclear (Poly or Polys)	%
Stab neutrophile (has unsegmented nucleus) (written as Stab)	%
Segmented neutrophile (Segs)	%
Lymphocyte (Lymph)	%
Monocyte (Mono)	%
Eosinophile (Eos)	%
Basophile (Baso)	%
Sedimentation Rate (Sed. Rate)	/mm hr.
Platelets	/cmm or /cu.mm
Reticulocytes	%
Bleeding Time	min.
Capillary Coagulation Time (Coag. Time)	min.
Lee-White Clotting Time (Clot. Time)	min.

URINALYSIS

Physical Appearance: Clear Hazy Cloudy
Color: Yellow Straw Amber
Volume: cc
Specific Gravity (Sp.Gr.): 1.0
Reaction: pH (acidity)
Protein (albumin) (alb.)
Sugar
Ketones
Microscopic:

RBC /hpf (per high powered field)
WBC /hpf
Epith (epithelial cells) /hpf

Bacteria	many	few	none
Mucous threads	many	few	none
Urates (crystals)	many	few	none
Phosphates	many	few	none

Casts

Hyaline	/hpf or	/lpf (per low powered field)
Fine Granules (gran.)	/hpf or	/lpf
Coarse Granules (gran.)	/hpf or	/lpf
Broad (casts)	/hpf or	/lpf

SPECIAL URINE CHEMISTRY TESTS

Porphyrin	negative or positive (neg. or pos.)
Porphobilinogen	" "
Uroporphyrin	" "
Coproporphyrin	" "
Urobilinogen	mg/24 hrs.
Bile	negative or positive
Calcium	gm/24 hrs.
Occult (altered) Blood	
Bence-Jones Protein	

ABBREVIATIONS FOR PATIENT CARE

Abbreviations of routine medical terms prove invaluable as time is such an important factor in the care of the patient and because complete information is absolutely necessary for everyone concerned in the care of the patient.

While the abbreviations are quite standard there is a certain amount of disagreement regarding the use of capital letters or lower case letters, whether or not to put periods between the capital letters and just how much to include in the abbreviation of the word or phrase. These conflicts are not of major importance as the personnel working with doctors quickly learn how each doctor writes those particular abbreviations.

This list is only a portion of the number of abbreviations used in medicine. Each speciality has so many of its own and as new ones are constantly being added it was decided to give the more basic, routine abbreviations to avoid confusion. The majority of abbreviations can be found in any of the medical dictionaries if there is any question about those not occurring in this list.

ABBREVIATION	ENGLISH TRANSLATION
A	
A-2	aortic second sound
AJ	ankle jerk
AP	anteroposterior
AP & Lat	anteroposterior and lateral
AB	abortion
accom.	accommodation
acid p'tase	acid phosphatase
adm.	admission
alb.	albumin
alk. p'tase	alkaline phosphatase
as tol.	as tolerated
A/V	arteriovenous ratio
B	
B.	bacillus
Ba	barium
Ba. enema	barium enema
B.B.A.	born before arrival
BJ	biceps jerk
BM	bowel movement
B.O.A.	born on arrival
B.P. or BP	blood pressure
B.P.H. or BPH	benign prostatic hypertrophy
B.R.P.	bathroom privileges
B.S.P.	bromosulphalein
BUN	blood urea nitrogen
baso	basophile
bili	bilirubin
bl. cult.	blood culture
br. sounds or B.S.	breath sounds
B & S	Bartholin's and Skene's glands
C	
CA or Ca	carcinoma
CBC	complete blood count
CC	chief complaint
chol.	cholesterol
chol. est.	cholesterol esters
C.I.	color index
CNS	central nervous system
CO_2	carbon dioxide
C-R	cardiorespiratory
CSF	cerebrospinal fluid
CVA	costovertebral angle or cerebrovascular accident

ABBREVIATION	ENGLISH TRANSLATION
D	
d.c.	discontinue
D & C	dilatation and curettage
diag.	diagnosis
disch.	discharge
DL	danger list
DOA	dead on arrival
E	
ECG	electrocardiogram
EEG	electroencephalogram
EMG	electromyogram
ENT	ears, nose and throat
EOM	extraocular movement
F	
fetal positions and presentations	
LOA	left occiput anterior
LOT	left occiput transverse
LOP	left occiput posterior
ROA	right occiput anterior
ROT	right occiput transverse
ROP	right occiput posterior
LSA(RSA)	left(right)sacrum anterior
LST(RST)	" " " transverse
LSP(RSP)	" " " posterior
LFA(RFA)	" " frontoanterior
LFT(RFT)	" " frontotransverse
LFP(RFP)	" " frontoposterior
LMA(RMA)	" " mentoanterior
LMT(RMT)	" " mentotransverse
LMP(RMP)	" " mentoposterior
FH	family history
F.H.S. or f.h.s.	fetal heart sounds
F.H.T.	fetal heart tone
for. body	foreign body
F.P.	flat plate
fract.	fracture

ABBREVIATION	ENGLISH TRANSLATION
G	
GA	general appearance
GB	gall baldder
gc or GC	gonorrhea
G-I	gastro-intestinal
gm%	grams per 100 milliliters of serum or blood as specified
Gold sol.	colloidal gold curve
Grav.I, Grav.II	primigravida, secundigravida, etc.
H	
HCl	hydrochloric acid
H.C.V.D.	hypertensive cardiovascular disease
Hct.	hematocrit
Hgb or Hb	hemoglobin
/hpf	per high powered field
H_2O	water
H.V.D.	hypertensive vascular disease
I	
I & D	incision and drainage
IM	intramuscular
in extremis	at the point of death
I & O	intake and output
IQ	intelligence quotient
IV	intravenous
IVP	intravenous pyelogram
K	
KJ	knee jerk
KUB	kidney, ureter, bladder
L	
lat.	lateral
LBCD	left border cardiac dullness
LCM	left costal margin
LKS	liver, kidney, spleen
LLQ (abdomen)	left lower quadrant
LUQ "	left upper quadrant

ABBREVIATION	ENGLISH TRANSLATION
LMP	last menstrual period
LP	lumbar puncture
l & w	living and well
lymphs	lymphocytes

M

ABBREVIATION	ENGLISH TRANSLATION
M-1	mitral first sound
MCHC	mean corpuscular hemoglobin count
MCL	midclavicular line
MCV	mean corpuscular volume
mEq (meq/L)	milliequivalents (per liter)
M & F l & w	mother and father living and well
MH	marital history
MI	mitral insufficiency
ml.	milliliter or milliliters
MLD	minimal lethal dose
MM	mucous membrane
MOM	milk of magnesia
mono	monocyte
M.S.	mitral stenosis

N

ABBREVIATION	ENGLISH TRANSLATION
n.b.	note well
NM	neuromuscular
noct.	nocturnal
NPN	nonprotein nitrogen
N.P.O.	nothing by mouth (per os)
N/S	normal saline

O

ABBREVIATION	ENGLISH TRANSLATION
O_2	oxygen
O_2 cap.	oxygen capacity
O_2 sat.	oxygen saturation
ol.	oil (oleum)
OOB	out of bed

P

ABBREVIATION	ENGLISH TRANSLATION
P	pulse
P-2	pulmonic second heart sound
P & A	percussion and auscultation
P-A	posteroanterior
Para I	primipara (a woman having born one child; unipara)
Para II	secundipara (a woman having born two children; bipara)
PBI	protein bound iodine
PE	physical examination
Pelvic Measurements:	
DC	diagonal conjugate
OC	obstetrical conjugate
bisp.	bispinous or interspinous diameter
IT	intertuberous
Ant.(or) Post.Sag.D.	anterior or posterior sagittal diameter
A-P D.	anteroposterior diameter
Trans D.	transverse diameter
per	through; by
pH	acidity
PH	past history
PI	present illness
P.I.D.	pelvic inflammatory disease
PMB	polymorphonuclear basophilic leukocytes
PME	polymorphonuclear eosinophilic leukocytes
P.M.I.	point of maximum impulse
PMP	previous menstrual period
p.o.	orally (per os)
polio	poliomyelitis
polys	polymorphonuclear leukocytes
post-op	postoperative
PPA	palpation, percussion and auscultation
pre-op	preoperative
prep.	prepare for
p.r.	per rectum
p.r.n.	whenever necessary (pro re nata)

ABBREVIATION	ENGLISH TRANSLATION
prothr. cont.	prothrombin content
prothr. time	prothrombin time
P.S.P.	phenolsulfonphthalein test (kidney)
pulv.	powder
PX	pneumothorax (may also be used for physical examination)
Q	
quant	quantitative or quantity
R	
R	respiration
RBC	red blood cell or corpuscle
RH	rhesus blood factor
ROS	review of systems
r.r.e.	round, regular and equal (of pupils)
react to 1 & a	react to light accommodation (pupils)
RLQ (abdomen)	right lower quadrant
RUQ "	right upper quadrant
RV	retroversion
RVO	relaxed vaginal outlet
RKS	retrograde kidney study
S	
sat.	saturated
sed. rate	erythrocyte sedimentation rate
SH	social history
SMR	submucous resection
S.M.W.D. Sep.	single, married, widowed, divorced, separated
s.o.s.	repeat once if urgently needed (si opussit)
spec.	specimen
sp.gr.	specific gravity
sq.cell ca.	squamous cell carcinoma

ABBREVIATION	ENGLISH TRANSLATION
SR	system review
SS enema	soapsuds enema
Staph.	staphylococcus
stab	neutrophilic leukocyte with unsegmented nucleus
stat	at once; immediately
stet	let it stand
stillb. or stb.	stillborn or stillbirth
Strep.	streptococcus
sympt.	symptoms
strab.	strabismus
T	
T	temperature
T & A	tonsillectomy and adenoidectomy
tbc	tuberculosis; tubercle bacillus
tbsp	tablespoon
temp.dext.	right temple (tempus dextra)
temp.sinistr.	left temple (tempus sinister)
TJ	triceps jerk
T.O.	telephone order
T.P.	total protein
T.P.R.	temperature, pulse and respiration
tsp	teaspoon
TURP	transurethral resection of prostate
U	
U	unit
U.C.H.D.	usual childhood diseases
ur.	urine
URI	upper respiratory infection
U.S.P.	United States Pharmacopoeia

ABBREVIATION	ENGLISH TRANSLATION	ABBREVIATION	ENGLISH TRANSLATION
	V		**W**
VD	venereal disease	Wass.	Wasserman
V.F.	focal fremitus	WBC	white blood cell or corpuscle
VC or vit.cap.	vital capacity	W.F.	white female
viz	namely (videlicet)	W.M.	white male
V.O.	verbal order	wd	well developed
		wn	well nourished

LATIN AND ENGLISH NUMERALS

NUMERALS IN LATIN*			NUMERALS IN ENGLISH*
unus	i	I	1
duo	ii	II	2
tres	iii	III	3
quattuor	iv	IV	4
quinque	v	V	5
sex	vi	VI	6
septem	vii	VII	7
octo	viii	VIII	8
novem	ix	IX	9
decem	x	X	10
undecim	xi	XI	11
duodecim	xii	XII	12
tredecim	xiii	XIII	13
quattordecim	xiv	XIV	14
quindecim	xv	XV	15
sedecim	xvi	XVI	16
septendecim	xvii	XVII	17
duodeviginti	xviii	XVIII	18
undeviginti	xix	XIX	19
viginti	xx	XX	20
viginti unus	xxi	XXI	21
viginti duo	xxii	XXII	22
trigenta	xxx	XXX	30
quadraginta	xl	XL	40
quinquaginta	l	L	50
sexaginta	lx	LX	60
septuginta	lxx	LXX	70
octaginta	lxxx	LXXX	80
nonaginta	xc	XC	90
centum		C	100

**The Latin numerals are commonly called "Roman" numerals. The English numerals are also called "Arabic" numberals.*

METRIC TABLES WITH AVOIRDUPOIS EQUIVALENTS

METRIC	AVOIRDUPOIS
LENGTH	
1 millimeter (mm.)	0.0394 inch (in.)
1 centimeter (cm.)	0.3937 inch
1 meter (m.)	39.37 inches
1 kilometer (km.)	0.6214 mile
WEIGHT	
1 milligram (mgm.)	0.0154 grain (gr.)
1 centigram (cgm.)	0.1543 grain
1 gram (gm.)	15.43 grains
1 kilogram (kg.)	2.2 pounds
CAPACITY	
1 cubic centimeter (cc.)	0.061 cubic inch
1 litre (l.)	0.908 dry quart or 1.0567 liquid quarts

APOTHECARIES' WEIGHTS

20 grains = 1 scruple

3 scruples = 1 dram (dr.)

8 drams = 1 ounce (oz.)

12 ounces = 1 pound (lb.)

PHARMACEUTICAL ABBREVIATIONS

The advent of manufactured medications is bringing about a change in the type of Latin abbreviations used by doctors when making out prescriptions. The abbreviations shown here are considered to be those most frequently in use today. This does not mean, however, that they are the only ones being used.

Although every physician has personal preferences, a large percentage of these abbreviations survive because their use is mandatory.

The Latin phrases from which these abbreviations have been taken, have been eliminated here because they are important only to the doctors and the pharmacists who must use them constantly. However, these phrases may be found in the appendices of most of the medical dictionaries.

LATIN ABBREVIATION	ENGLISH TRANSLATION
a, aa	equal parts of each
a.	before
a.c.	before eating
ad	to, up to
ad gr. acid	to an agreeable acidity
ad lib.	at pleasure; as much as is needed
ad sat.	to saturation
agit.	shake, stir; let it be shaken or stirred
agit. bene.	shake well
alt. noc.	every other night
aq., aqua	water
aq. bull.	boiling water
aq. dest.	distilled water
aq. ferv.	hot water
aq. frig.	cold water
aq. menth. pip.	peppermint water
aq. pur.	pure water
arg.	silver
bib.	drink
b.i.d.	twice daily
bis	twice
b.p.	boiling point
bull.	let it boil

LATIN ABBREVIATION	ENGLISH TRANSLATION
c̄	with (from the Latin "cum")
cap., caps.	a capsule, capsules
cat.	a poultice
chart.	paper, powder
cito disp.	let it be dispensed
cong.	a gallon
contra	against
cont. rem.	let the medicines be continued
c.v.	tomorrow night
cyath.	glassful
cyath. vinos	wineglassful
D.	dose
d.d. in d.	from day to day
decub.	lying down, having gone to bed
dieb. alt.	on alternate days
dil.	dilute
dim.	one-half
dis.	dissolve
div.	divide
div. in p. aeq., div. in par. aeq.	divide into equal parts
d.t.d.	give of such doses
elix.	elixir
e.o.d.	every other day
eq.	equal
ex. aq.	in water
exhib.	let it be given
ext.	extract
Fahr, F.	Fahrenheit (temperature scale)
Fe	iron
fl.	fluid
fl. dr. ʒ	fluid dram
fl. oz. ℥	fluid ounce
f.m.	make a mixture
f.p.	make a pill
ft.	let it be made

LATIN ABBREVIATION	ENGLISH TRANSLATION
ft. garg.	make a gargle
ft. in fus.	make an infusion
ft. mist.	make a mixture
ft. pulv.	make a powder
ft. ung.	make an ointment
garg.	a gargle
Gm., gm.	gram, grams
gr.	grain, grains
gtt.	a drop, drops
h.n.	tonight
h.s.	at bedtime or hour of sleep
in aq.	in water
ind.	daily
inf.	an infusion
inj.	an injection
liq.	a liquor; solution
lot.	a lotion
m.	mix (misce)
m.ft.	mix together
m.f.m.s.a. (misce fiat mistura secundum artem)*	mix a mixture by skill
min.	minim
mist.	a mixture (mistura)
mod. praes.	as prescribed
noct.	night
non rep.	do not repeat or refill
O.	a pint
O.D.	right eye (oculus dexter)
o.m.	every morning
o.n.	every night
O.S.	left eye (oculus sinister)
O.U.	each eye (oculus uterque)
oz.	ounce

*This is sometimes spelled out on the prescription as shown.

LATIN ABBREVIATION	ENGLISH TRANSLATION
part aeq.	equal parts
p.	after
p.c.	after eating
p.r.	by the rectum (per rectum)
p.r.n.	as needed; as often as necessary
pt.	let it be continued
pulv.	a powder
p.v.	by the vagina (per vagina)
q.i.d.	four times a day
q.o.d.	every other day
q.h.	every hour
q.n.	every night
q 4 H, q 6 H, etc.	every 4 hours, every 6 hours, etc.
q 2 day	every 2 days
q.l.	as much as is wanted
q.s.	a sufficient quantity
q.s. ad	a sufficient quantity
Rx	take (thou)
rep.	let it be repeated
rep. sem.	let it be repeated once only
sol.	solution
$\bar{s}$	without (from Latin "sine")
$\overline{ss}$	one-half (1/2)
stat.	at once
sum.	let him take or let it be taken
s.v.	spirits of wine
syr.	syrup
tab.	a tablet, tablets
t.i.d.	three times daily
tinct., tr.	tincture
t.w.	twice a week
U.	unit
u.d.	as directed
ung.	ointment
ur.	urine

SPECIAL NUMERALS AND SYMBOLS

LATIN ABBREVIATION	ENGLISH TRANSLATION
i, ii, iv, viii, etc.	1, 2, 4, 8, etc.
5", 10", 15", etc.	5 minutes, 10 minutes, 15 minutes, etc.
5', 10', 15', etc.	5 hours, 10 hours, 15 hours, etc.
ʒ (dr.)	dram (drachm)
℥ (oz.)	ounce

PRESCRIPTION FORMAT

Each prescription written by a doctor to a pharmacist contains specific components. These elements compose a format and the classification of these specific parts is shown below.

NAME OF PHARMACY OR DOCTOR

Phone Number — Registry Number
Street Address — City, State, Zip

PATIENT'S NAME ________ DATE ________

ADDRESS ________

SUPERSCRIPTION — the "order recipe": ℞

INSCRIPTION — contains names and quantities of ingredients:

Salicylic Acid	5%
Benzoic Acid	10%
Wool Fat	6 gm.
White Petrolatum	q.s. ad 60 gm.

SUBSCRIPTION — directions to the pharmacist: m. ft. ung.

TRANSCRIPTION or SIGNATURE — directions to the patient: Sig: Apply u.d.

Refill ____ times ________ M.D.

EXAMPLES OF PRESCRIPTIONS

For a better understanding of the directions given in prescriptions the following examples contain abbreviations used by doctors and pharmacists.

Locate the abbreviation in the listing of Pharmaceutical Abbreviations. Then rewrite the prescription using the English translation instead of the abbreviation.

Example No. 1

Penicillin 200,000 U.

#24

Sig: ii stat, i q 4 H

Example No. 2

Sterozalidin Caps

#15

Sig: i t.i.d. p.c.

Example No. 3

Benzalkonium Cl.	1:5000
aq.pur. q.s. ad	30 cc

Sig: gtt. i O.D. q 4 H

Example No. 4

Atropine Sulfate 1/4 gr.
Dis. aq. q.s. ad fl.ʒ i

m. ft. sol.

Sig: gtt. ii ex.aq. 10' a.c.

Example No. 5

Salicylic Acid	5%
Benzoic Acid	10%
Wool Fat	6 gm.
White Petroleum q.s.ad	60 gm.

m. ft. ung.

Sig: apply u.d.

Example No. 6

Belladonna Ext.	0.004
Pentobarbital Na	0.010
Acetylsalicylic Acid	0.150

m.ft. Cap i d.t.d. #iv

Sig: i Cap. 1 h before dental appointment

Example No. 7

Chloral Hydrate	ʒ viii
Sodii. Bromide	ʒ x
Syr. Rubi Idiac	fl.℥ iii
Aqua q.s.ad	fl.℥ viii

m.f.m.s.a.

Sig: i fl.ʒ q 3 or 4 H p.r.n. stomach

EXAMPLES OF CASE HISTORIES

The two case histories and physical examinations presented here are representative of two areas which differ slightly. Case No. 1 is a history as taken in a doctor's office of a patient who is consulting the specialist about a specific ailment. Case No. 2 concerns an industrial accident in which the doctor has been called in to see the patient on an emergency basis.

CASE NO. 1

CHIEF COMPLAINT: Anuria for the past two days.

PRESENT ILLNESS: This patient was referred to my office by her private physician because of anuria for the past two days. Patient also had nausea, anorexia, dry itchy skin, and swelling of her legs.

PAST HISTORY: The patient had a total hysterectomy, bilateral oophorectomy and salpingectomy in 1951, for carcinoma of fundus uteri. Her postoperative course was uneventful. In 1952 she was given 12 x-ray treatments on her abdomen for bilateral enlarged inguinal nodes. Six months later patient developed anuria of 36 hours duration and had bilateral ureteral catheterization for 14 days. Upon removal of the catheters the patient was able to void. The patient was discharged from the hospital and moved to this state to live with relatives. Menopause was at age 42.

FAMILY HISTORY: Not contributory.

INVENTORY BY SYSTEMS: Patient denied any cardiac or pulmonary disease.

PHYSICAL EXAMINATION

GENERAL APPEARANCE: Patient appeared toxic, pale and weak when seen in the office.

HEAD: No abnormalities noted.

EENT: Pupils round and equal. React poorly to light and accommodation. Tongue is dry and coated, "uremic odor" to breath.

NECK: No tenderness, masses or rigidity.

CHEST: Lungs clear to percussion and auscultation.

HEART: Regular sinus rhythm, soft systolic murmur at apex. A-2 equals P-2.

ABDOMEN: Soft. Liver palpable one finger down below the right costal margin. Kidneys and spleen not palpable. No costovertebral angle tenderness. No suprapubic tenderness or masses. Well healed suprapubic scar. Telangiectasia of the lower abdomen. Peristalis hypoactive.

GENITALIA: Atrophic vaginal vault. Cervix, fundus and adnexae are not palpable but there is marked induration and tenderness. Urethral meatus slightly inflamed. A #14 Robinson catheter passed into the bladder with ease. No urine obtained.

RECTAL: Marked induration and fibrosis in the cul-de-sac.

EXTREMITIES: Marked edema of both legs. No other abnormalities noted.

REFLEXES: Sluggish. None pathological.

SKIN: Warm and dry.

Because this industrial accident case concerns the individual's future ability to earn a living the doctor's first and subsequent reports to the insurance carrier must be as detailed as possible. A facsimile of the first accident report form with the information it should contain has been reproduced following the detailed report.

(All names of patient, doctors, employers, insurance carriers and hospitals are fictitious and any resemblance to anyone living or dead is purely coincidental. All dates have also been changed.)

In re: Emp - Universal Paper Co., Inc.
Inj - Mr. Harry Andrews
Date- July 10, 1968

EXAMINATION AND REPORT

HISTORY:

The examinee, Mr. Harry Andrews, was first seen by me at Community Hospital on July 10, 1968 at 11:45 A.M. He had suffered an injury earlier that morning at about 9:30 A.M. when a bale of paper fell about eight feet striking him on the back of his head and shoulders and knocking him to the ground. Apparently, he had suffered a severe acute flexion of the spine. He was, according to him, unconscious for awhile. He tells me he was immediately unable to move his lower extremities. He was taken to Community Hospital.

PAST HISTORY:

The past history is essentially negative. He never before had any injuries to his back and he never before had any paralysis of his lower extremities. He has been in general good health. He did have a urethral stricture in 1961 which was taken care of at the County Hospital.

EXAMINATION:

Examination on entrance revealed a well developed negro male who was alert and cooperative. He did not appear to be in any great pain although he had had medication for pain. The heart tones were good. Pulse was 96. Respiration was 20. Blood pressure was 60/40. He was perspiring and in general was in a degree of shock. He was extremely tender over the lower left thorax and there was limited expansion of the left chest. The abdomen showed tenderness in the flanks especially on the right upper. Peristalsis was checked and found to be present but hypoactive.

The neurological examination showed a complete paralysis of both lower extremities and a loss of sensation from the level of the umbilicus to the toes. Upper extremity neurological was entirely negative. Central nervous system neurological was negative. Pupils were equal, regular and reacted to light and to accommodation. The ocular and facial motions were normal.

X-RAYS:

X-rays were taken on admission and these revealed a severe compression fracture of the ninth dorsal vertebra, the vertebra being fractured in the middle and one portion driven backwards into the region of the spinal cord and the other portion being driven forwards. All in all there was narrowing of this vertebra. The transverse process of T 10 is also fractured on the left side and there is also possible fracture of the left transverse process of T 9.[1] The transverse processes of L 1 and 2[2] on the left are fractured with partial separation. The left lung showed haziness and punctate markings probably due to small hemorrhages in the lung. There is a hematoma along the left side of the mediastinum behind the heart extending laterally for a distance of about five centimeters. The left tenth, eleventh and twelfth ribs are avulsed and displaced laterally, the tenth to a slight degree and the eleventh and the twelfth for a distance of about two centimeters. There also appears to be a fracture of the anterior end of the left ninth rib without displacement.

1. T 9 refers to the ninth thoracic vertebra. The abbreviation of the vertebrae used in this manner may be written with a space between the letter and the number or the space may be left out. Both methods are used in the transcription copy appearing in this text.

2. L 1 and 2 refers to the first and second lumbar vertebrae.

LABORATORY:

A catheterized specimen of urine was obtained which was quite bloody indicating that probably there was a kidney, bladder or other damage along the urogenital system.

A blood count taken upon arrival showed a hemoglobin of 10.9 grams 72% with a hematocrit of 33 volumes percent. This indicated that severe hemorrhage had taken place and was probably still going on.

DIAGNOSIS:

A general diagnosis was, therefore, made of a major compression fracture of the ninth dorsal vertebra with displacement into the region of the spinal canal, avulsion of the lower left ribs, transverse process fractures of the ninth, tenth, and of the first and second lumbar all on the left, and last but not least is a paraplegia from the waist down. In addition, there is kidney damage which is subsequently determined to be on the left side with hemorrhage and a severe hemorrhage into the left lung plus an additional hemorrhage retroperitoneally.

CONSULTATIONS:

Dr. Booth, urologist, was called in consultation and he did an intravenous pyelogram. He felt there was damage to the left kidney but the right kidney was intact and functioning normally. Dr. Jackson, internist, was called in and he made certain recommendations medically which were subsequently of value. Dr. Southfield, neurosurgeon, was also called in consultation.

It was decided that this man's condition was too serious to be handled in the ordinary hospital room so he was moved to the surgical care unit. Intravenous fluids were started and subsequently units of blood were administered. The chest condition caused considerable concern so the thoracic surgery department of the hospital was called upon for consultation. Dr. Zachary responded. He felt there was a great deal of hemorrhage in this left chest and placed a tube in the left chest from which a large quantity of blood was evacuated.

Finally, Dr. Brownley, surgeon, was called in consultation because of the retroperitoneal hematoma.

In general, the consultants agreed that this man's condition was too serious to stand any surgery either on the spine or the abdomen and a period of intensive treatment was initiated. The initial condition of this man is exceedingly grave and there is some question as to whether he will survive. It is felt by both myself and Dr. Southfield that this man has most likely a severed spinal cord but this is pure conjecture. It will be necessary at a later date to do a laminectomy and find out the condition of the spinal cord at this D 9 level. The chances are that if this man survives, there will be a permanent life time disability.

DOCTOR'S FIRST REPORT OF WORK INJURY

STATE OF CALIFORNIA
DEPARTMENT OF INDUSTRIAL RELATIONS
DIVISION OF LABOR STATISTICS AND RESEARCH
P. O. Box 965, San Francisco, Calif. 94101

Immediately after first examination mail one copy **directly** to the Division of Labor Statistics and Research. Failure to file a report with the Division is a misdemeanor. (Labor Code, Sections 6407-6413.) Answer all questions fully.

A. INSURANCE CARRIER General Accident Insurance Company, 1000 Blair Ave., Los Angeles, Calif

Do not write in this space

1. **EMPLOYER** Universal Paper Company, Inc.
2. Address (No., St. & City) 1700 Jackson St., Vernon, Calif. 90058 731-0023
3. Business (Manufacturing shoes, building construction, retailing men's clothes, etc.) Paper company

4. **EMPLOYEE** (First name, middle initial, last name) Harry M. Andrews Soc. Sec. No. 000-00-0000
5. Address (No., St. & City) 20768 Hampton Street, Los Angeles, Calif. 90067 296-4310
6. Occupation Truck driver Age 35 Sex M
7. Date injured July 10, 1968 Hour 9:00A.M. Date last worked July 10, 1968
8. Injured at (No., St. & City) 1700 Jackson St., Vernon, Calif. County Los Angeles
9. Date of your first examination 7-10-68 Hour 12:00A.M. Who engaged your services? employer
10. Name other doctors who treated employee for this injury

11. **ACCIDENT OR EXPOSURE:** Did employee notify employer of this injury? yes Employee's statement of cause of injury or illness:
Heavy bale or roll of paper fell striking this man across his upper dorsum and squashing him to the ground or floor. He suffered immediate painful injuries and lost the use of his lower legs.

12. **NATURE AND EXTENT OF INJURY OR DISEASE** (Include all objective findings, subjective complaints, and diagnoses. If occupational disease state date of onset, occupational history, and exposures.)
Examination reveals loss of sensation and paralysis from the waist down.

Diagnosis: Compression fracture 9th dorsal vertebra extending into neural canal, left 11th and 12th ribs torn loose from vertebral attachment, pneumonitis left lower lobe, subperitoneal hematoma posteriorly.

13. X-rays: By whom taken? (State if none) Community Hospital
Findings: Show severe compression fracture of the 9th dorsal vertebra extending into the neural canal area. X-ray also reveals a tearing loose of the left 11th and 12th ribs from their vertebral attachment. X-ray reveals a pneumonitis of the left lower lobe.
14. ~~Treatment~~ There is also a subperitoneal hematoma posteriorly. Condition is critical. Laminectomy may be required. Prognosis is poor.
Treatment: 7-10-68: Examination, hospitalized
15. Kind of case (Office, home or hospital) Hospital If hospitalized, date 7-10-68 Estimated stay undetermined
Name and address of hospital Community Hospital, 1200 Barlow St., Los Angeles, Calif. 90054
16. Further treatment (Estimated frequency and duration) many months and possibly life time
17. Estimated period of disability for: Regular work many months and possibly life time Modified work
18. Describe any permanent disability or disfigurement expected (State if none) probable high degree of permanent disability
19. If death ensued, give date —
20. **REMARKS** (Note any pre-existing injuries or diseases, need for special examination or laboratory tests, other pertinent information.)

Name (Type or print) Degree PERSONAL SIGNATURE OF DOCTOR

Date of report Address (No., St. & City)

FORM 5021

Use reverse side if more space required

EXAMPLES OF RADIOLOGICAL, PATHOLOGICAL AND SURGICAL REPORTS

Every examination performed on a patient is committed to a written report which is placed in the patient's files at the hospital and at the doctor's office. Eventually this information will be computerized but a knowledge of medical terminology will still be required to prepare the coding.

Until widespread use of computers is reached typewritten reports will continue to be needed and will probably continue to be used in connection with the computers.

This has resulted in the installation of extensive and expensive transcription departments in hospitals, clinics and medical secretarial services. Trained transcribers are always in demand. There are three major requirements for transcribing: 1. a good working knowledge of medical terminology, 2. the ability to spell correctly and 3. the ability to type well.

The following reports which cover the specialties of x-ray, pathology and surgery are representative of material dictated in these fields.

While most of the medical terms used in these reports have appeared in the text material, it will be noted that new terms still occur. This is one of the reasons these reports have been included. It cannot be more clearly emphasized that no matter how much medical terminology the individual learns there are always more terms to be encountered.

There is, however, one reassuring thought for those who wish to become transcribers. Each specialist favors the use of certain medical terms and, as the transcriber learns which these are, it simplifies transcription of his reports.

The reports used here cover two different cases. Each case starts out with the x-ray findings, then the transcript of the surgical findings and procedure, and ends with the pathologist's findings of the tissue and/or specimen removed.

CASE NO. 1
RADIOLOGY REPORT

LUMBAR SPINE: (AP AND LATERAL)

The 12th ribs are somewhat hypoplastic. There is slight narrowing of the L5-S1[1] disc space with marginal sclerosis at this site. There are no fractures or destructive lesions noted. The remaining disc spaces appear intact.

LUMBAR MYELOGRAM:

The examination was performed by Dr. David. Spinal puncture was performed at the L3-L4 level and 9cc of Pantopaque was introduced into the subarachnoid space. There is an extradural type defect causing somewhat of an hour glass deformity at L5-S1 with the indentation being most prominent on the left side, however, there is an indentation on the right side and also ventrally. The contrast column was run to the thoracolumbar region and there are no intradural type defects noted and there are no other extradural type indentations demonstrated.

The contrast was removed and the patient was returned to the ward in satisfactory condition.

IMPRESSION:

Narrowing at L5-S1 with extradural type defect bilaterally and ventrally but most pronounced on the left side. These findings are felt to be indicative of a herniated disc at L5-S1.

1. L5-S1 indicates the space between the fifth lumbar vertebra and the first sacral vertebra.

SURGERY REPORT

PREOPERATIVE DIAGNOSIS: Herniated disc and degenerated disc, lumbar spine

POSTOPERATIVE DIAGNOSIS: Same

OPERATION PERFORMED: Laminectomy

FINDINGS AND PROCEDURE: FINDINGS: A bulging disc was found at L5-S1 on both sides. There was marked narrowing of the interspace of L4-5-S1.

PROCEDURE: After the usual preparation, under general anesthesia, a midline incision was made and curved below the left part of the sacrum. By subperiosteal dissection then the lamina of facette joints and sacrum were exposed. Bleeding throughout the procedure was controlled with electrocautery. The interspinous ligament was removed between L5-S1 and L4-5. The interspace at the L4-5 was explored on the left side and was found to be normal. The ligamentum flavum was then removed from L5-S1 bilaterally and the disc was removed from both sides. Following this the lamina of facette joints, sacrum and spinous processes were skived[1] up down to bleeding cancellous bone.

The left posterior iliac crest was exposed through the same incision and bone was removed from this structure. An H-type graft was formed and cancellous strips placed between L5 and S1. Following this dilute Kantrex was introduced into the wound and the wound was closed using interrupted #0 chromic on the deep fascia layers, #000 chromic on the subcutaneous fascia, and the skin was closed with continuous #00 nylon.

The patient withstood the procedure well and was returned to the ward in good condition.

PATHOLOGY REPORT

SPECIMEN: Lumbar disc

GROSS EXAMINATION: Specimen consists of a 35 x 25 x 8 mm. aggregate of irregular white-tan rubbery segments of tissue. Representative sections.

MICROSCOPIC EXAMINATION: Sections show fragments of cartilage and of nucleus pulposus with a few fragments consistent with ligament. The cartilaginous matrix is frayed and focally mucoid and some of the chondrocytes are not well preserved. A few small bone spicules are included.

Evidences of neoplasia are not noted.

DIAGNOSIS: Fragments of cartilage, nucleus pulposus, ligament and bone, consistent in appearance with stated origin from herniated intervertebral disc.

CASE NO. 2
RADIOLOGY REPORT

RETROGRADE PYELOGRAM: The collecting system appears essentially unchanged when compared with the previous study of 8-10-67. The right ureter is well outlined and normal. There is some extravasation of contrast in the distal ureter on the left.

IMPRESSION: Essentially negative retrograde pyelogram.

CHEST: The pulmonary calcification and fibrosis as well as cardiac enlargement appear essentially unchanged when compared with the previous study of 8-10-67. The diaphragm and bony thorax appear essentially intact and normal.

IMPRESSION:
1. Cardiomegaly, predominantly left ventricular chamber of minimal degree.
2. Pulmonary fibrosis and calcification.

1. "skived" means "to shave or pare the surface of, as leather; to slice"

SURGERY REPORT

PREOPERATIVE DIAGNOSIS: Recurrent bladder tumor

POSTOPERATIVE DIAGNOSIS: Same

OPERATION PERFORMED: Cystoscopy; retrograde pyelogram and fulguration and biopsy of bladder tumors

FINDINGS AND PROCEDURE: Under general anesthesia, the urethra and prostate were examined with the #24 panendoscope. The urethra bled rather easily but no gross abnormalities were noted. The prostate showed some hypertrophy, mostly of the left lateral lobe, very little median and very little obstruction, about Grade I to I½. The bladder, examined with a #24 Brown-Buerger, showed two papillary tumors arising from the right lateral wall of the bladder at about 11 o'clock.[1] The larger one measured about 1½ cms in diameter. These tumors were biopsied and then fulgurated. The tissue around and beneath this area was soft, mushy, and the electrode went quite deep. The rather wide area was fulgurated and further inspection of the bladder showed possible tumor arising from the right lateral wall adjacent to and just above the right interureteric ridge, but proximal to the ureteral orifice and this was lightly fulgurated. Also there were two lesions on the left lateral wall at about 3 o'clock, which were lightly fulgurated. The ureteral orifices were in their usual locations and a #4 catheter passed easily up the right side. A pyelogram was made but a urine was not collected. Urine was collected from the bladder for culture and sensitivity. The left ureter could not be catheterized for more than about 2 cms, apparently due to angulation, so a #12 Brash-bulb was inserted and the dye was injected retrograde and a pyeloureterogram was obtained. No catheter was inserted. The postoperative condition was satisfactory.

PATHOLOGY REPORT

SPECIMEN: Biopsy of bladder

GROSS DESCRIPTION: The specimen consists of a slightly irregularly shaped nodule of grayish-white tissue measuring 0.2 cm in maximum dimension. The tissue is relatively firm.

SECTIONS: All.

MICROSCOPIC DESCRIPTION: Microscopic examination reveals a small fragment of bladder wall. The mucosa is intact, but is composed of malignant transitional cells. The cells show moderate variation in size with nuclear atypism, hyperchromatism, but no mitotic figures. The tumor cells invade into the superficial submucosa in several areas. The stroma in these areas shows a moderate inflammatory reaction consisting mainly of lymphocytes and histiocytes.

DIAGNOSIS: 1. Superficially infiltrating transitional cell carcinoma A.F.I.P.[2] Class III.

1. This is a commonly used method to designate specific location of lesions, tumors, etc. and is based on the position of the numerals on the face of a clock.

2. A.F.I.P. is an abbreviation for Armed Forces Institute of Pathology.

STUDY 10 LESSONS

for

MASTERING MEDICAL TERMINOLOGY

By Verlee E. Gross

NOTE: For convenience the pages of the Study Section are perforated so they can be removed from the book. They are also drilled for use in a loose-leaf binder.

TO REMOVE PAGES: Fold each page at the perforation before tearing it out. This will prevent tearing of the paper outside of the perforation at the binding.

STUDENT STUDY

These study lessons are not difficult to complete. All answers are in the textbook and appear in the same continuity as the text material. A combination of conscientious reading of the text material and a degree of common sense is all that is needed to locate the answers. Space has been allowed for these answers to be written in longhand. If you have a typewriter or access to one it is excellent practice to type in the answers. For those who wish to specialize in transcribing this is almost a "must."

Because this is a text dealing with the language of medicine, emphasis has been placed on working with the medical terms. However, as these terms are also used in close relationship with the area of the body in which they occur, it, therefore, follows that a knowledge of anatomy and its related diseases and surgeries will also be acquired.

The last question of each study lesson covers a list of medical terms to be translated. These English translations will be found by referring to the Index which is placed at the end of each chapter. The Index gives the page and line number on which the term occurs. For translation of suffixes use the list of suffixes with their translations on Page iv at the beginning of the book.

All illustrations are duplications of those in the text to simplify identification of the organs indicated.

It is important that you keep your textbook and study lessons as neat as possible. You may wish to show them as proof of your medical terminology education. Untidy, careless entries will create a bad effect with prospective employers.

CHAPTER I
INTRODUCTION
STUDY LESSON

1. What are the two divisions of biology?

   A. Anatomy B. Physiology

2. Anatomy belongs to what group of biological sciences?

   morphology

3. What is gross anatomy?

   Can be seen with naked eye; large; macroscopic

4. When body structures (cells, tissues, organs) are diseased in what branch of medicine do they belong?

   Pathology

5. The function and activity of cells, tissues and organs is known as Physiology.

6. The period of growth and development before birth is known as Embryology.

7. Give the cell's relationship to the body.

   smallest unit of anatomy and physiology

8. Groups of cells make up tissue. The type of tissue is determined by the type of specialized cells.

9. What makes up an organ?

   tissues with the same function

10. Organs are arranged into systems.

11. What is a system?

    Organs concerned with the same function

12. List the systems of the body.

Skeletal	Vascular	Digestive
Endocrine	Nervous	Excretory
Muscular	Respiratory	Senses

13. Name the Senses and the organs belonging to each.

hear - ear   taste - tongue   smell - nose

see - eye   touch - skin and appendages

14. What is the Genito-Urinary System?

____

15. Give the correct terminology for the following:

A. The side containing the backbone is dorsal or posterior.

B. The abdominal side is ventral or anterior.

C. The head end is cranial or superior or cephalad.

D. The tail end is caudal or inferior.

E. A part above another part is superior.

F. A part below another part is inferior.

G. The body is divided into right and left sides by the sagittal plane. It is also referred to as the midsagittal plane.

H. The body is divided into front and back parts by a frontal or Coronal plane.

I. Those parts nearest the midsagittal plane are medial (mesial).

J. Those parts farthest from the midsagittal plane are lateral.

K. The walls of cavities or hollow viscera are known as ______________ and ______________.

L. The position nearest the central portion of the body is called ______________.

M. The position farthest away from the center of the body is called ______________.

15. (cont'd)

N. What term is used to indicate the area between medial and lateral?

_______________________.

O. Use the illustration on Page 4 for reference and fill in the directional terms on the illustration shown below.

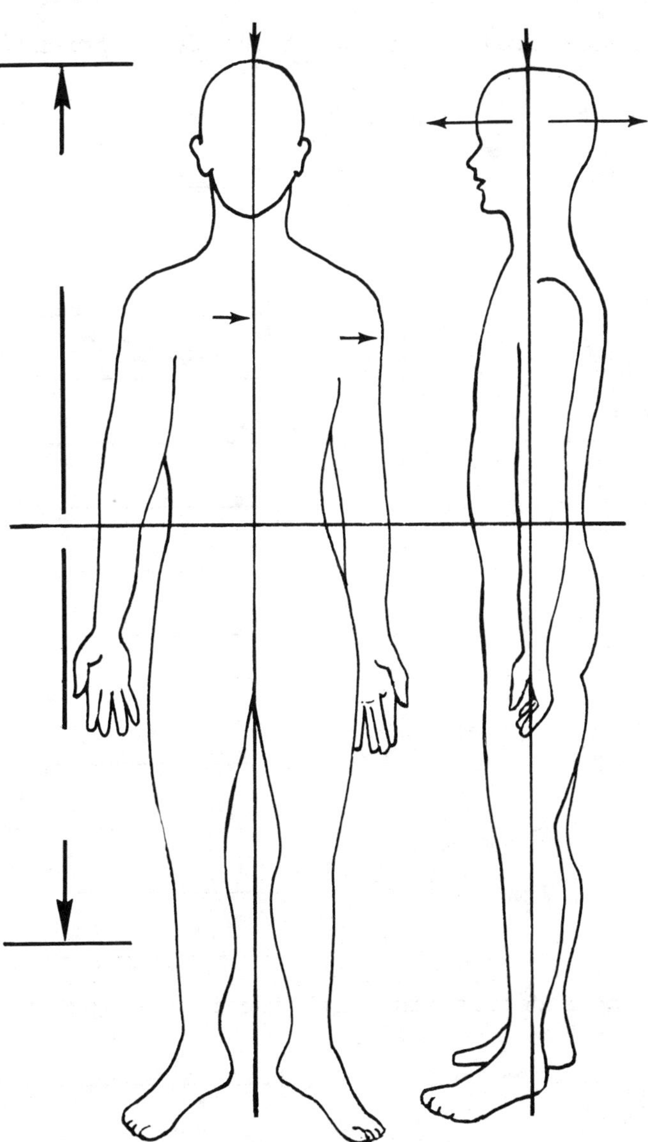

15. (cont'd)

P. The walls enclosing the body cavity or surrounding organs are known as ________________.

Q. Organs within the body cavity are called ______________.

R. What terms indicate the outside or surface of a body or an organ?

__________________ __________________

S. Away from the surface is designated as ____________.

T. Near the surface is designated as ______________.

16. List the different bone projections and their descriptions.

_________________ or _____________ ________________________________

_________________ ________________________________

_________ ________________________________

_________________ ________________________________

____

_____________________ ________________________________

________ ________________________________

____

____

____

_______ ________________________________

_______ ________________________________

_______ ________________________________

__________ ________________________________

17. List the different bone depressions with their descriptions.

__________ ________________________________

__________ ________________________________

__________ ________________________________

_______________ ________________________________

18. What are the three perforations: Describe each.

_______________ ________________________________

____

_____________ ________________________________

____

_______________ ________________________________

19. A cavity within a bone is known as a __________ or ______________.

20. What are the two types of materials used for sutures?

A. ____________________ B. ________________________

21. Which of the two suture materials does not have to be removed after the wound has healed?

____

22. Which of the above materials are these sutures? Use "A" for absorbable and "NA" for non-absorbable.

Cotton ________________ Surgical gut ______________________

Metal clips ____________ Artificial silkworm gut ____________

Silkworm gut ___________ Tantalum wire _____________________

Fascia lata ____________ Silk ______________________________

Nylon _________________

Metal wire _____________

23. What is the finest gauge in suture materials? _________________

24. List the other gauges.

______, _____, ______________. ____________, __, __, __, __, __, __.

25. Suture materials may also be designated as ______, _________, ____________.

26. The following sutures are used routinely in a majority of surgical procedures. List the name of the suture technique after each of the following descriptions.

A. A type of suture in which the surgeon ties each stitch separately.

____

26. (cont'd)

B. A suture in which the two ends are fastened by passing them through a split shot which is then compressed. ____________________

C. A continuous stitch passed in and out through the skin encircling the wound ____________________________

D. A "running" type of stitch in which the surgeon ties the first and last stitches only. ___________________

E. A suture in which the stitches are made through two strips of adhesive tape applied along each edge of the wound. ____________

F. A suture that is applied back and forth through both edges of a wound. __________________

G. Sutures placed at a short distance from the primary suture line. ___________ or __________

H. A suture for the stomach and intestines. ____________________

27. Name the tissues which comprise the scar or cicatrix.

A. ____________________ B ______________________ C ______________________

28. List the six terms used to describe the healing process.

A. __________________________________ D. __________________________________

B. __________________________________ E. __________________________________

C. __________________________________ F. __________________________________

29. What are the five stages of the exudative phase?

A. ____

B. ____

C. ____

D. ____

E. ____

30. What are the three causes of wound infection?

A. ___________________ C. __________________

B. ___________________

31. Describe the procedure of debridement.

____

____

32. What is chemotherapy?

____

33. How does chemotherapy aid healing of wounds?

____

____

____

____

34. Describe each of the following terms.

avulsion ______________________________________

____

dehiscence ____________________________________

____

eventration ___________________________________

____

evisceration __________________________________

____

35. A number of surgical instruments are routinely used in most doctors' offices.

Give the description for the following:

forceps _______________________________________

____

speculum ______________________________________

____

trocar ____

____

____

35. (cont'd)

bougie ______________________________

____

____

curette or curet ______________________________

____

sound ______________________________

____

catheter ______________________________

____

____

hemostat ______________________________

tenaculum ______________________________

cannula ______________________________

____

36. What are the four stages of anesthesia?

A. ______________

B. ______________

C. ______________

D. ______________

37. How are volatile substances administered? ______________

38. What are the two types of volatile substances? A. ______________ B. ______________.

39. How are nonvolatile substances administered? ______________ or ______________.

40. Name the topical anesthetics.

A. ______________ C. ______________

B. ______________ D. ______________

41. What is general anesthesia?

____

____

42. Name the four methods of administering general anesthesia.

A. ______________________ C. ______________________

B. ______________________ D. ______________________

43. What is local and regional anesthesia?

____

____

44. Give the seven methods of administering local and regional anesthesia.

A. ______________________ E. ______________________

B. ______________________ F. ______________________

C. ______________________ G. ______________________

D. ______________________

45. What are coramine, caffein and metrazol?

____

46. What is an antinarcotic?

____

47. Tapping of the eyelid to evoke its immediate closure is a guide to determine the depth of anesthesia. What is it called? ______________________

48. Curare and anectine are drugs that block the passage of motor impulses. They are known as ______________________.

49. IPPB is known as ______________________________________.

50. Refer to the alphabetical index beginning on Page 24 to find the Line and Page number for the following words. Then write the English translation beneath each word component in each of these medical terms.

P E R I / P H E R Y

H E M O / R R H A G E

E / V E N T R / A T I O N

F I B R O / P L A S I A

T U B E R / C L E

R E / S P I R A T / O R Y

A N / A L G E S / I A

P A R I E T / A L

C E P H A L / A D

A D / R E N / A L

E P I / C O N D Y L E

N E C R / O S I S

H Y P O / T H E R M / I A

S A G I T T / A L

V A S O / C O N / S T R I C T O R S

A / V U L S I O N

S U B / A R A C H N / O I D

B I / C E P S

E X / U D A T I V E

V E S / I C L E S

CHAPTER II
THE SKELETAL SYSTEM
STUDY LESSON

1. List the bones of the skull. Include the small bones of the ear. Also give the name of the bone found in the neck just above the Adam's apple.

A. ____________ G. ____________ M. ____________

B. ____________ H. ____________ N. ____________

C. ____________ I. ____________ O. ____________

D. ____________ J. ____________ P. ____________

E. ____________ K. ____________ Q. ____________

F. ____________ L. ____________ R. ____________

2. Name the bones of the trunk.

A. ____________ B. ____________ C. ____________

3. How many vertebrae in the adult? ____________

4. Give the different types of vertebrae and the number of each which compose the vertebral column.

A. ____________ C. ____________ E. ____________

B. ____________ D. ____________

5. A. What happens to the vertebrae in the sacral and coccygeal regions in the adult?

A. ____

____

B. What are these two (2) bones called?

____

6. Which of these two bones is the terminal bone of the vertebral column?

____

7. What is the sternum and how long is it?

____

8. How many ribs are there? ____________________

9. What are the spaces called between the ribs?

____

10. List the bones found in the upper extremity.

A. __________ D. __________ G. __________

B. __________ E. __________ H. __________

C. __________ F. __________

11. How many bones in the carpus or wrist joint? ______

12. Name the carpal bones in the proximal row.

A. __________ C. __________

B. __________ D. __________

13. Name the carpal bones in the distal row.

A. __________ C. __________

B. __________ D. __________

14. What are the phalanges of the hand?

____

15. A. How many phalanges in each finger? ______

B. How many phalanges in the thumb? ______

C. How many phalanges in each hand? ______

16. List the bones of the lower extremities.

A. __________ E. __________

B. __________ F. __________

C. __________ G. __________

D. __________ H. __________

17. Name the three parts which form the hip bones in the adult.

A. __________ B. __________ C. __________

18. What is the socket joint called into which the head of the femur fits?

____

19. A. What is the kneecap called? __________ B. What type of bone is it?

____

20. The inner and outer projections of the ankle are known as the medial ____________________ and lateral ________________.

21. Name the seven tarsal bones.

A. ____________________ C. ____________________ E. ____________________

B. ____________________ D. ____________________ F. ____________________

G. ____________________

22. The sole or instep of the foot is called the ________________.

23. How many phalanges in the great toe? ________ in each of the other toes? ____________.

24. Wherever two bones glide over one another, articulations permitting movement arise. They are known as ______________.

25. When an imperfect joint is produced by a fracture which has not united properly, it is called a "false joint" or ____________________.

26. What is the purpose of the synovial fluid?

____

____.

27. What is the function of the bursae?

____

28. What is the cause of bursitis?

____. This results in a condition known as ________________.

29. Immovable joints are called ________________________.

30. Where do they occur? A. ____________________ B. ________________________ ____________.

31. Slightly movable joints are called ______________________. Name their two (2) divisions.

A. __________________________________ B. ________________________________

32. Where does the symphysis occur?

A. _____________________ B. _________________ C. ________________________

33. Where does syndesmosis occur? ____________________

34. Freely movable joints are called ____________________.

35. Give the six (6) types of freely movable joints and where they occur.

A. ____________________ D. ____________________

B. ____________________ E. ____________________

C. ____________________ F. ____________________

36. Read the description of each of the joint movements given below and then put in the name of that movement.

A. ankle movement that turns foot inward ____________________

B. movement toward the midline of the body ____________________

C. forward movement ____________________

D. movement that raises the bone, muscle and limb ____________________

E. movement away from the midline of the body ____________________

F. movement that reduces the angle between the bones, as in bending the arm at the elbow ____________________

G. backward movement ____________________

H. ankle movement that turns the foot outward ____________________

I. clockwise movement of the hand, turning the palm forward ____________________

J. movement opposite to elevation ____________________

K. counterclockwise movement of the hand, turning the palm backward ____________________

L. movement that bends the part beyond the position taken in extension ____________________

M. circular movement as in a circular swinging of the arm ____________________

N. movement that increases the angle between bones and is thus opposite to flexion ____________________

O. movement that flexes the foot toward the sole ____________________

Use the illustrations on page 28, 30, 31, 35, 38, 40 and 41 in the textbook for reference. Write in the identification on all drawings on this page and the following two pages.

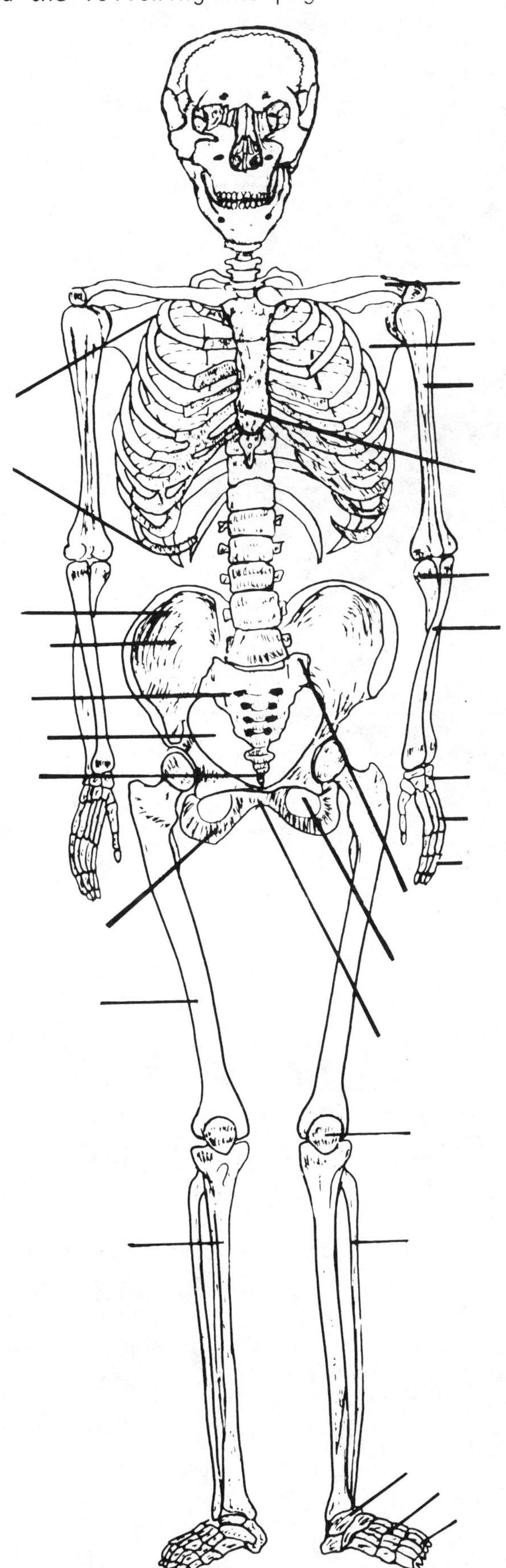

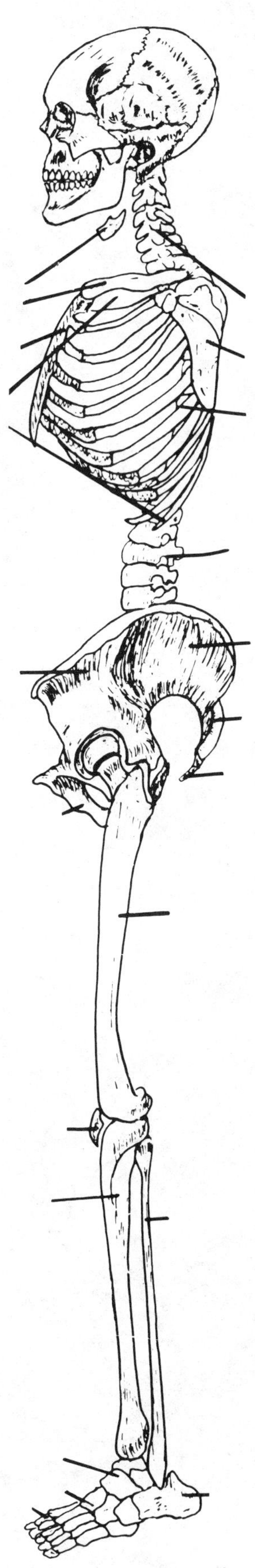

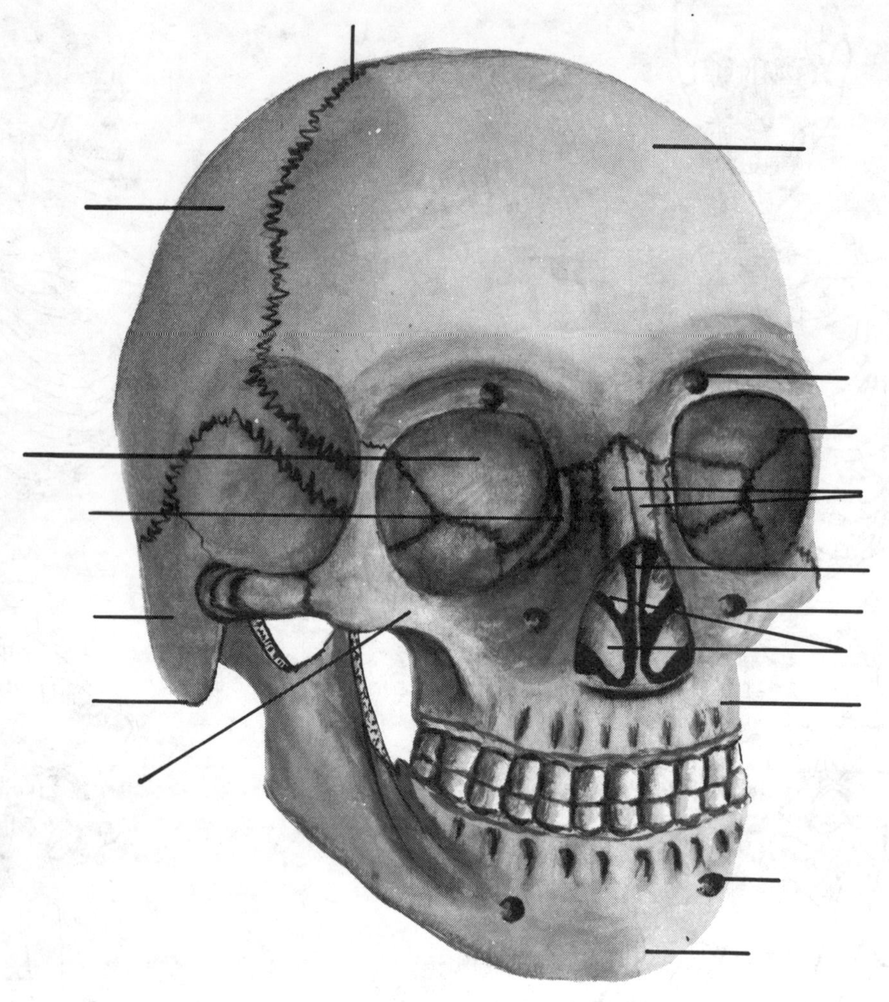

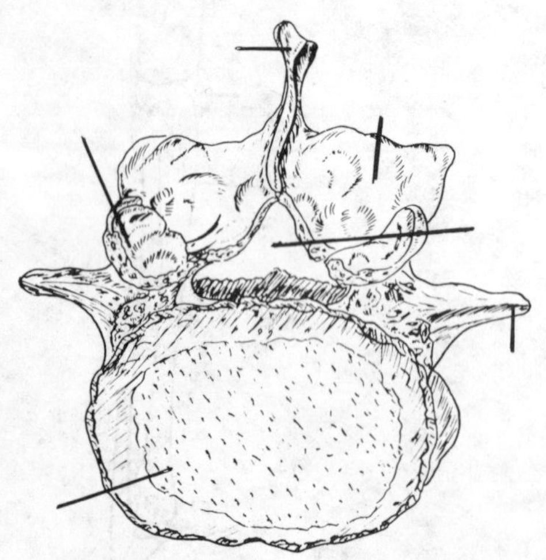

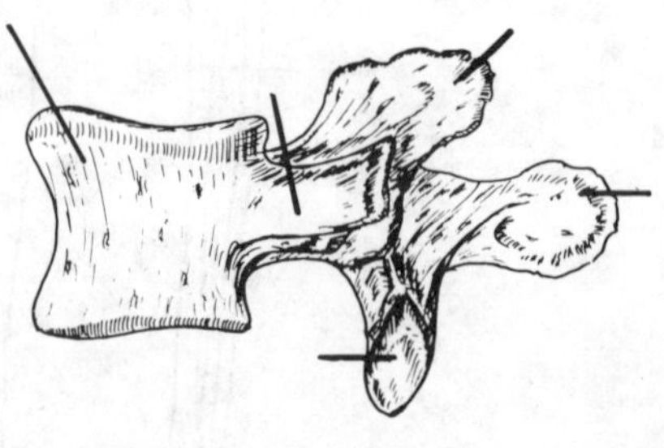

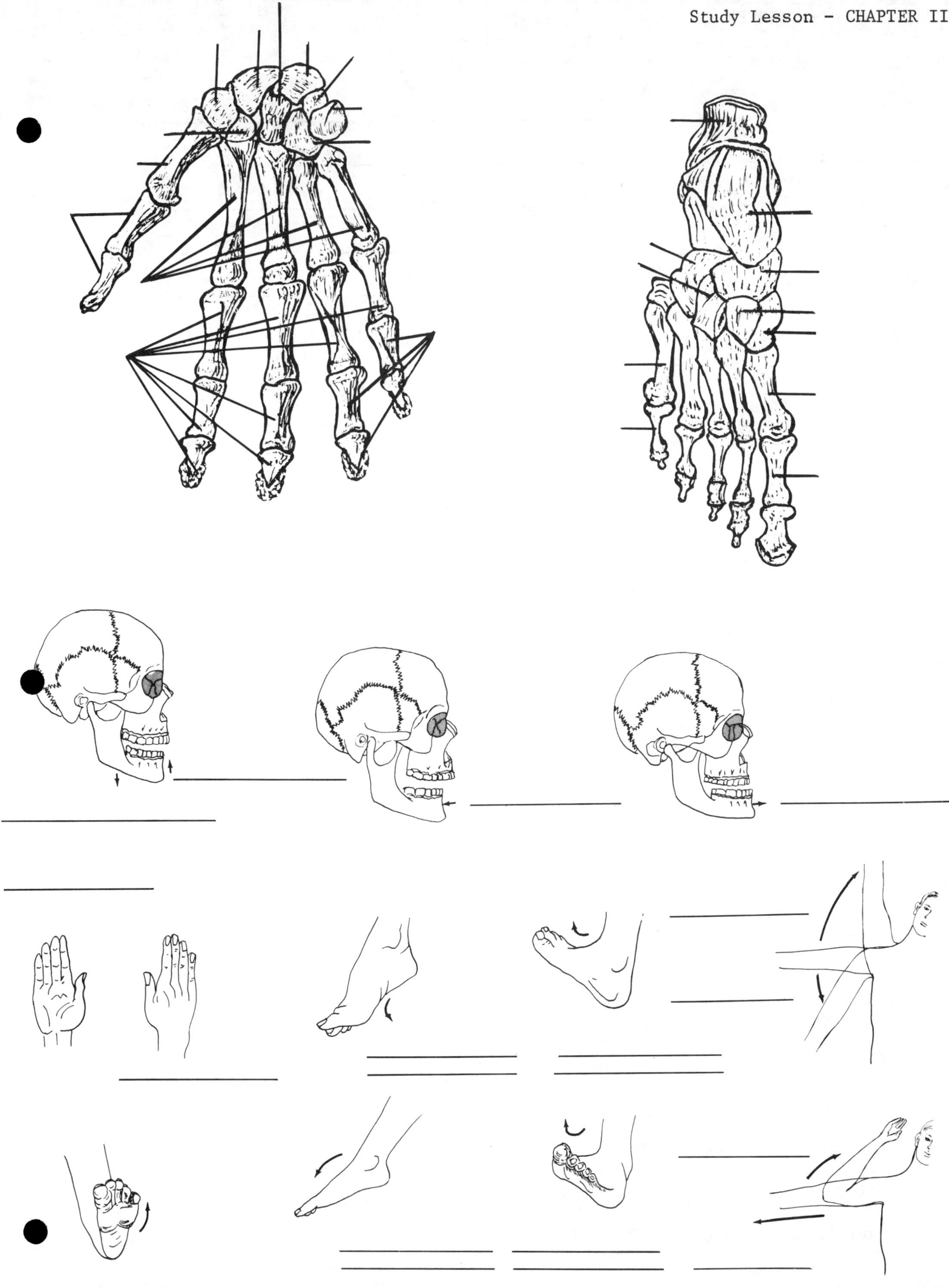

37. Name the four (4) types of fractures and explain each.

A. ____

____

B. ____

____

C. ____

____

D. ____

____

38. Describe what causes a sprain.

____

____

39. Describe what causes a dislocation.

____

____

____

____

40. What terms describe incomplete or partial dislocation?

____________________ and ____________________

41. Give the medical terms for the diseases and anomalies described below.

A. necrosis or death of a bone without the presence of infection

____

B. inflammation of bone and cartilage ____________________

C. flattening of the upper femoral epiphysis under the influence of weight bearing muscle pull ____________________

D. inflammation of bone marrow ____________________

E. joint affection characterized by the partial detachment of a fragment of cartilage and underlying bone from the articular surface

____

F. Give the other term for von Recklinghausen's disease of the bones.

____

G. a disease of childhood in which the bones become crooked and deformed and their earthy salts diminished ____________

H. knock knees ____________

I. bowlegs ____________

J. affections of bones induced by endocrine disturbances are ____________ ____________ or ____________, ____________, ____________ ____________, and ____________ ____________

K. Enlargement, softening and distortion of the bones is known as ____________ ____________ or ____________

L. abnormal curvature of the vertebral column in which the spinal column curves to one side ____________

M. an abnormal curvature of the spine with convexity backward (often called hunchback or humpback) ____________

N. a forward displacement of one vertebra over another

____

42. Give the six main benign osteogenic tumors.

A. ____________ D. ____________

B. ____________ E. ____________

C. ____________ F. ____________

43. Three malignant osteogenic tumors are: ____________

B. ____________ C. ____________

44. What is the most common malignant tumor of joints? ____________

45. List the five congenital deficiencies of bone as given in the text.

A. ____________

B. ____________ D. ____________

C. ____________ E. ____________

46. What is the main disease of the joints? ________________

47. List the different types of acute and chronic arthritis.

A. ____________ C. ____________ E. ____________

B. ____________ D. ____________

48. A. Chronic inflammatory disease of the joints and tissues around them is known as ____________

B. A chronic, non-inflammatory disease of the joints which occurs mostly in old people is known as ____________

49. Give the medical term for the following surgical procedures:

A. manual or surgical breaking of bone ____________

B. the operative fastening of the ends of a fractured bone by mechanical means ____________

C. surgical refracture of a bone in cases of malunion ____________

D. reconstruction or repair of bone ____________

E. excision of bone ____________

F. surgical removal of a piece of dead bone ____________

G. spinal fusion ____________

H. surgery for decompression of spinal cord ____________ and ____________

I. taking out bits of bone from the lamellar arch to widen the space ____________

J. removal of the transverse process with adjacent portions of the ribs ____________

K. types of drainage performed for abscesses in the lumbar spine ____________ and ____________

L. excision of the fifth lumbar transverse process ____________

M. surgery performed for coccygodynia ____________

N. removal of loose bodies (joint mice) ____________

O. reconstruction of ankylosed or stiffened joints ____________

50. Refer to the alphabetical index beginning on Page 56 to find the Line and Page number for the following words. Then write the English translation beneath each word component in each of these medical terms.

I N T E R / C O S T / A L

C H O N D R O / M Y X O / S A R C / O M A

E P I / P H Y S I S

P T E R Y G / O I D

S E P T I C / E M I A

T A L I P E S

C O C C Y G O / D Y N I A

A R T H R O / P L A S T Y

P Y O / G E N / I C

X I P H / O I D

E X / O S T / O S I S

S P O N D Y L O / L I S T H / E S I S

P E R I / O S T E U M

H Y P E R / N E P H R / O M A

F E N E S T R / A T I O N

M E T A / S T A T / I C

C E R E B R O / S P I N / A L

CHAPTER III
THE MUSCULAR SYSTEM
STUDY LESSON

1. A. What is the special function of muscles when they are stimulated?

   ____

   B. What other functions do muscles have?

   ____________________, ____________________, ____________________

2. What percentage of body weight is muscular tissue? ____________________

3. Name the three types of muscle fibers.

   A. ______________________________

   B. ______________________________

   C. ______________________________

4. In what part of the body do striated muscles occur?

   ____

5. Muscles which can be made to operate by an individual's will are called

   ____________________ muscles.

6. What is the function of skeletal muscles?

   ____

7. Muscles over which we have no control are known as ____________________ muscles.

8. These muscles occur in the ____________, ____________, ____________________ and are called ______________ or ____________________.

9. The muscle which forms the heart is ______________________________.

10. The end of the muscle attached to less movable bone is the ______________; the attachment of the muscle to a bone which moves in the ordinary activity of the body is the ________________.

11. What is a tendon?

    ____

12. What is an aponeurosis?

    ____

13. The property of muscle tissue whereby a steady, partial contraction varying in degree is maintained is called __________.

14. Most skeletal muscles occur in __________ and are usually arranged so they __________ each other.

15. If the flexors cause the arm to bend, what do the extensors do?

____

16. Give the name of the muscle which fits the following muscular action.

A. rolls eyeball outward __________________

B. raises the upper lid and opens the eye ________________________________

C. raises the mandible and closes the mouth ____________________

D. raises the mandible and closes the mouth; assists in protruding mandible

____

E. compresses the cheeks and retracts the angles of the mouth _______________

F. draws angle of mouth causing an expression of grinning __________________

G. raises and retracts the tongue ____________________

H. wrinkles skin of neck; depresses lower jaw and lower lip _________________

I. depresses and rotates head; flexes head on chest or neck

____

J. draws humerus downward and backward, rotates it inward __________________

____

K. retracts and elevates the scapula ____________________

L. depresses arm to side, adducts and draws it forward, rotates it; helps to raise ribs in forced inspiration ____________________

M. compresses abdomen and flexes vertebral column __________________________

N. tenses linea alba; aids in inspiration _______________________

O. flexes and rotates thigh outward; flexes thigh on pelvis; abducts and flexes lumbar spine ________________________

P. flexes arm at shoulder ___________________________

Q. flexes middle and proximal phalanges _____________________________________

Use the illustration on page 67 as reference. Write in the names of the muscles indicated on the drawings below.

MUSCLES OF THE BODY

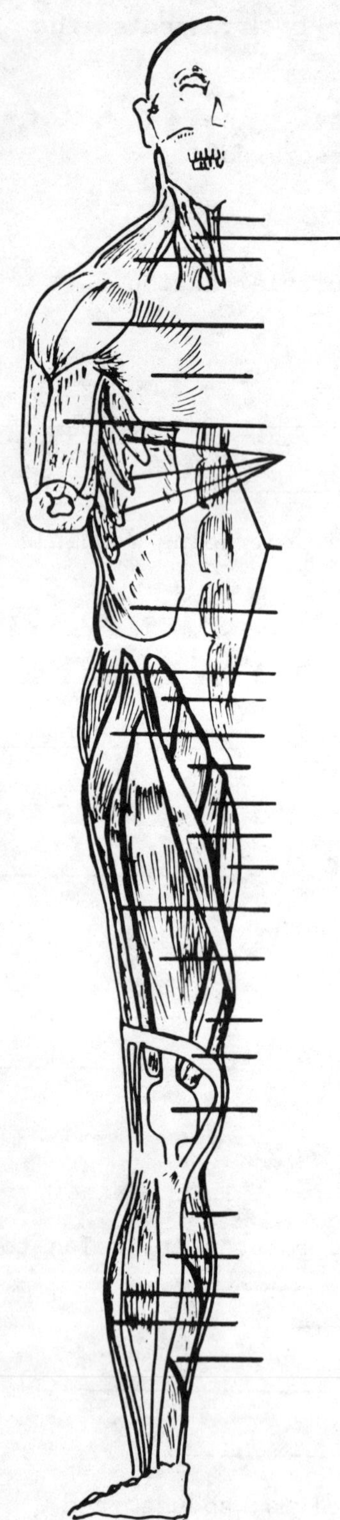

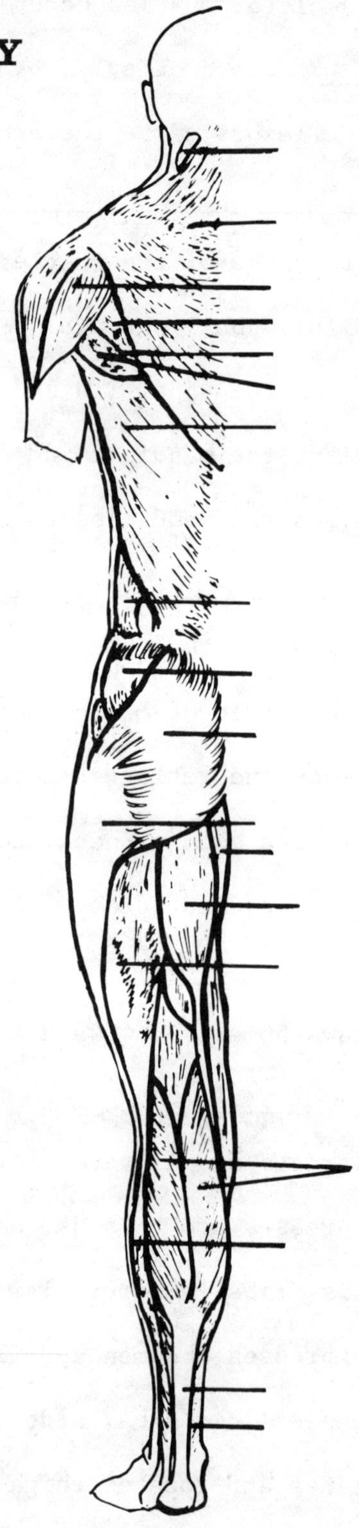

16. (continued)

R. extends little finger ______________________________

S. extends index finger ______________________________

T. flexes leg on thigh and thigh on pelvis; abducts and rotates thigh outward

____

U. rotates leg inward ______________________________

V. extends foot at ankle; flexes femur upon tibia ______________________________

W. flexes foot at ankle and elevates inner border of foot ______________________________

____

X. assists flexor digitorum longus in flexing the toes ______________________________

____

Y. extends last phalanges of toes and flexes the first phalanges

____

Z. flex proximal and extend middle and distal phalanges; abduct 2nd, 3rd and 4th toes ______________________________

17. Name the different types of bursitis using the medical term.

A. ______________________________ G. ______________________________

B. ______________________________ H. ______________________________

C. ______________________________ I. ______________________________

D. ______________________________ J. ______________________________

E. ______________________________ K. ______________________________

F. ______________________________ L. ______________________________

18. What is the medical term for "wry neck?"

____

19. Inflammation of the skeletal muscles with pus formation is called ______________________________; without pus formation the condition is called ______________________________.

20. Give the five types of nonsuppurative myositis.

A. ______________________ D. ______________________

B. ______________________ E. ______________________

C. ______________________

21. Hereditary and familial conditions with marked weakness of muscles are called ______________________ .

22. Give two other muscle affectations.

A. ______________________ B. ______________________

23. List the conditions for which surgery is performed on muscles, tendons or tendon sheaths.

A. ______________________

B. ______________________

C. ______________________

D. ______________________

E. ______________________

F. ______________________

G. ______________________

H. ______________________

I. ______________________

J. ______________________

K. ______________________

24. Give the medical term for the following procedures.

A. ____________ and ____________ ____________ is done for release of contracture.

B. ______________________ is tendon suture and repair for torn muscles, separation of tendons from bone, ruptured tendons.

C. ______________________ is tendon sheath plasty for trigger finger.

D. ______________________ or ______________________ is performed for stenosing tenosynovitis.

24. (continued)

E. _______________ is the suturing of the end of a tendon to the skeletal attachment.

F. __________________________ is the removal of a tendon and its sheath.

G. _________________ is the surgical repair of a muscle by free muscle graft or pedicle graft.

H. ___________________ is the suturing of a muscle.

I. ___________________ is the stretching of a muscle.

25. Refer to the alphabetical index on page 80 for the line and page number of the following words. Under each word component write the English translation.

MY/ASTHENIA

INTER/STITIAL

PSEUDO/HYPER/TROPHIC

GASTRO/CNEMIUS

TENO/SYNOV/ITIS

QUADRI/CEPS

OSSI/FICATION

PIRI/FORMIS

AB/DUCTOR

STERNO/CLEIDO/MAST/OID

BRACHIO/RADI/ALIS

TORTI/COLLIS

25. (continued)

P Y O / G E N / I C

C A R T I L A G I N / O U S

H A L L U C I S

A P O / N E U R O S I S

S T Y L O / G L O S S U S

N A S O / L A B I / A L

S U B / C L A V I U S

I S C H I O / G L U T E / A L

CHAPTER IV
THE NERVOUS SYSTEM
STUDY LESSON

1. What are the two main divisions of the central nervous system?

   A. ______________________ B. ______________________________

2. What is the abbreviation for the central nervous system? ____________

3. Give the names of the two groups of nerves which make up the peripheral nervous system.

   A. ______________________ B. ______________________________

4. Give the total number of cerebrospinal nerves.

   ____

5. How are they divided and to what part of the nervous system are they attached?

   A. ____

   B. ____

6. The cerebrospinal nerves are associated with what type of bodily movements?

   ____

7. The autonomic nervous system transmits impulses which ___________________

   ____

   _______________________________.

8. What three membranes protect the medulla spinalis?

   A. _______________ B. ________________ C. __________________

9. What are the divisions of the 31 spinal nerves and how many nerves in each division?

   A. _______________ C. ________________ E. __________________

   B. _______________ D. ________________

10. Name the components of the brain.

    A. _______________________ C. ________________________

    B. _______________________ D. ________________________

Use the illustrations on Pages 85, 86 and 87 for reference. Then write the proper identifications on the drawings shown on this page and page 31, of the various organs which make up the nervous system.

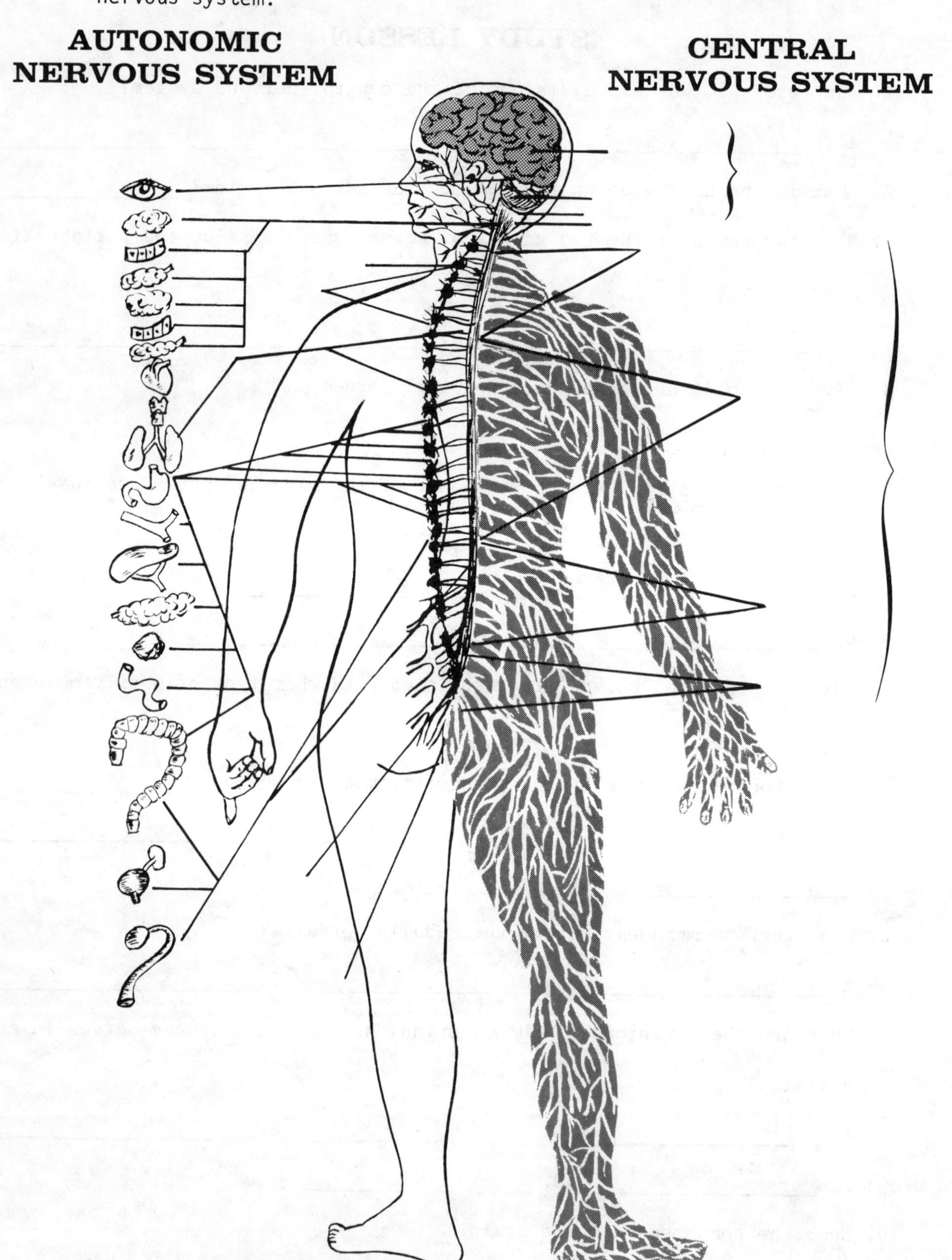

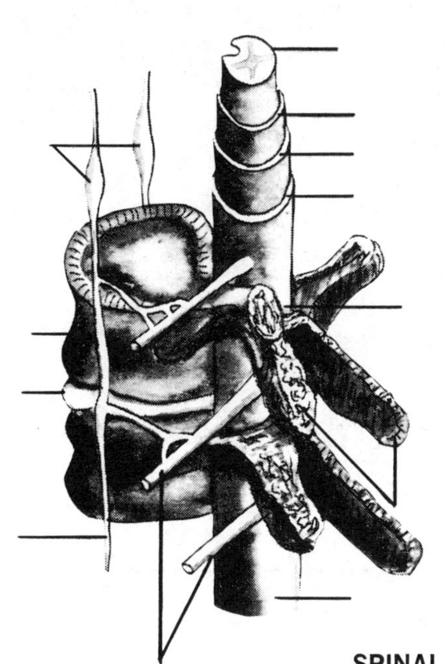

SPINAL CORD AND MENINGES

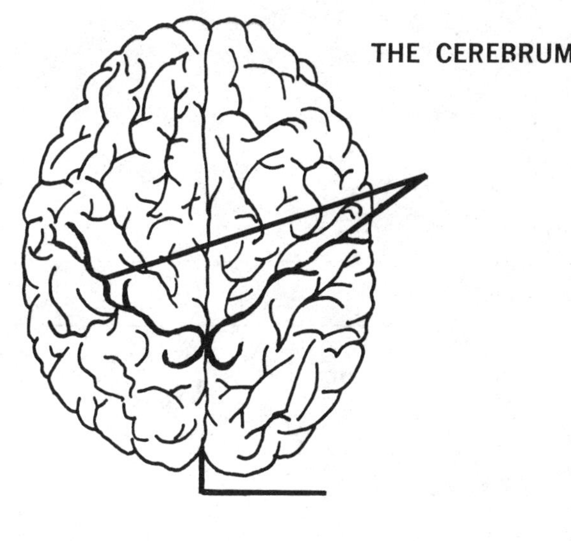

THE CEREBRUM

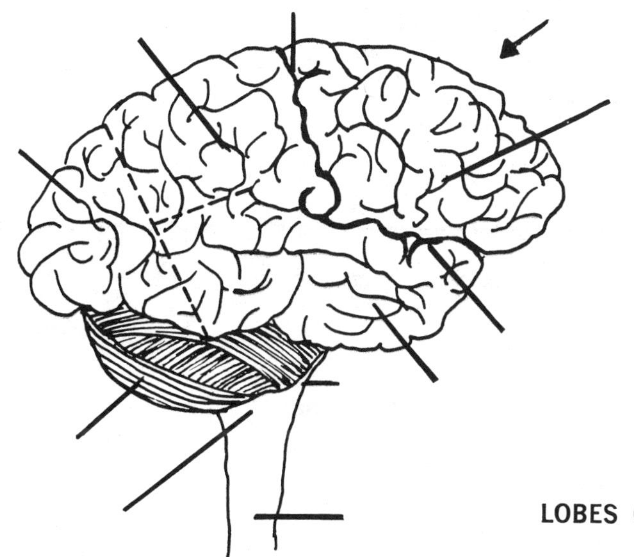

LOBES OF THE BRAIN

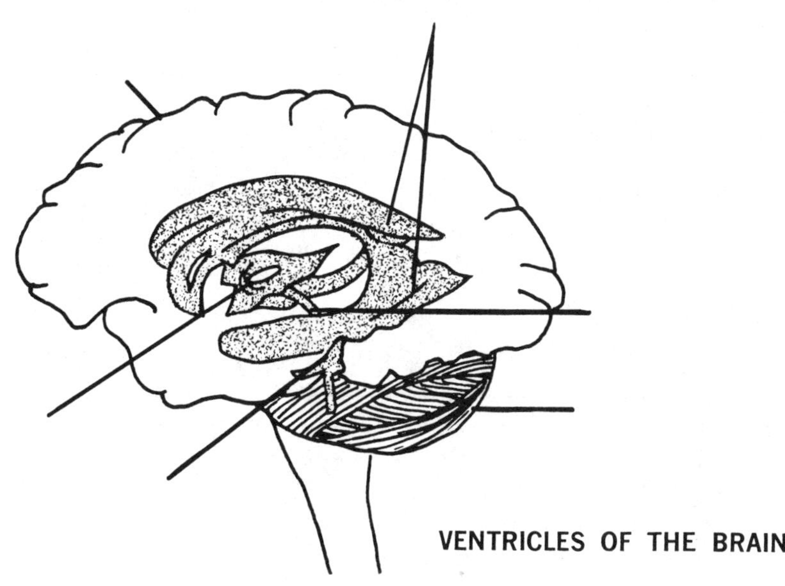

VENTRICLES OF THE BRAIN

11. Name the fissures of the brain.

    A. ____________________ C. ____________________

    B. ____________________

12. How many lobes in the cerebrum and what are their names?

    A. ______________ C. ______________ E. ______________

    B. ______________ D. ______________ F. ______________

13. How many ventricles in the brain and what are they called?

    A. ____________________

    B. ____________________ } which form the ____________________

    C. ____________________ }

    D. ____________________

    E. ____________________

14. The two halves of the cerebellum are known as ______________. The central portion is called the ______________.

15. What parts of the nervous system does the medulla oblongata connect?

    ____

16. Where is the pons located? ____________________.

17. What is the purpose of the cerebrospinal fluid?

    ____

    ____________________.

18. What are the two divisions of the autonomic nervous system?

    A. ____________________ B. ____________________

19. What is the function of these divisions?

    ____________________.

20. List the cranial nerves in numerical order with their Roman numerals.

__________________ __________________

__________________ __________________

__________________ __________________

__________________ __________________

__________________ __________________

__________________ __________________

21. Name the three groups which cover the symptoms and signs of disease of the nervous system.

A. __________________

B. __________________

C. ____________________________

22. A. The involuntary response of an individual to a given type of stimulation applied to a specific area is called a __________.

B. The two general types of reflexes are ______________ and ________________.

23. After each of the following reflexes write whether it is "deep" or "superficial."

A. plantar reflex __________

B. biceps and triceps reflexes __________

C. Achilles reflex or ankle jerk __________

D. abdominal reflex __________

E. corneal reflex __________

F. patellar reflex or knee jerk __________

G. jaw or masseter reflex __________

H. cremasteric reflex __________

24. What other important tests are part of the physical examination of the nervous system?

A. ________________________ B. ________________

25. List the x-ray and other procedures from the text.

A. ____________ D. ____________

B. ____________ E. ____________

C. ____________

26. What are the main causes of disease of the cerebral cortex?

A. ________ B. ____________ C. ________ D. ________

27. Give another medical term for Parkinson's disease. ____________

28. A lesion in the anterior portion of the external capsule of the white matter of the cerebrum causes paralysis of the entire opposite side of the body -- face, arm and leg -- and is known as ____________.

29. A lesion in the posterior portion causes loss of sensation in the opposite side of the body and is known as ____________.

30. Hemorrhage due to rupture of the ____________ branch of the middle cerebral artery in patients with high blood pressure causes a condition known as ________ or ________.

31. What are the common causes of cerebellar disease?

A. ____________ C. ____________

B. ____________ D. ____________

32. A lesion of the medulla causes ____________.

33. Large lesions in the midbrain or pons may cause paralysis of both arms and legs a condition called ____________.

34. Inflammation of the meninges is called ________.

35. What are the important organisms which causes meningitis?

A. ____________ E. ____________

B. ____________ F. ____________

C. ____________ G. ____________

D. ____________ H. ____________

36. A chronic disease characterized by attacks of brief or prolonged loss of consciousness and frequently accompanied by convulsions is called

_______________.

37. Major attacks of epilepsy are called _______________.

38. Minor attacks of epilepsy are called _______________.

39. Specific infections of the spinal cord are ______________________ and

____________________.

40. What is the most common cause of disease of individual nerves? _____________

41. Nutritional deficiency is the most frequent cause of what nervous disease?

____

42. Pain over the course of a nerve or over its cutaneous distribution is called

__________________.

43. Name the five layers which cover the skull.

A. ______________ D. ______________________________

B. ______________________ E. ______________________________________

C. ___________________________

44. List the methods used for control of brain hemorrhage.

A. ____

B. _______________________

C. ____

D. ____

45. List the types of grafts used to cover dural defects.

A. ___________________________ D. ______________________

B. ___________________________ E. ______________________

C. ___________________________

46. What are the benign tumors of the skull?

A. ______________________ D. ______________________

B. ______________________ E. ______________________

47. Methods of radiographic diagnosis of brain tumors consist of

A. ______________________________

B. ______________________________

C. ______________________________

D. ______________________________

48. What two surgical procedures may be performed for internal hydrocephalus, obstructive, noncommunicating.

A. ______________________ B. ______________________

49. A procedure performed for Parkinson's disease is called ______________ or ______________.

50. Psychosis of chronic agitated depression may require a surgical procedure called ______________________ or ______________.

51. In cases of irritable carotid body with the resulting conditions ______________________ is performed.

52. A number of procedures are performed for intractable or intolerable pain. What are they?

A. ______________________________

B. ______________________________

C. ______________________________

D. ______________________________

E. ______________________________

F. ______________________________

G. ______________________________

H. ______________________________

I. ______________________________

J. ______________________________

K. ______________________________

53. What is the medical term for "milk leg?" ______________________

54. Cervical spine dislocations are reduced by the use of ____________________ ___________.

55. The surgical procedure performed for herniated _______________________ is called _________________________________.

56. Where adequate decompression of the cord is needed from extradural tumors a ______________________ with removal of the tumor is performed.

57. An accumulation of fluid which eventually forms a cyst in the central canal of the spinal cord causing compression is called ____________________________.

58. What are the common intracranial nerve disorders?

A. ______________________________________

B. _________________________

C. _____________________

D. ______________________________________

E. _______________________________

59. The following are procedures performed for peripheral nerve damage caused by trauma. Give the medical term for each.

A. the suture of an injured nerve ______________________

B. the freeing of a nerve of adhesions ___________________

C. the joining of nerve ends _________________________

D. the transection of a nerve _____________________

E. the plastic repair of a nerve ____________________

F. the excision of a nerve _____________________

G. the excision of a ganglion _______________________

60. Use the alphabetical index on page 108 to find the line and page numbers of the following words. Then write the English translation below each word component of these medical terms.

C R A N I O / T O M Y

E N C E P H A L O / G R A P H Y

H E M I / P L E G I A

D E / S Y M / P A T H / E C T O M / I Z E

N E U R / A L G I A

A / S Y / S T O L E

O L F A C T / O R Y

M E N I N G O / C O C C U S

R A D I O / I S O / T O P E

C E R E B E L L U M

A / T R O P H Y

T R I / G E M I N / A L

V E N T R I C / U L O -/U R E T E R O / S T O M Y

A U T O / N O M / I C

S Y M / M E T R / I C A L

D E / N E R V / A T I O N

R H I Z O / T O M Y

CHAPTER V
THE CIRCULATORY AND LYMPH VASCULAR SYSTEM
STUDY LESSON

1. The circulatory system is made up of four functionally different parts. Give the name of each after its description.

   A. a muscular pump ______________

   B. the conducting and distributing vessels ________________ and ________________; the functional part ________________; the collecting vessels ________________________ and ________

   C. the circulatory fluid ____________________

   D. The auxiliary system for returning fluid from tissue spaces is the ________________________ also called the ____________________________.

2. What are the three coats which make up the walls of the heart?

   A. ____________________

   B. ____________________

   C. ____________________

3. What is the sac in which the heart is lodged?

   ____

4. The superior and inferior venae cavae empty into the _________ ____________ or ___________ of the heart.

5. The pulmonary arteries leave from the ___________ ____________ or _________________ and always contain ____________ blood.

6. The four pulmonary veins empty into the _______ _________ and always contain ______________ blood.

7. The aorta leaves from the ________ ____________ and always contains ________________ blood.

8. There are two valves between the auricles and ventricles. The valve on the right side is the ___________ valve; the valve on the left side is the _____________ or _________ valve.

Using the illustration on page 112 as reference identify the components of the circulatory system marked on this drawing.

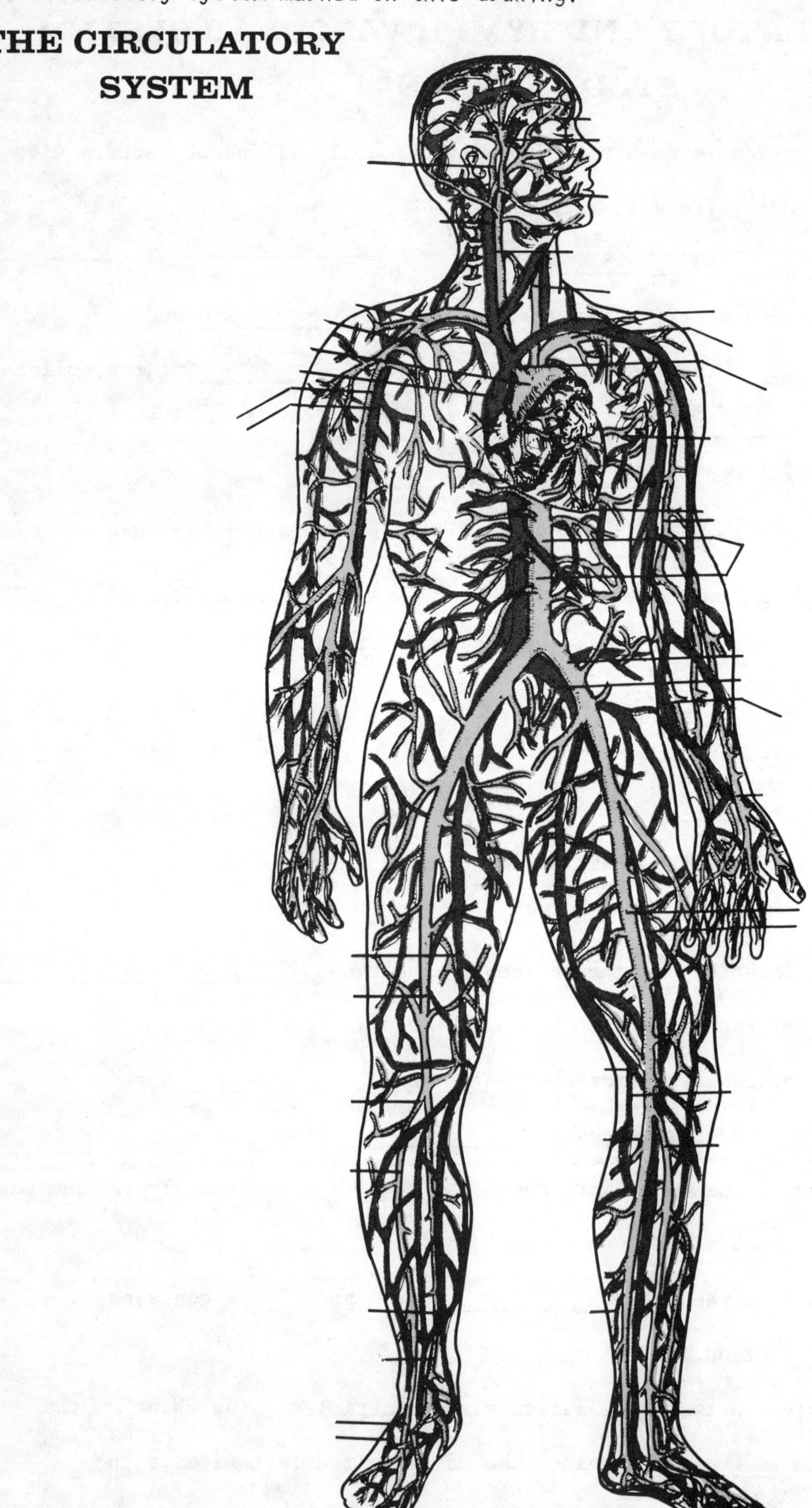

Using the illustration from page 116 as reference identify the areas of the heart marked on this drawing. On the lines below copy the material on the circulation of blood from page 116.

CIRCULATION OF BLOOD THROUGH THE HEART

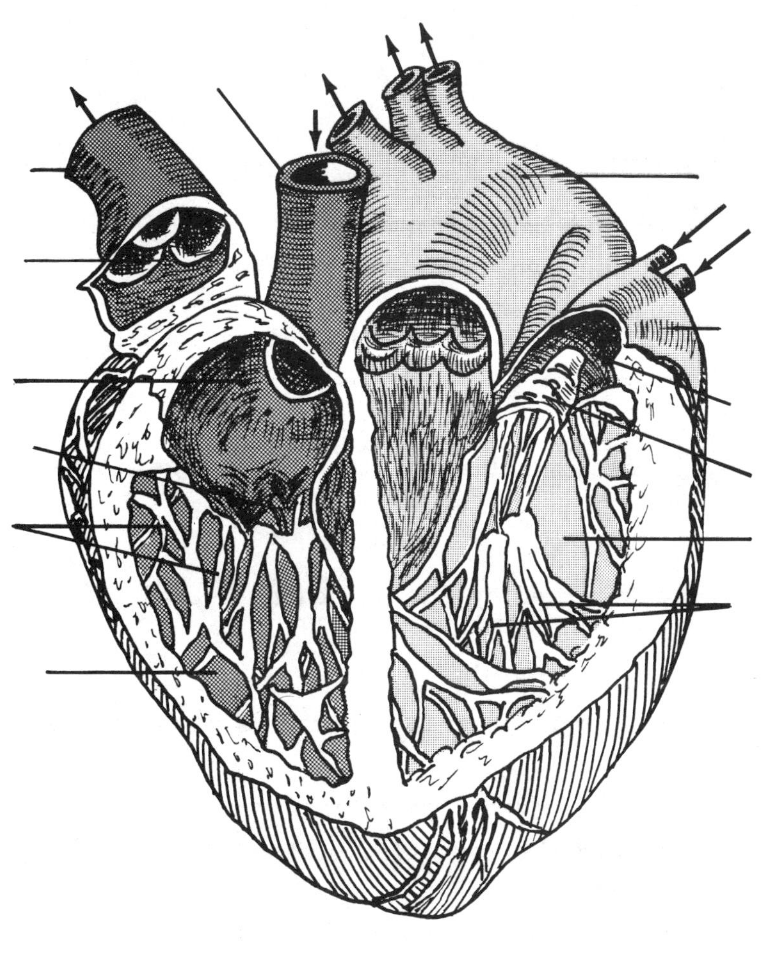

9. The strong cords attached at one end to the border of the valves are called the ____________ ________________. The fleshy columns to which they are attached at their other end are the ______________ muscles.

10. The arteries which encircle the heart like a crown and which supply the substance of the heart with blood are the ______________arteries.

11. The walls of larger blood vessels are nourished by small blood vessels called ________ ______________.

12. What are the three coats which make up the arterial walls?

    A. the inner coat, the ________ __________ or ________

    B. the middle coat, the ________ __________

    C. the outer coat, the __________ __________ or ______________

13. Complete the following to show how some of the blood vessels are formed and the functions some of them perform.

    A. The small arteries formed by the branching out of the arteries are called ____________.

    B. The microscopic vessels formed by the branching out of the arterioles are called the _________________.

    C. There is only one place where the blood performs its function of nourishing the tissues. It is in the _________________.

    D. The larger tubes formed by the reuniting of the capillaries are known as the _________________.

    E. The merging of the venules results in vessels called ____________.

14. The blood is composed of ____________ and ____________.

15. The solids in the blood are composed of

    A. red blood cells or _______________,

    B. white blood cells or _______________,

    C. platelets or ___________________.

Using the illustration on page 117 as reference identify the various types of blood cells. Write the names of the cells on the lines provided in the drawing.

NORMAL BLOOD CELLS

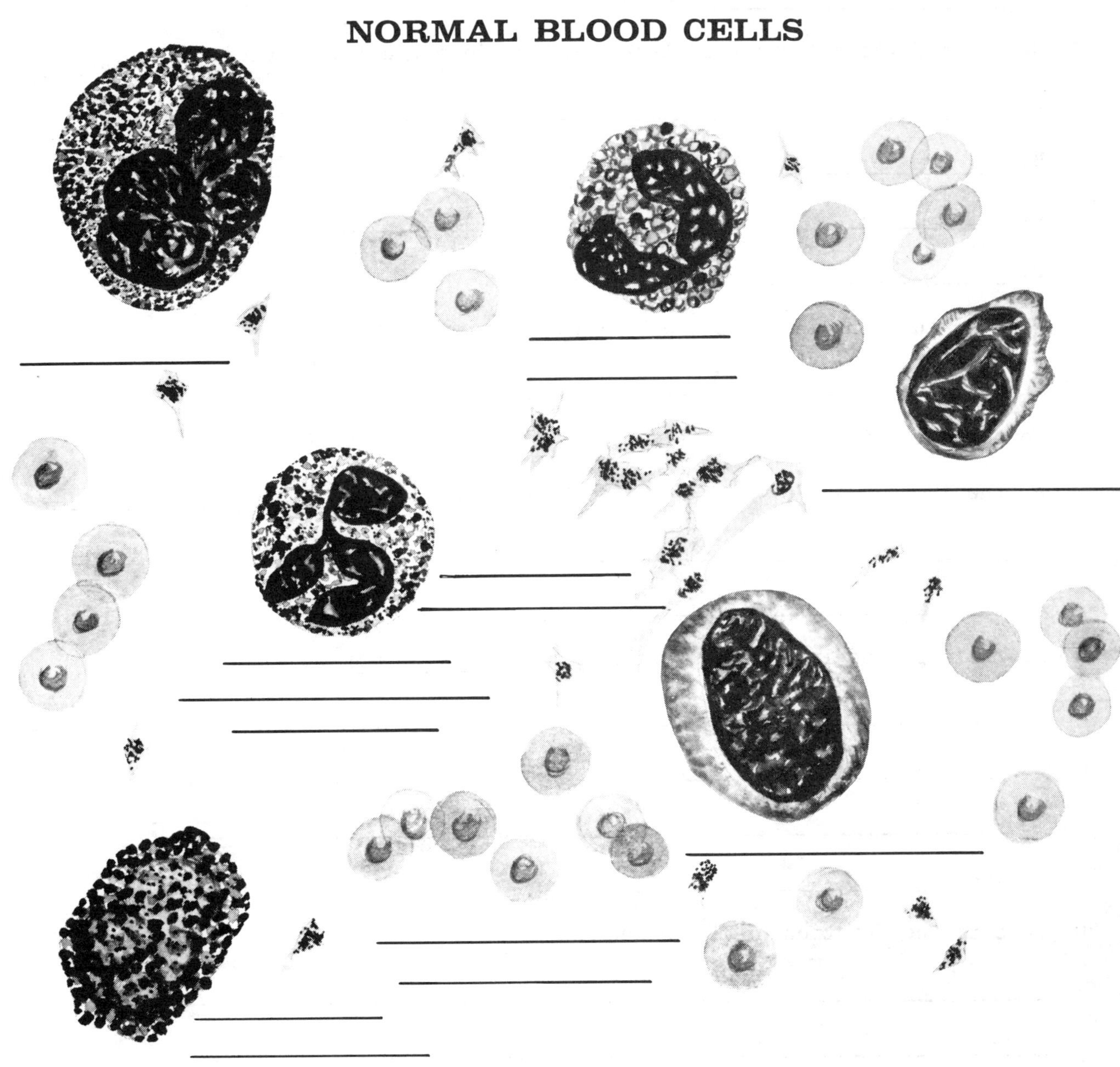

16. Give the normal amount of red blood cells (RBCs) and white blood cells (WBCs) in a cubic millimeter of healthy blood for men and women.

    A. ____________________ RBC for men

    B. ____________________ RBC for women

    C. ____________________ WBC or leukocytes

17. Name the different types of leukocytes besides the lymphocytes.

    A. ________________________ or ________________________

    B. ________________________ or ________________________

    C. ________________________ or ________________________

    D. ________________________

18. What is the function of the platelets or thrombocytes?

    ____

19. Complete the following listing of the three lymphatic divisions.

    A. the lymph vessels which are made up of the ________ __________,
    ______________, ____________ ______, ______ ___ ________
    ______, ______________:

    B. the expanded lymph spaces made up of the ________ ________, ____
    ________ ________, ___ ______________ ________, ____
    ____________ ________, ____ __________ ________ ___
    ____ ____ ____ ____, ______ __________ ______;

    C. the ________ ______.

20. What is the function of the lymphatics?

    ____

    ____

21. Fill in the following material on the lymph nodes.

    A. Where are the lymph nodes found?

        1. Around the ______________________________muscle draining the back of the tongue;

21. (continued)

    2. the ____________, ____________ cavities, __________ of the ____________, and ____________;

    3. under the __________ of the ____________ draining the floor of the __________.

    B. When the lymph nodes in these areas become inflamed as a result of infection it is called _________________.

    C. In the lower extremities the greatest number of lymph nodes are massed in the ______________.

22. An excessive amount of lymph in the tissues results in a condition known as ___________ or ___________.

23. What are some of the causes of heart disease?

    A. __________________

    B. _________________________

    C. ______________________________

    D. _____________________________________

    E. _____________________________________

24. What are the most important diseases of the arteries?

    A. _________________________

    B. ______________________________

25. What are the principal causes of disease of the veins?

    ____

26. Name the most frequent etiologic types of heart disease.

    A. ______________________

    B. ______________________

    C. ______________________________

    D. ____________________

27. What are the lesions found in congenital heart disease?

    A. ______________________________

    B. ____

    C. ______________________________________

    D. ____

    E. ____________________________________

    F. ___________________________

Refer to the illustration on page 119 as a guide in identifying the component parts of the lymph vascular system indicated on this drawing.

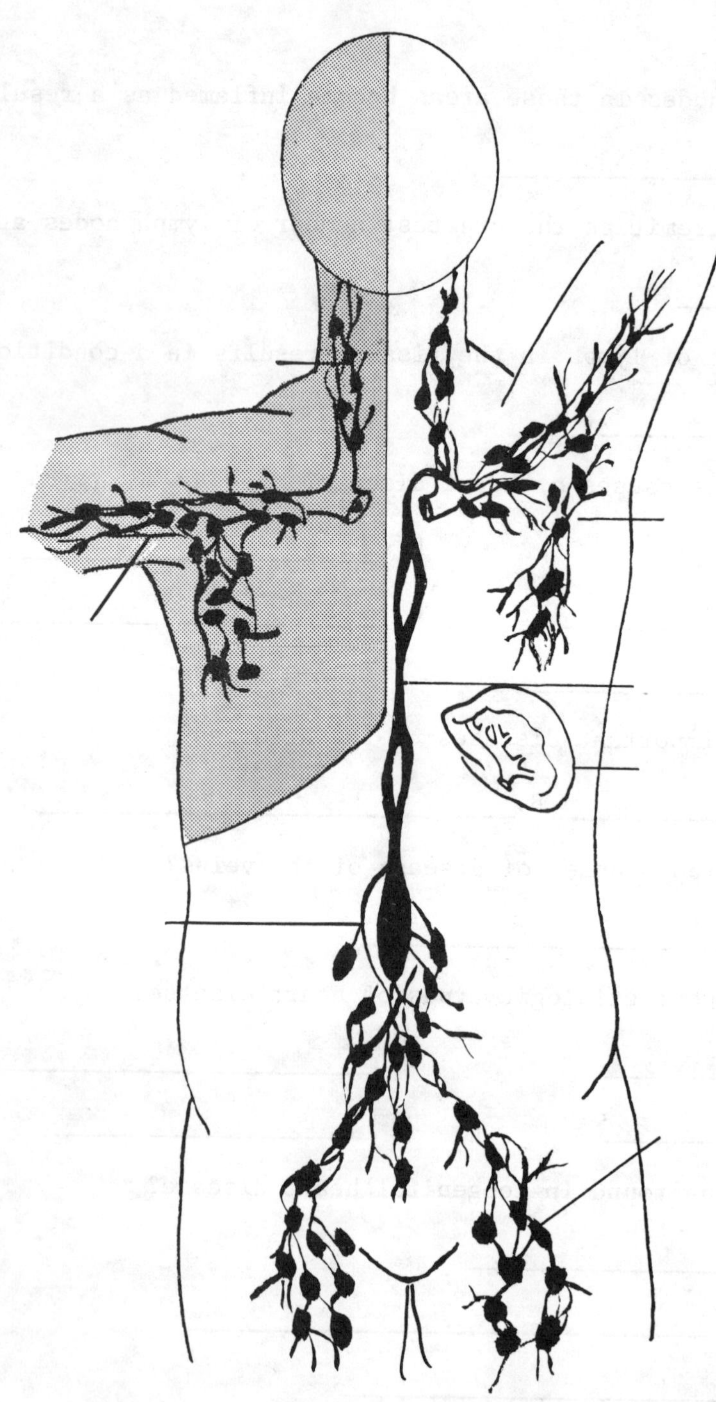

LYMPH VASCULAR SYSTEM

28. When a sinus rhythm is unusually rapid it is called sinus __________________; when it is unusually slow it is called sinus ____________________; when it is irregular it is called sinus _____________________.

29. What are the most important ectopic rhythms?

   A. ______________________________

   B. _________________________________

   C. ______________________________

30. Give the medical term for these diagnoses:

   A. Heart block is known as _____________________________ block.

   B. Pain due to coronary narrowing is called __________________________.

   C. The formation of a blood clot within a blood vessel is known as ___________________.

   D. The obstruction of the blood vessel by the lodging of some particle floating in the blood stream is called ___________________.

31. A. The localized dilation of an artery is known as an _______________.

   B. Give the two types of aneurysms.

      1. _________________________

      2. _________________________

32. Rare diseases of the arteries include:

   A. _____________________________________ or ____________________________

   B. _________________________________

   C. ______________________________ or ___________________________________

   D. _____________________________

   E. _____________________________________

33. High blood pressure is called _____________________; low blood pressure is called ________________________.

34. List the three conditions which may affect the veins.

   A. ______________________   C. ______________________________

   B. ______________________________

35. A. What is anemia?

____

____

B. Name some of the primary anemias.

1. ____________________ 4. ____________________

2. ____________________ 5. ____________________

3. ____________________

36. Give the medical term for each of these diseases of the blood.

A. An increase above normal of the number of erythrocytes per unit of circulating blood is called ____________________.

B. Diseases characterized by the presence of abnormal white cells in the blood and an unusually high white cell count are called the ____________________.

C. A decrease of granulocytes in the blood is called ____________________. It is also known as ____________________ and ____________________.

D. Spontaneous bleeding into the skin and mucous membrane is called ____________________.

E. A hereditary disease in which the blood clots very slowly, which only affects males but is transmitted through females is known as ____________________.

37. Give the medical term for the following lymphatic diseases and conditions.

A. Inflammation of the lymph vessels ____________________.

B. Obstruction by parasites ____________________.

C. Obstruction of lymphatics ____________________.

D. Chronic swelling due to lymphatic obstruction ____________________

E. Inflammation of the lymph nodes ____________________

38. A by-passing of the heart by diverting the blood around the heart and lungs to obtain an almost bloodless operating field is known as ____________________ ____________________.

39. A. What terms are used to designate cessation of heart action?

    1. ____________________ 3. ____________________

    2. ____________________

    B. What is the name of the treatment given?

    ______________________________ and ______________________

40. A procedure of diagnostic value is cardiac ______________________.

41. List the acquired heart lesions amenable to surgery.

    A. ____________________ F. ____________________

    B. ____________________ G. ____________________

    C. ____________________ H. ____________________

    D. ____________________ I. ____________________

    E. ____________________

42. List the congenital heart lesions amenable to surgery.

    A. ____________________ D. ____________________

    B. ____________________ E. ____________________

    C. ____________________

43. Separation of the leaflets of a valve is a surgical procedure known as

    ____________________ or ______________________________.

44. Give the surgical procedures performed for the following diagnoses:

    A. serofibrinous pericarditis ____________________

    B. hemorrhagic pericardial effusion ______________________ and

    ____

    C. suppurative pericarditis and infected serofibrinous pericarditis

    ____________________ with ______________________,

    ______________________________ and ____________________

    ____

    D. chronic constrictive pericarditis ____________________ and

    ____

44. (continued)

E. subacute or acute bacterial endocarditis

1. ______________________________

2. ______________________________

F. coronary arterial disease ____________________________ or ______________

____

G. removal of obstructing area within the lumen of the vessel ________________

____

H. aortic regurgitation or insufficiency ______________________________________

I. pulmonic stenosis ____ and

____

J. tricuspid atresia with hypoplasia of right ventricles __________________

or ______________________________

K. diverticula or aneurysms of the heart ______________________________

45. List the types of malignant tumors of the heart.

A. ______________________________ F. ______________________________

B. ______________________________ G. ______________________________

C. ______________________________ H. ______________________________

D. ______________________________ I. ______________________________

E. ______________________________ J. ______________________________

46. In obliterative disease or Leriche's syndrome what procedure is used to remove the clot and plaque from the artery?

____

47. Give the two methods used for treatment of varicose veins.

A. ____

____

B. ____

48. Give the conditions for which a splenectomy is performed.

A. ______________________________

B. ______________________________

C. ______________________________

D. ______________________________

E. ______________________________

F. ______________________________

G. ______________________________

H. ______________________________

I. ______________________________

J. ______________________________

K. ______________________________

49. What three surgical procedures are performed for portal hypertension?

A. ______________________________

B. ______________________________

C. ______________________________

50. Use the alphabetical index on page 142 to find the line and page numbers of the following words. Then write the English translation below each word component of these medical terms.

C O M / M I S S U R O / R R H A P H Y

E N D / A R T E R / E C T O M Y

I N F U N D I B U L / A R

E R Y T H R O / M E L / A L G I A

P E R I / C A R D I O / C E N T E S I S

A U R / I C U L O / V E N T R / I C U L / A R

L Y M P H O / C Y T E S

P H L E B O / T H R O M B / O S I S

P A N / H E M A T O / C Y T O / P E N I A

V A S A   V A S O R U M

A D A M A N T I N / O M A

C O / A R C T / A T I O N

A / G R A N U L O / C Y T O S I S

D I M I N U / T I O N

A R / R H Y T H M / I A

C A R D I O / P E R I / C A R D I O / P E X Y

D I P H T H E R I A

A T H E R O / S C L E R / O S I S

L E I O / M Y O / S A R C / O M A

H E M O / S T A S I S

CHAPTER VI
THE ENDOCRINE SYSTEM
STUDY LESSON

1. A. If glands are classified according to structure they are

   1. ______________ and 2. ______________

   B. If classified according to function, glands are

   1. ____________________ and 2. ____________________

   C. The secretory glands are of two types: one type is provided with

   _____________, and the second type is called ________________

   or ____________________ glands.

2. Name the glands which secrete external secretions.

   A. ________________ E. ________________ H. ____________________

   B. ________________ F. ________________ I. ____________________

   C. ________________ G. ________________ J. ____________________

   D. ________________

3. List the seven ductless (endocrine) glands.

   A. ____________________________ E. ________________ or ________________

   B. ____________________________ F. ________________ or ________________

   C. ____________________________ G. __________ (__________ and __________)

   D. ________________ or ________________

4. What other organs have special cells which function as ductless glands?

   A. ____________________________

   B. ____________________________

   C. ____

5. What is the name of that part of the thyroid gland which connects its two lobes?

   ____

6. What health essential (hormone) does the thyroid gland furnish?

   ____

7. What is the general effect of the thyroid gland?

   ____

Use the illustration on page 148 as reference for identification of the endocrine glands indicated on this drawing.

THE ENDOCRINE SYSTEM

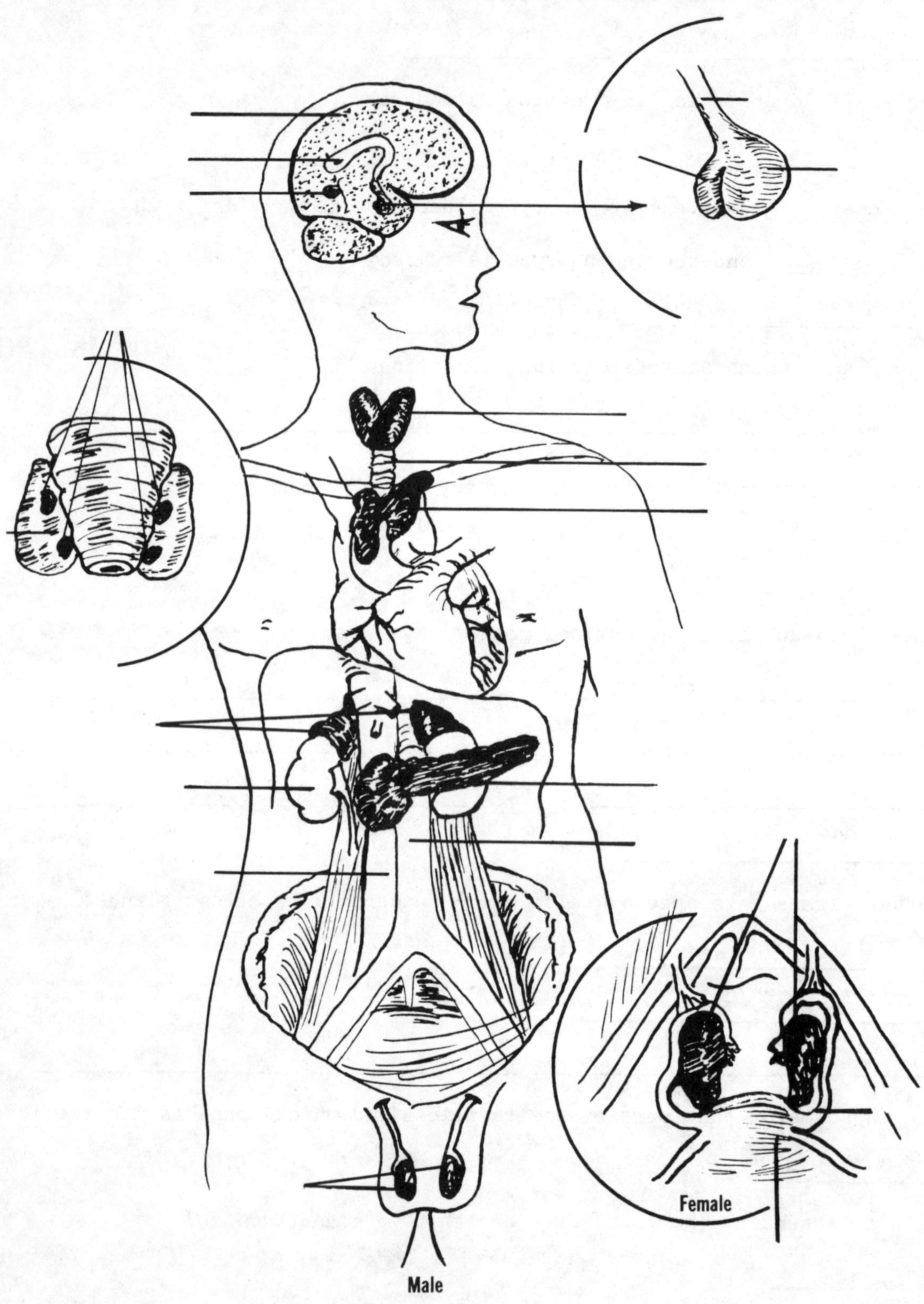

8. A. What are the small glands located between the posterior borders of the lateral lobes of the thyroid gland?

____

B. How many are there?

____

9. What gland is only a temporary organ and diminishes after puberty?

____

10. There are two small, yellowish bodies which are placed above and in front of the upper end of each kidney. They are called the __________________glands or _________________. These glands are composed of two parts: the _________ and the ____________. The medulla secretes a substance called ______________.

11. A. What gland is situated at the base of the brain?

_______________________ or ______________________

B. What is the term for the saddle-like depression in which this gland is lodged? ________________________

C. How many lobes does this gland have and what are they?

______________. They are the _________________ and the ____________________.

D. What substance is extracted from the posterior lobe? ______________________

E. What medical specialty is this substance used in and for what reasons?

________________ ____

____

12. This gland is a small reddish body that is attached to the roof of the ventricle. It decreases in size after puberty. It is the _______________________ or

__________________.

13. The ovaries produce _________ and two internal secretions. One secretion is formed by the _______________ ____________ and is called ____________. The second secretion is formed by the cells of the ____________ ____________ and is known as _________________ or _________________.

14. The testes produce ____________________ and the ______________ cells produce an internal secretion ____________________.

15. What two substances does the liver form? ________________ and _________.

16. A special group of cells in the pancreas called the islands of ______________________ furnish an internal secretion containing ____________ which is essential in sugar _______________.

17. When there is a decrease in the iodine content of the thyroid gland as a result of atrophy or removal of the gland it is called ____________________.

18. Give the pathological conditions which result from this condition.

A. __________________

B. __________________

C. __________________

19. Over-activity of the thyroid gland is called _______________________ and produces a condition called ____________________ or ____________________ ________________.

20. Benign tumor of the thyroid is known as _______________ of the thyroid (______________________________ or ______________goiter).

21. Adenoma of the parathyroids causes _________________________________. This causes a condition known as ______________ ___________ ___________.

22. Lack of parathyroid secretion causes _______________________________.

23. Hypersecretion of the adrenal cortex leads to a combination of symptoms called ____________ _____________.

24. Hypofunction of the adrenal cortex leads to a syndrome called _______________ ______________.

25. Name the two primary medullary tumors of the adrenals.

A. ____________________________ B. ___________________________________

26. These tumors are also known as ___________________________________.

27. Lack of descent of the testes into the scrotum is called ____________________.

28. Failure of establishment of the menses or their sudden stoppage is known as

_______________________.

29. What is the medical term for "change of life?" _____________

30. Substances with estrogenic effects such as ________________, ________________ are used to give relief from menopausal symptoms.

31. What condition of the bones may occur from 10 to 20 years after the menopause?

____

32. Malignant tumors believed to arise from rests of testicular cells in the ovary are ______________________________.

33. When bones become thicker and heavier due to hypersecretion of the eosinophile cells of the _____________ body a condition called _____________ results.

34. Simmond's disease or ____________ ___________ results from severe _____________________________ in adults.

35. Name four types of pituitary tumors.

A. _________________________________ C. _________________________________

B. _________________________________ D. _________________________________

36. The inability of the body cells to utilize glucose results in a condition known as _______________ ______________.

37. What are the symptoms of this condition?

A. _______________________________ D. _______________________________

B. _______________________________ E. _______________________________

C. _______________________________

38. What condition is the reverse of diabetes mellitus?

_______________ ________________ This condition is also called

_______________________________.

39. The chemical changes that take place within the cells and tissues of the body as it carries on its life processes are known as ____________________.

40. When the body fluids shift to the acid side it is _________________. The reverse condition is _________________.

41. Bronze diabetes or ______________________ results from the deposition of

________________.

42. Pigmentation of the skin due to deposition of an unidentified black pigment results in ________________.

43. When excessive quantities of organic pigments called ________________ are formed in the body a condition known as ________________ occurs.

44. Gout is a disorder of __________ ________________ characterized by inflammation of the joints and sometimes by deposition of ____________ __________ in the ____________________ tissues.

45. The deposition of an unidentified substance known as ______________ in the organs or tissues is called ____________________.

46. A. Obscure disturbances of fat and lipoid metabolism which occur in children are known as _________________________.

B. List the names of these diseases which include the names of the doctors who first described them.

1. ____________________________ 3. ______________________________

2. ____________________________ 4. ______________________________

C. What is another term for Tay-Sach's disease? ________________________

_______________.

47. List the indications for a subtotal or total removal of the thyroid gland known as ____________________.

A. _____________________________________

B. ____

C. _____________________________________

D. ____

E. ____

F. ____

G. __________________________________

48. Parathyroid surgery is indicated in cases of ______________________________.

49. What surgeries are performed on the adrenal glands?

A. ____

B. ____

C. ____

D. ____

50. Refer to the index on page 160 for the line and page number of the following words. Under each word component write the English translation.

P A T H O / L O G I C / A L

C R Y P T / O R C H I D / I S M

H Y P O / P H Y S I S

T A C H Y / C A R D / I A

A R R H E N O / B L A S T / O M A S

E X / O P H T H A L M / I C

P A N / C R E A S

P A R A / G A N G L I / O M A

S P E R M A T O / Z O A

A / M E N O / R R H E A

M Y X / E D E M A

A M Y L / O I D / O S I S

H Y P E R / P A R A / T H Y R / O I D / I S M

P O L Y / P H A G I A

N E P H R O -/ A D / R E N A L / E C T O M Y

S E L L A T U R C I C A

O S T E O / P O R O S I S

A C R O / M E G A L Y

H E M O / C H R O M A T / O S I S

O C H R O N / O S I S

CHAPTER VII
THE RESPIRATORY SYSTEM

STUDY LESSON

1. A. When the blood is brought into contact with the air in the lungs it takes up ____________ and gives up __________ ____________.

   B. As the blood circulates to the tissues and the cells it gives up ____________ and takes on __________ ____________.

   C. This exchange is known as __________________.

2. A. The external opening of the nasal cavities are the _____________ or anterior ___________.

   B. The lateral wall of each external opening is called the ________ of the nose.

   C. The nasal cavities are separated by the __________ ____________.

   D. The three scroll-like processes of bone attached to the lateral wall of each nasal cavity are called the nasal __________ or _______________.

3. Air is transmitted from the nose or mouth to the larynx by way of the ____________.

4. What is the medical term for that part of the respiratory system which is called the "voice box?"

   ____

5. Give the names of the three single and the three paired cartilages of the larynx.

   A. __________________________ D. __________________________

   B. __________________________ E. __________________________

   C. __________________________ F. __________________________

6. The thyroid cartilage consists of two square plates which form by their union the ______________ ______________ or "__________ ___________."

7. The windpipe, which is cylindrical in shape, is called the _____________.

8. Into what does the trachea divide?

   ____

Use the illustrations on pages 164, 166, 168 and 169 for reference. Then identify the areas indicated on the drawings on this page and the following two pages.

UPPER RESPIRATORY TRACT

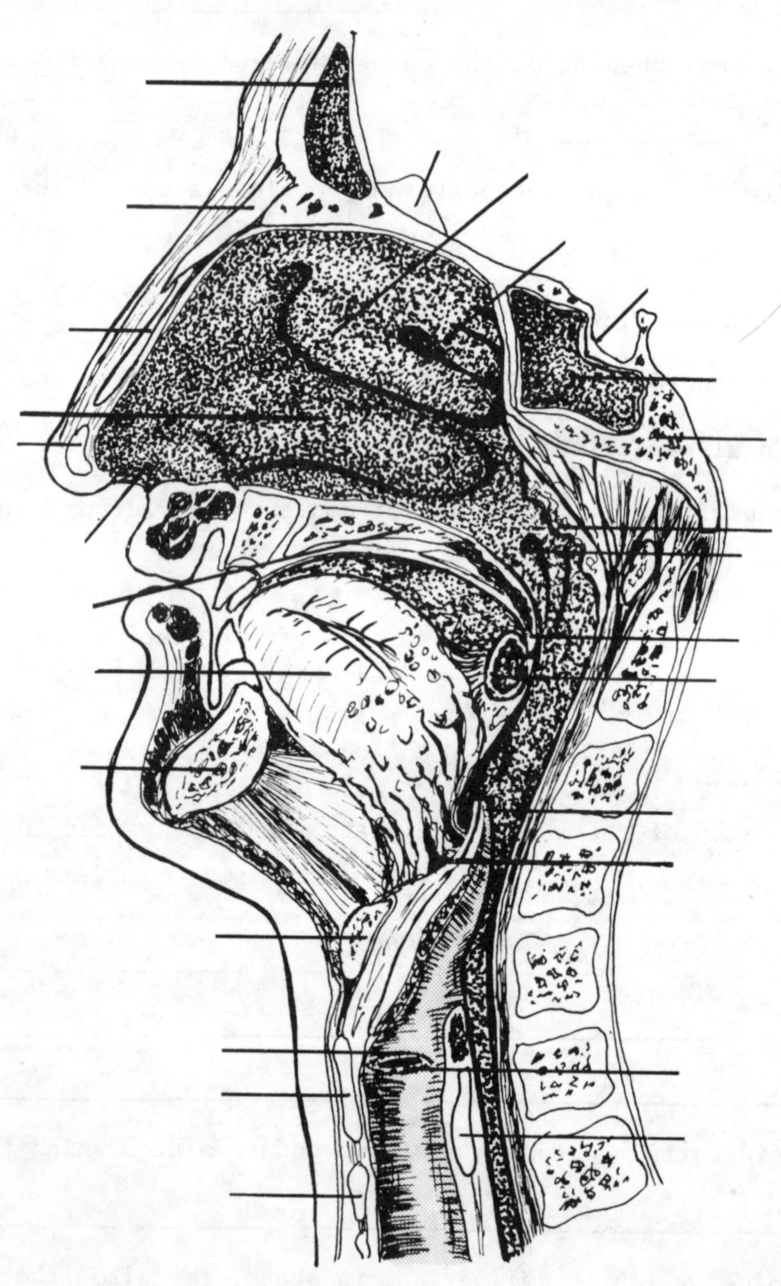

THE RESPIRATORY SYSTEM

Use the illustrations on pages 166, 168 and 169 as reference. Then identify the areas shown on this drawing and the two drawings on page 64.

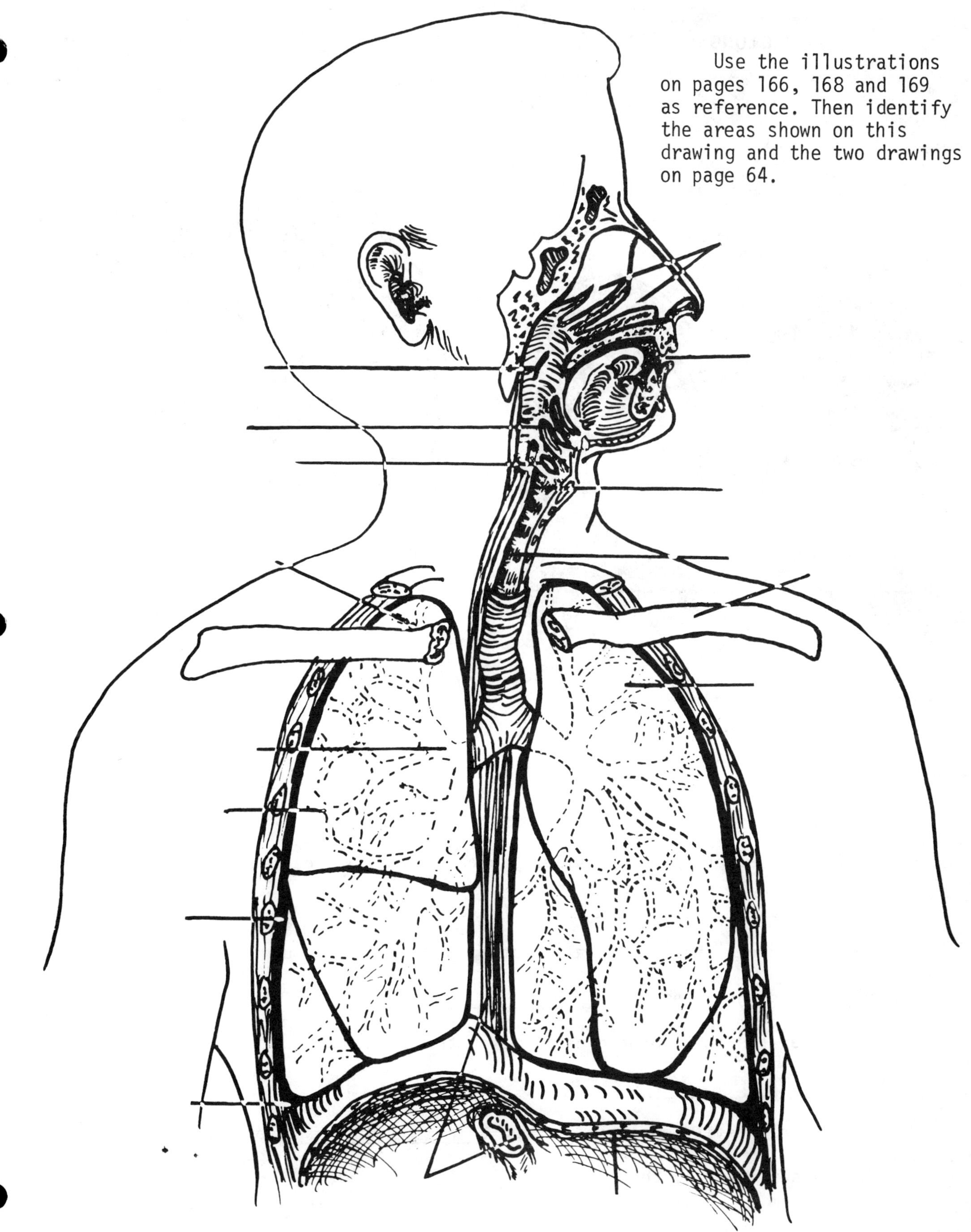

THE LUNGS

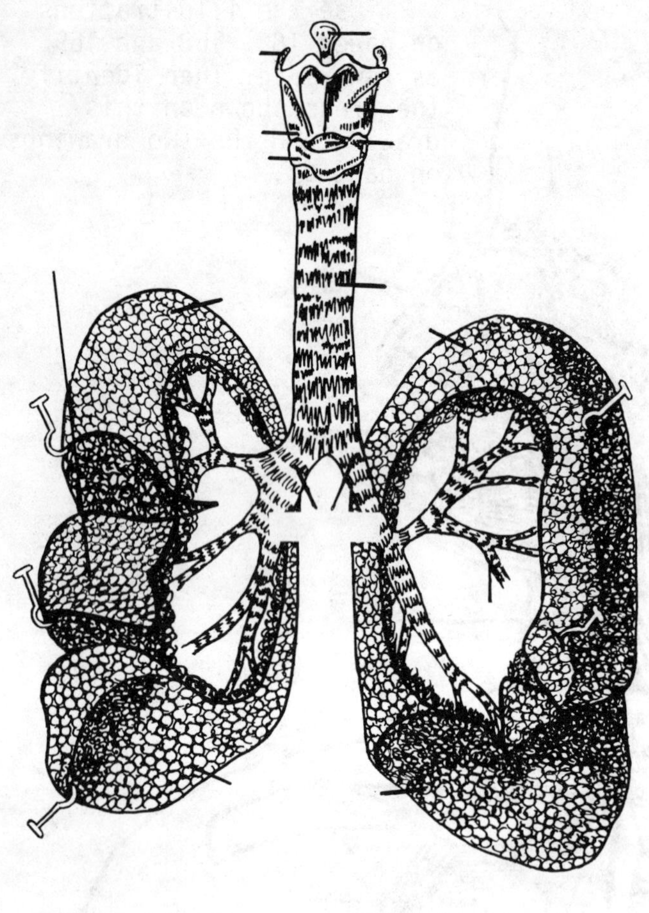

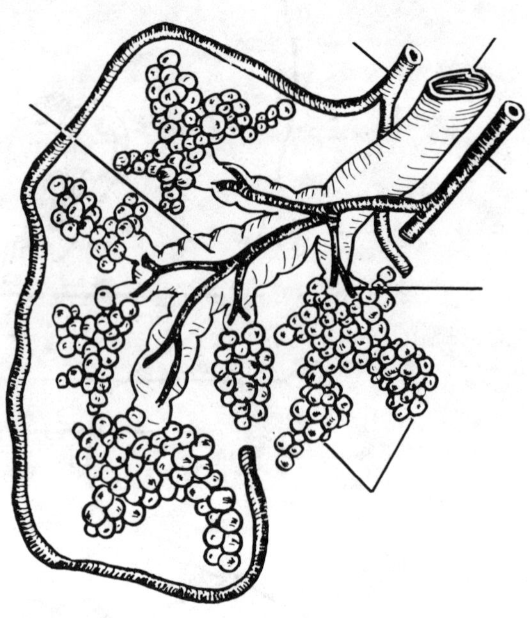

PRIMARY LOBULE OF THE LUNG

9. The bronchi break up into smaller branches which are called ________________ tubes or ____________________.

10. Each bronchiole ends in a small duct or ____________ upon which are small, irregular projections, the ______________ or air cells.

11. What separates the thoracic cavity from the abdominal cavity?

____

12. The thoracic cavity encloses the two ______________ cavities which are completely separated by the ________________.

13. Give the contents of the mediastinum.

A. ____________________ H. ____________________

B. ____________________ I. ____________________

C. ____________________ J. ____________________

D. ____________________ K. ____________________

E. ____________________ L. ____________________

F. ____________________ M. ____________________

G. ____________________ ____________________

14. The pleura closely adherent to the walls of the chest is called the ____________________ and the pleura which closely covers the lung is called ____________________ or ____________________.

15. Each lung is connected to the heart and trachea by the

A. ____________________ E. ____________________

B. ____________________ F. ____________________

C. ____________________ G. ____________________

D. ____________________ H. ____________________

16. The above structures constitute the root of the lung and enter the lung substance through the ____________________.

17. What is the main cause of respiratory diseases? ____________________

18. List the specific infectious diseases which cause respiratory disease.

A. ____________________ E. ____________________

B. ____________________ F. ____________________

C. ____________________ G. ____________________

D. ____________________

19. Give the most important symptoms of respiratory disease.

A. ____________________ C. ____________________

B. ____________________ D. ____________________

____

20. What methods are used to examine the chest?

A. ______________________________ C. ______________________________

B. ______________________________ D. ______________________________

21. A. Acute inflammation of the nose is called ______________.

B. Give the different types.

1. ________________________

2. ________________________

3. ________________________

4. ________________________

22. Nasal _________ are rounded, _______________, _________________ benign tumors attached to the lateral walls of the nose.

23. Inflammation of the mucous membrane of the paranasal sinuses is called _________________.

24. Inflammation of the pharynx is called ___________________.

25. Typical acute tonsillitis is caused by ________________ _________________.

26. Atypical or milder forms of tonsillitis may occur in the absence of detectable _______________ organisms, in ______________ ________________ and Vincent's _________________.

27. The tonsils are involved in most cases of ______________.

28. Severe acute inflammation of the soft tissues of the palate adjacent to the tonsil is called __________________ _____________ or ______________.

29. A. Inflammation of the larynx is called ___________________.

B. Benign tumors of the larynx give rise to persistent hoarseness and ______________________ cough.

C. If a foreign body passes the vocal cords it nearly always passes down as far as the ___________________ of the trachea.

30. What are the most important diseases of the bronchi?

A. ______________________________ C. ______________________________

B. ______________________________

31. A. Give the causes of acute pneumonia.

_____________________ and _____________________

B. Collapse of the lung so that the air sacs become smaller is called

____

C. Overdistension of the lungs is _____________________. It is the reverse of _____________________.

D. Continued inhalation of certain mineral dusts results in _____________________.

E. Valley fever, desert fever or San Joaquin Valley fever is also known as _____________________. It is caused by inhaling the spores of the fungus _____________________.

32. A. Using the medical term from the text give the three principal diseases of the pleura.

1. _______________ 2. _____________________ 3. _______________

B. Give the three types of pleurisy.

1. _____________________ 3. _____________________

2. _____________________

33. What are the important diseases of the mediastinum?

A. _____________________ C. _____________________

B. _______________

34. Give the surgical procedure used for the following indications:

A. nasal deformities including rhinophyma _____________________

B. polyposis _______________ _______________ or _______________

C. deviations of nasal septum _______________ _______________

D. Chronic sinusitis which does not respond to conservative treatment is treated by several procedures. List all.

1. _____________________ 4. _____________________

2. _____________________ 5. _____________________

3. _____________________

35. What are four forms of neoplasms which can occur on the tongue.

A. ______________________ C. ______________________

B. ______________________ D. ______________________

36. What does I & D mean? ______________________

37. Give the indications for tonsillectomy.

A. ______________________ E. ______________________

B. ______________________ F. ______________________

C. ______________________ G. ______________________

D. ______________________ ______________________

______________________ H. ______________________

____

38. A. The growth of normal adenoid tissue in the pharyngeal vault is called ______________ of the ______________ tonsil. The surgery for this condition is called ______________.

B. What does T & A mean? ______________________

39. What are the procedures performed for tuberculosis of the larynx?

A. ______________________ E. ______________________

______________________ F. ______________________

B. ______________________ G. ______________________

C. ______________________ H. ______________________

D. ______________________

40. What are the indications for tracheotomy?

A. ______________________ F. ______________________

B. ______________________ G. ______________________

C. ______________________ ______________________

D. ______________________ H. ______________________

E. ______________________ I. ______________________

J. ______________________

41. For tumors of the larynx that are not accessible by direct means a ______________ or ______________ is performed.

42. What is the indication for a total laryngectomy?

____

43. What happens to patients who have this surgery?

____

44. List the indications for bronchoscopy.

A. ______________________________

B. ______________________________

C. ______________________________

D. ______________________________

E. ______________________________

F. ______________________________

G. ______________________________

H. ______________________________

I. ______________________________

J. ______________________________

K. ______________________________

L. ______________________________

M. ______________________________

N. ______________________________

O. ______________________________

____

45. A. The introduction of a needle into the chest wall for purposes of diagnosis and therapy is called ______________.

B. It is indicated for the following reasons:

1. ______________ 3. ______________

2. ______________ 4. ______________

46. A. The procedure performed for acute empyema is ______________________.

    B. For tuberculosis with cavitation an ________________ ______________ is performed.

47. Give the full medical term for the following abbreviations:

    A. C.A.O. ____

    B. C.O.L.D. ____

    C. C.O.P.E. ____

    D. I.P.P.B. ____

48. Lobectomy is performed for

    A. ____________________________ D. ____________________________

    B. ____________________________ E. ____________________________

    C. ____________________________

49. A. Total removal or _____________________ of the lung is called _______________________.

    B. One of the indications for this procedure is ______________________ carcinoma.

50. Refer to the index beginning on page 180 for the line and page number of the following words. Put the English translation beneath each word component.

D Y S / P N E A

Q U I N S Y

B R O N C H I / O L E S

M O N O / N U C L E / O S I S

P A R O X Y S M / A L

S E S S I L E

A T E L / E C T A S I S

B I F U R C / A T I O N

C O R P U L M O N A L E

M E D I A / S T I N U M

D I A / P H R A G M

A R Y T E N / O I D

H E M O / P T Y S I S

T H O R A C O / T O M Y

A / Z Y G O S

C O C C I D I O I D O / M Y C / O S I S

E X T I R P / A T I O N

H E M / A N G I O / E N D O / T H E L I / O M A

A U S C U L T A T I O N

R H I N O / P H Y M A

CHAPTER VIII
THE GASTRO-INTESTINAL SYSTEM

STUDY LESSON

1. What are the organs which make up the digestive system?

   A. ____________ C. ____________ E. ____________

   B. ____________ D. ____________ F. ____________

2. List the divisions of the alimentary canal.

   A. ______________________________

   ____

   B. ____________

   C. ____________

   D. ____________

   E. ______________________________

   ____

   F. ______________________________

   G. ____________

   H. ____________

3. What are the divisions of the colon?

   A. ____________ C. ____________

   B. ____________ D. ____________

4. A. What is the name of the small process which hangs from the middle of the lower border of the palate? ____________

   B. What is its English translation? ____________

5. A. Give the names of the two arches which occur on both sides of the uvula.

   ____________ and ____________ arches.

   B. What else are they called?

   ____________ and ____________

   ____

Refer to pages 184 and 189 for identification. Then identify the areas noted on these drawings from the original illustrations.

GASTRO-INTESTINAL SYSTEM

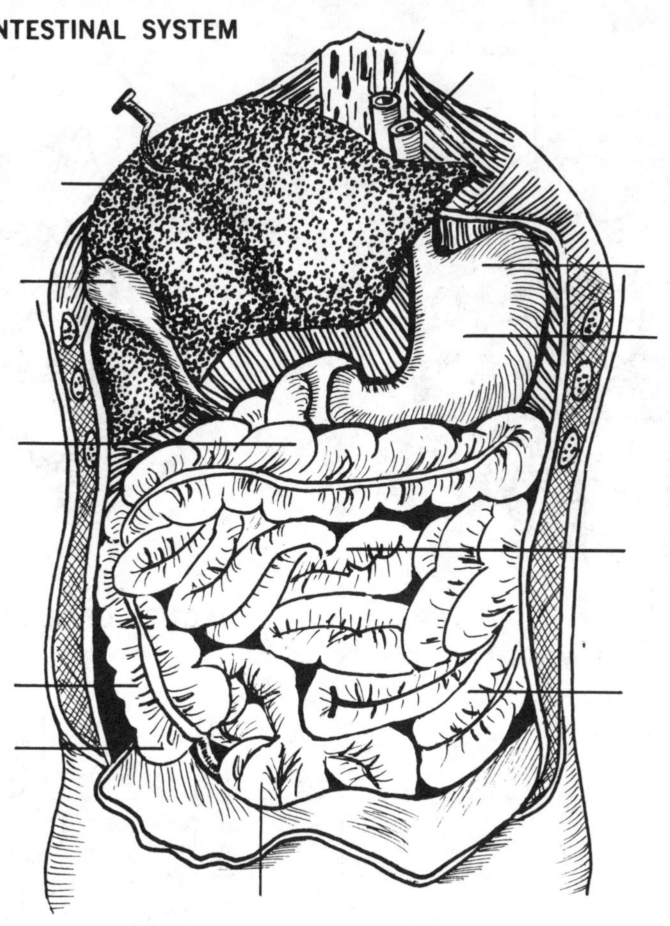

REGIONS OF THE ABDOMEN

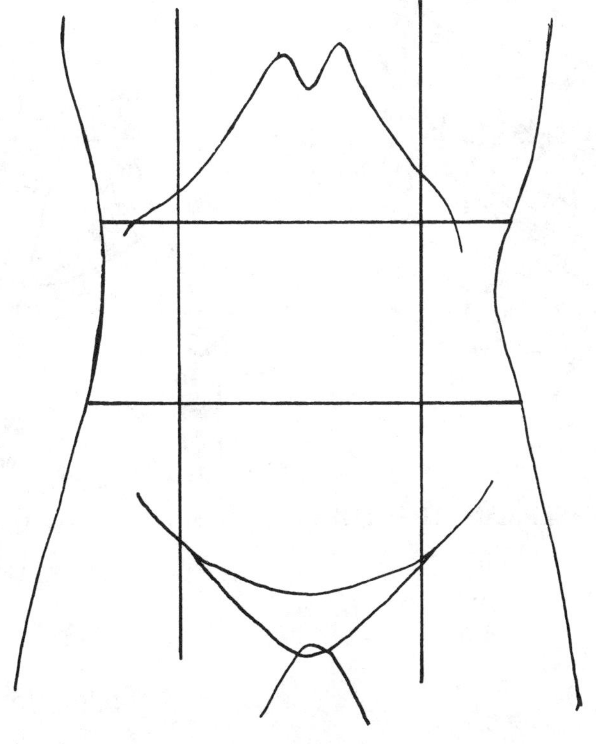

Use the illustrations on pages 186 and 187 to identify the areas indicated on these drawings.

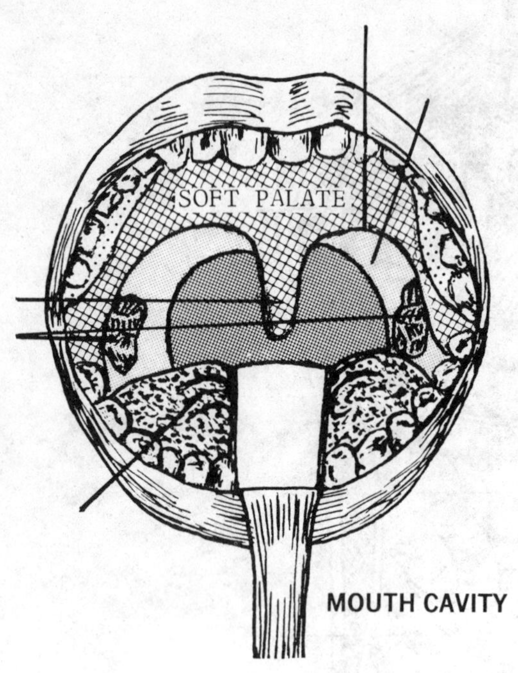

MOUTH CAVITY

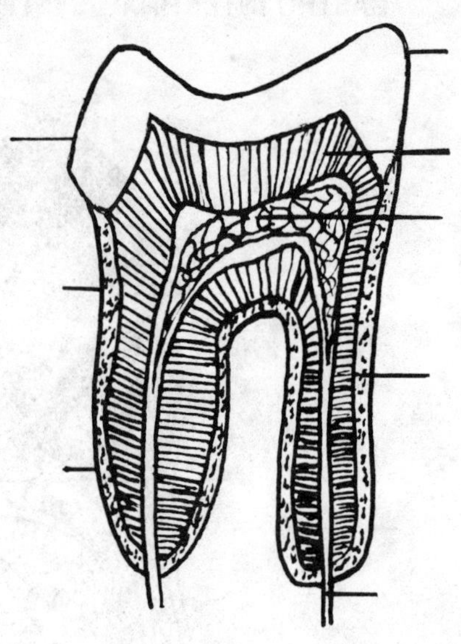
SECTION OF HUMAN MOLAR TOOTH

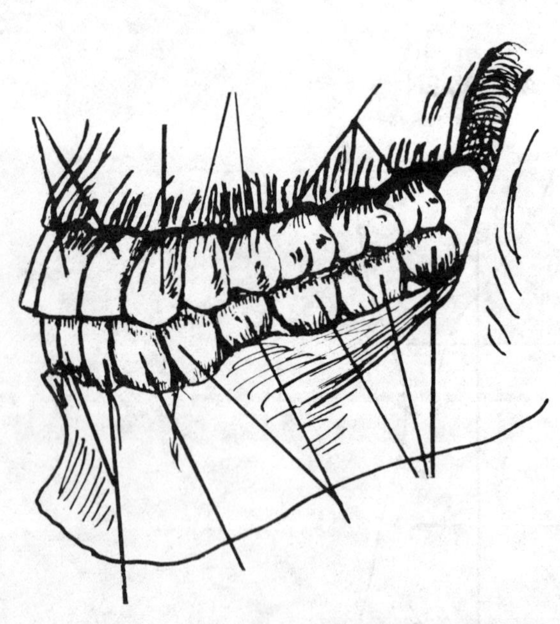
PERMANENT TEETH

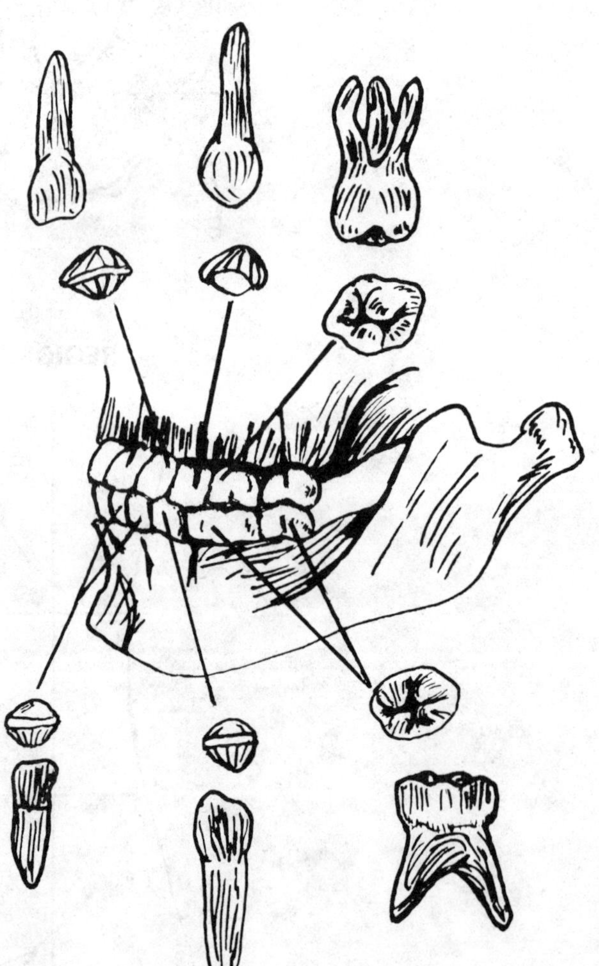
DECIDUOUS TEETH

6. What are the gastro-intestinal functions of the tongue besides taste?

   A. ______________ B. ______________ C. ______________

7. The sockets in which the teeth are lodged are found in the ______________ and the ______________. These sockets are known as ______________.

8. A. How many sets of teeth develop during life? __________

   B. Give their names. ______________ and ______________

9. A. How many teeth are there in each jaw in the first set? __________

   B. What are they and how many of each type in each jaw?

   ______________, ______________, ______________

10. A. How many teeth are there in each jaw in the second set? __________

    B. What are they and how many of each type in each jaw?

    ______________, ______________, ______________ or ______________, ______________

11. What is the tube called which connects the mouth to the esophagus?

    ____

12. Give the following information on the stomach.

    A. What is the purpose of the stomach? ______________

    B. Where is it situated? ______________

    ____

    C. How many openings does the stomach have? __________

    D. What are they? ______________ and ______________

    E. What is the blind rounded part of the stomach called? ______________

    F. What is the smaller or opposite end called? ______________

    G. What is the area between these two called? ______________

13. A. What is the name of the portion of the small intestine which extends from the pyloric end of the stomach? ______________

    B. What is the next portion of the small intestine called? ______________

    C. What is the last portion which extends to the large intestine called?

    ____

14. Attached to the end of the cecum is a narrow, worm-like tube called the

    ________________ ____________.

15. Enlargement of the veins of the anal canal causes what condition?

    ____________ or _________________________

16. What is the largest gland in the body? ___________

17. A. What is the chief bile pigment? ____________

    B. The chamber formed by the joining of the common bile duct and the pancreatic duct is known as the ______________ of _____________. The opening of this chamber is guarded by a ring of muscle called the ____________ of _______.

18. What is the function of the gall bladder?

    ____

19. The pancreas is known as what type of gland? _________________________

20. What are the cells called which furnish the internal secretion from which insulin is extracted? _________________________________

21. List the symptoms which occur in the following areas of the aigestive system:

    A. esophagus: _____________________________

    B. stomach: ____

    ____

    C. small intestine: ____

    ____

    ____

    D. large intestine: ____

22. A. What is one of the most important diseases of the liver? ___________

    B. Give the names only of the three types:

    1. _________________ 2. _________ or _____________ 3. _______________

    C. Obstruction of the portal circulation producing serum in the peritoneal cavity is known as ______________.

Use the illustration on page 193 to identify the organs indicated on this drawing.

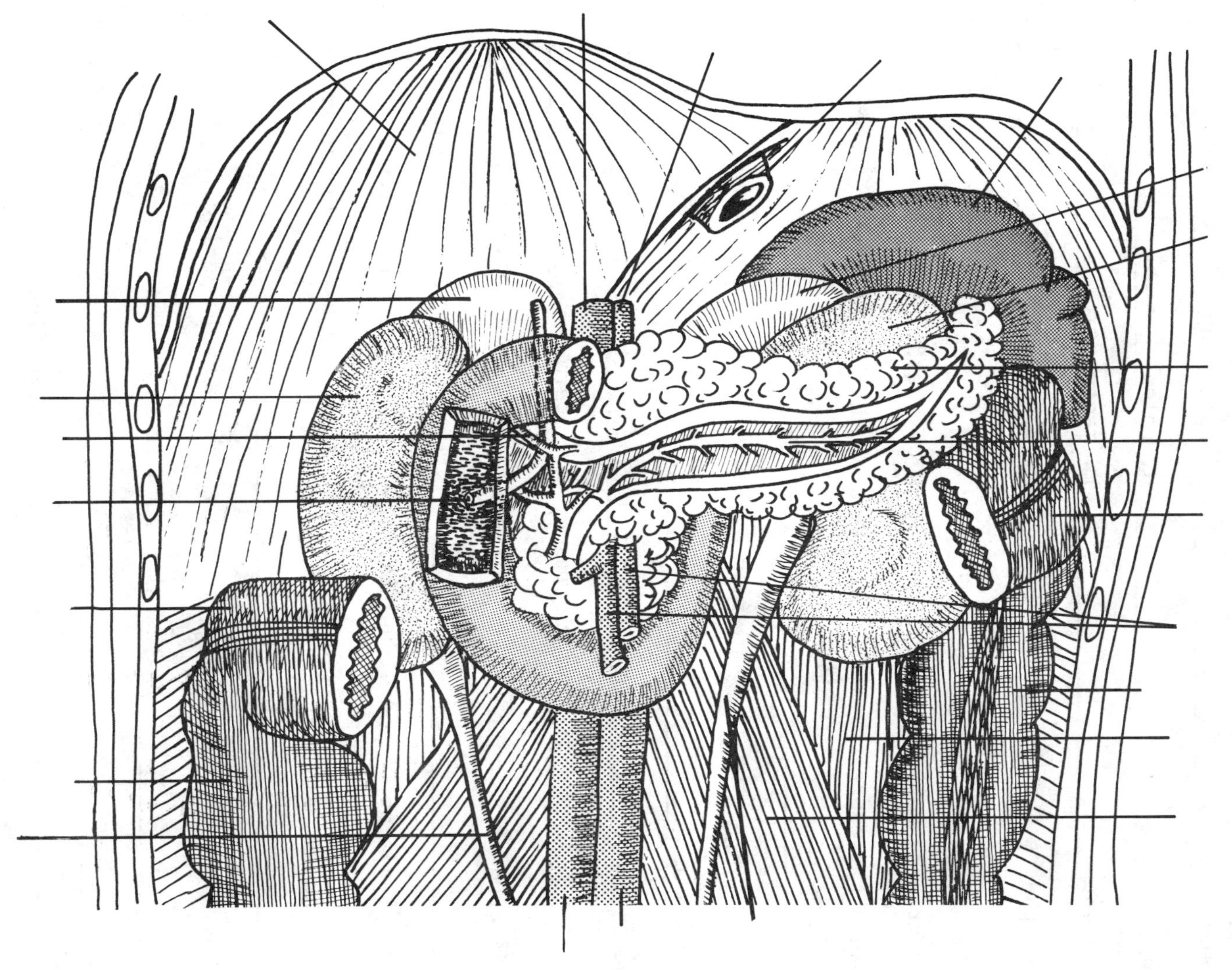

PANCREAS AND DUODENUM

23. Disease of the islands of Langerhans produces ________________ _____________

or _____________________________.

24. Give the names of the inflammatory diseases of these organs:

A. mouth _________________________ F. intestine _____________________

B. gums _________________________ G. colon _________________________

C. tongue ________________________ H. rectum ________________________

D. esophagus _____________________ I. appendix ______________________

E. stomach _______________________

25. What are the most common benign tumors of the digestive tract? ____________

26. A. When the esophagus ends in a blind pouch the anomaly is known as

_____________.

B. When the rectum is completely occluded at or near the anus the anomaly is known as _______________ _________.

27. A pouch or pocket leading off from a main cavity or tube is a

__________________. The pleural of this term is __________________.

28. A. Falling or prolapse of the digestive organs is called

_____________________________.

B. Displacement of individual organs of the digestive system due to tumors, paralysis of either side of the diaphragm, or to hernias is known as

____________________________ _____________.

C. Where the stomach herniates through the normal opening, called the

________________, in the diaphragm it is called ____________________ or

____________ ____________.

29. What are the causes of obstruction of the intestine?

A. ____

____

B. _________________________________

C. _________________________________

D. _________________________________

30. A. List the five most important diseases of the liver.

1. ______________ 4. ______________

2. ______________ 5. ______________

3. ______________

B. What other conditions may involve the liver?

1. ______________ 5. ______________

2. ______________ 6. ______________

3. ______________ 7. ______________

4. ______________ 8. ______________

31. The outstanding symptom of this disease is jaundice. The disease usually runs a benign course of four to six weeks. This disease of the liver is

______________ ______________.

32. Give the medical terms for these gall bladder conditions.

A. inflammation of the bile ducts ______________

B. inflammation of the gall bladder ______________

C. presence of stones in the gall bladder or bile ducts ______________

33. A. The surgical procedure performed for congenital short esophagus is

______________.

B. The operative procedure performed for diverticula is ______________.

C. The surgical procedure for cicatricial stenosis and cardiospasm is

______________ .

34. Surgeries performed for gastric ulcer consist of

A. ______________ and ______________

B. excision of a portion of the stomach containing the gastric ulcer and vagotomy in some cases combined with ______________ or

____

C. ______________ excision of the ulcer from the posterior wall of the stomach

D. ______________ resection of the stomach

35. Surgeries performed for duodenal ulcer include:

A. ____________ and ____________ with ____________;

B. ____________ with ____________;

C. ____________, Billroth I (____________)

or Billroth II (____________) with ____________.

36. Division of the vagus nerve for relief of ulcer distress and acid production is called ____________.

37. The procedure performed for stenosis of the pylorus is called ____________. It is also known as the ____________ operation.

38. Give the types of surgical procedures performed for the following mechanisms which cause small bowel obstruction.

A. strangulation of intestine: ____________ and ____________ ____________ and ____________

B. adhesions and adhesive bands: ____________ and ____________

C. intussusception: ____________. In recurrent conditions primary resection and ____________ ____________ is usually done.

D. removal of stones for gallstone obstruction: ____________

E. mesenteric venous thrombosis: ____________ ____________

F. gangrenous bowel: ____________

39. For relief of pain due to calcification in the pancreas ____________ and ____________ are performed.

40. Large pseudocysts of the pancreas are ____________.

41. A. Surgical incision into the gall bladder with drainage is called ____________.

B. Complete removal of the gall bladder is known as ____________.

Jse the illustrations on pages 196, 201, 202, 203 to indicate the areas marked on these drawings.

CONGENITAL ABNORMALITIES OF THE ESOPHAGUS

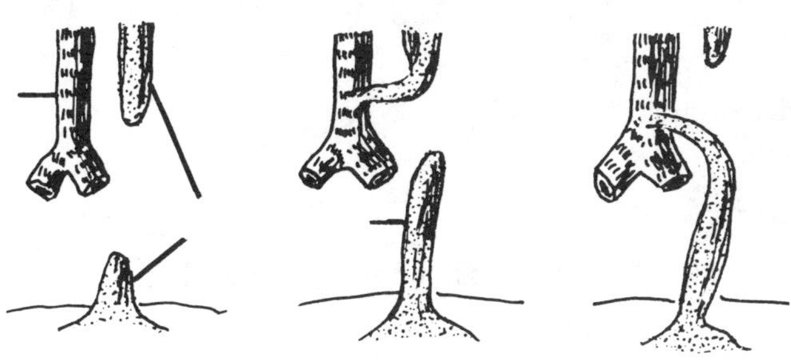

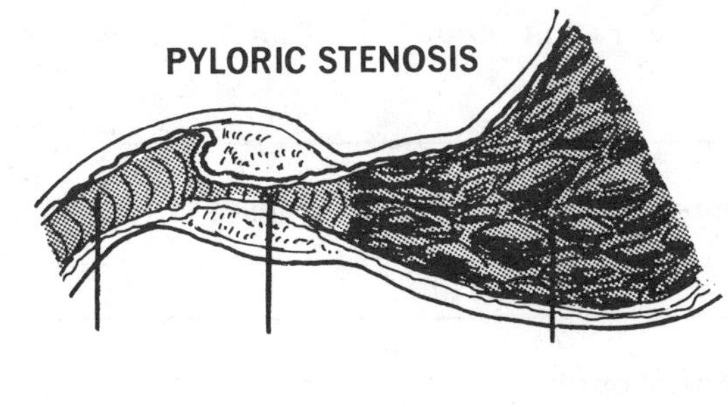

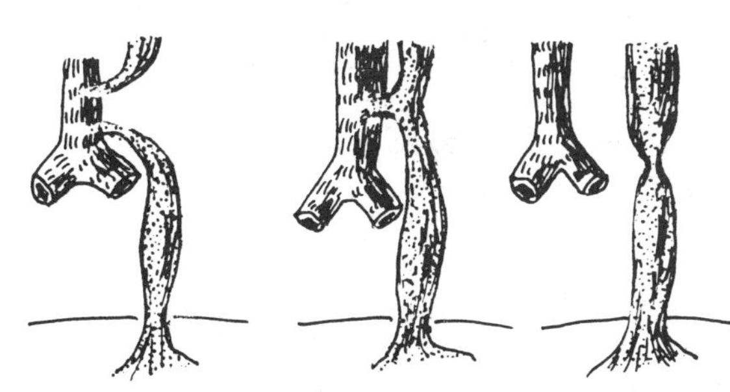

ANAL AND RECTAL ABNORMALITIES

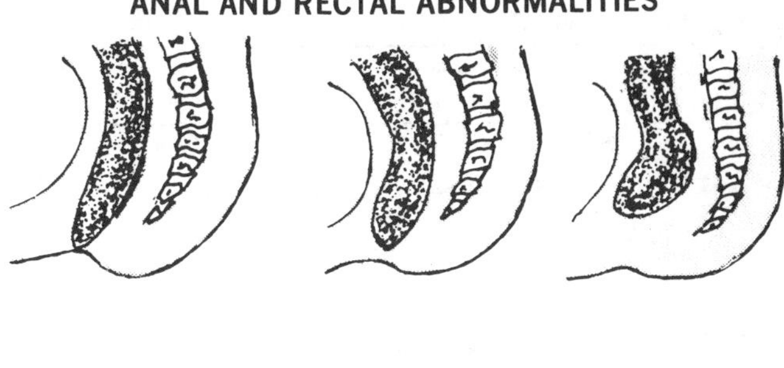

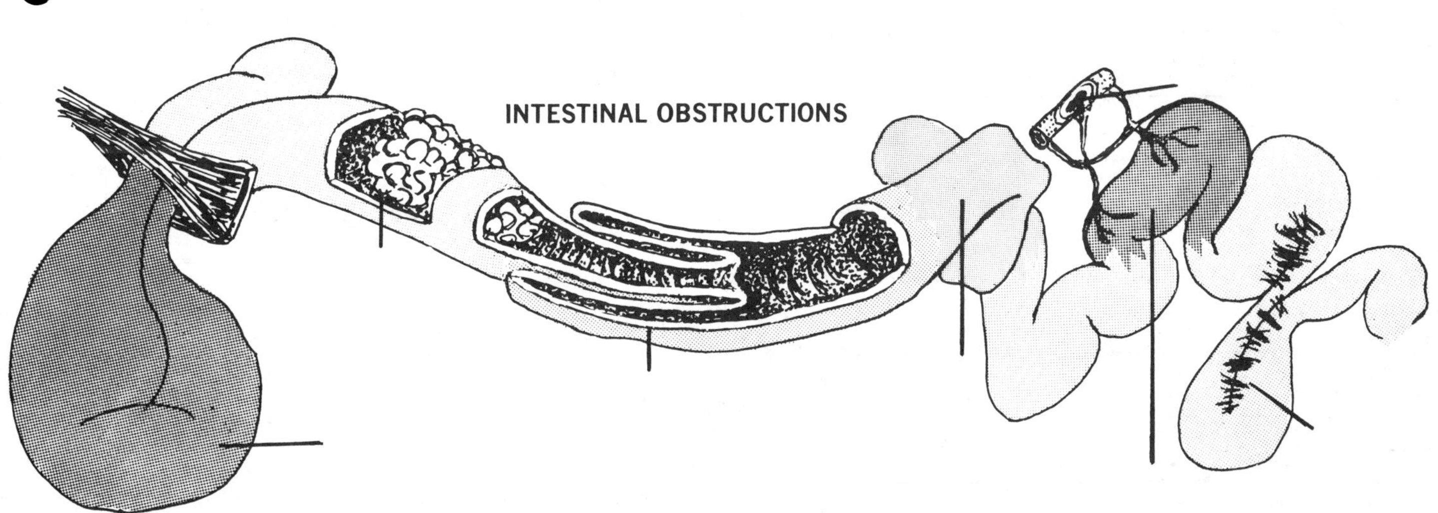

INTESTINAL ANASTOMOSIS PROCEDURES

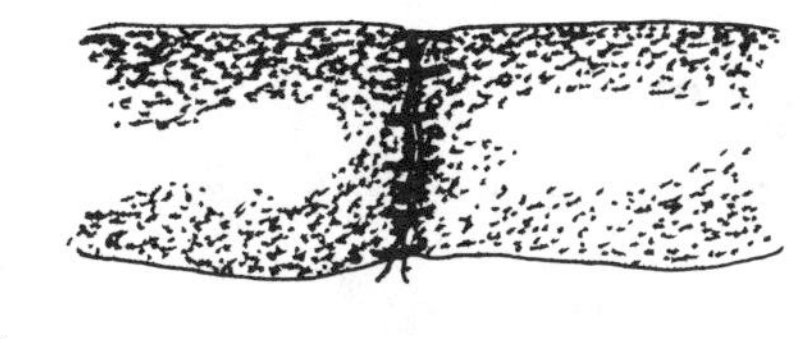

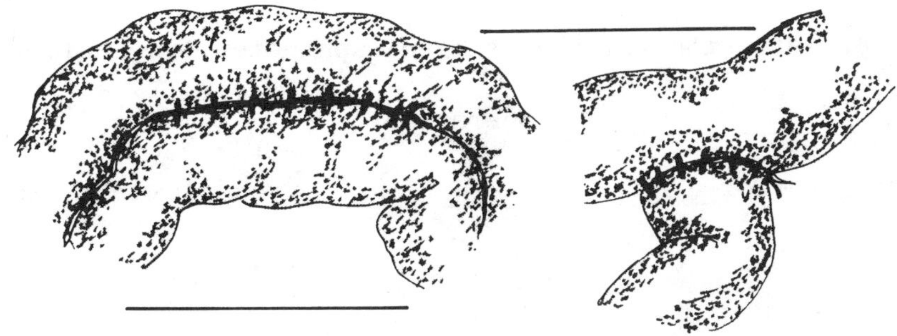

42. A. Two procedures are performed on the common bile duct for obstruction due to various causes. These procedures are ________________ and ________________.

B. Anastomosis of the common duct to the duodenum is called ________________________.

C. Anastomosis between the biliary tract and the intestinal tract is called ________________________.

43. What two procedures are performed for subphrenic abscess:

A. ________________________________

B. ________________________________

44. Surgical procedures performed for malignant neoplasms of the colon are ________________ or ________________.

45. Fill in the medical terms where indicated for the following surgical procedures for malignant lesions of the rectum and lower part of the sigmoid.

A. ________________ resection of rectum and sigmoid with permanent ____________;

B. ________________ and lower bowel resections;

C. anterior resection of the upper part of the rectum and lower portion of the sigmoid with preservation of intestinal continuity by ________________;

D. ________________ operations with ________________ or ________________ resection;

E. modified ________________ resection;

F. ________________ ________________ with preservation of the external sphincter (the pull-through or ____________ operation);

G. posterior ________________ and lower excision.

46. Fill in the terms where indicated for the following procedures for abscess and fistula of the anorectal regions.

    A. I & D for ______________ abscess

    B. ________________ of fistula in ano

    C. repair of defect in _____________________ fistula

    D. repair of _____________________fistula

47. Give the surgical procedures for the following conditions:

    A. prolapse of the rectum: ___________________________________ or ____________________________________

    B. hemorrhoids, internal, external or combined: ___________________ or _____________________________

    C. fissure in ano: ____________________

    D. pilonidal cysts or sinuses: __________________

    E. imperforate anus (infants): ___________________________ and ______________________________

48. What are the two phases in the operation for hernia?

    A. ____

    B. ____

49. A. What is the medical term for hernia repair: ____________________

    B. What are the indications for hernia repair:

    1. ___________________________ 4. _____________________________

    2. ___________________________ 5. _____________________________

    3. ___________________________ 6. _____________________________

    ___________________________ 7. _____________________________

    ____

50. Refer to the index beginning on page 210 for the line and page number of the following words. Then write the English translation beneath each word component.

C H O L E / D O C H O / D U O D E N O / S T O M Y

E X A C E R B / A T I O N

I N T U S / S U S C E P T I O N

P R O C T O / S I G M / O I D / E C T O M Y

V I S C E R O / P T O S I S

A N A S T O M O S I S

E X T R A / P E R I / T O N E / A L

H E M A T / E M E S I S

M E S / E N T E R Y

P H R E N I C O -/ E X E R E S I S

P Y L O R O / M Y O / T O M Y

V O L V U L U S

C H O L E / L I T H / I A S I S

C A U D / A T E

G I N G I V / I T I S

C O N / V O L U T E D

A S C I T E S

CHAPTER IX
THE GENITO-URINARY SYSTEM
STUDY LESSON

1. Name the organs and the number of each which comprise the female reproductive system.

   A. ______________________ D. ______________________

   B. ______________________ E. ______________________

   C. ______________________ F. ______________________

2. A. What is another term for fallopian tubes besides uterine tubes?

   ____

   B. At the distal end of the oviducts are many fringe-like processes called ______________. One of these ____________ is attached to each __________.

3. The ovaries furnish two internal secretions. What are they and what parts of the ovary produce each of the secretions?

   A. __________ produced by the ______________________

   B. __________ or ______________ produced by the ______________

4. What is the condition caused by an impregnated ovum remaining in a fallopian tube? ______________

5. Name the three parts of the uterus.

   A. __________ B. __________ C. __________

6. A. When the fundus of the uterus turns too far forward it is ______________.

   B. When the fundus turns too far backward it is ______________.

   C. If the body of the uterus bends forward it is known as ______________.

   D. If the body bends backward it is known as ______________.

7. A. The external genitals are known as the __________ or ______________.

   B. List the external genitals.

   1. ______________________ 4. ______________________

   2. ______________________ 5. ______________________

   3. ______________________ 6. ______________________

Use the illustration on page 214 as reference to identify the various organs of the female reproductive system depicted in this drawing.

FEMALE ORGANS OF REPRODUCTION

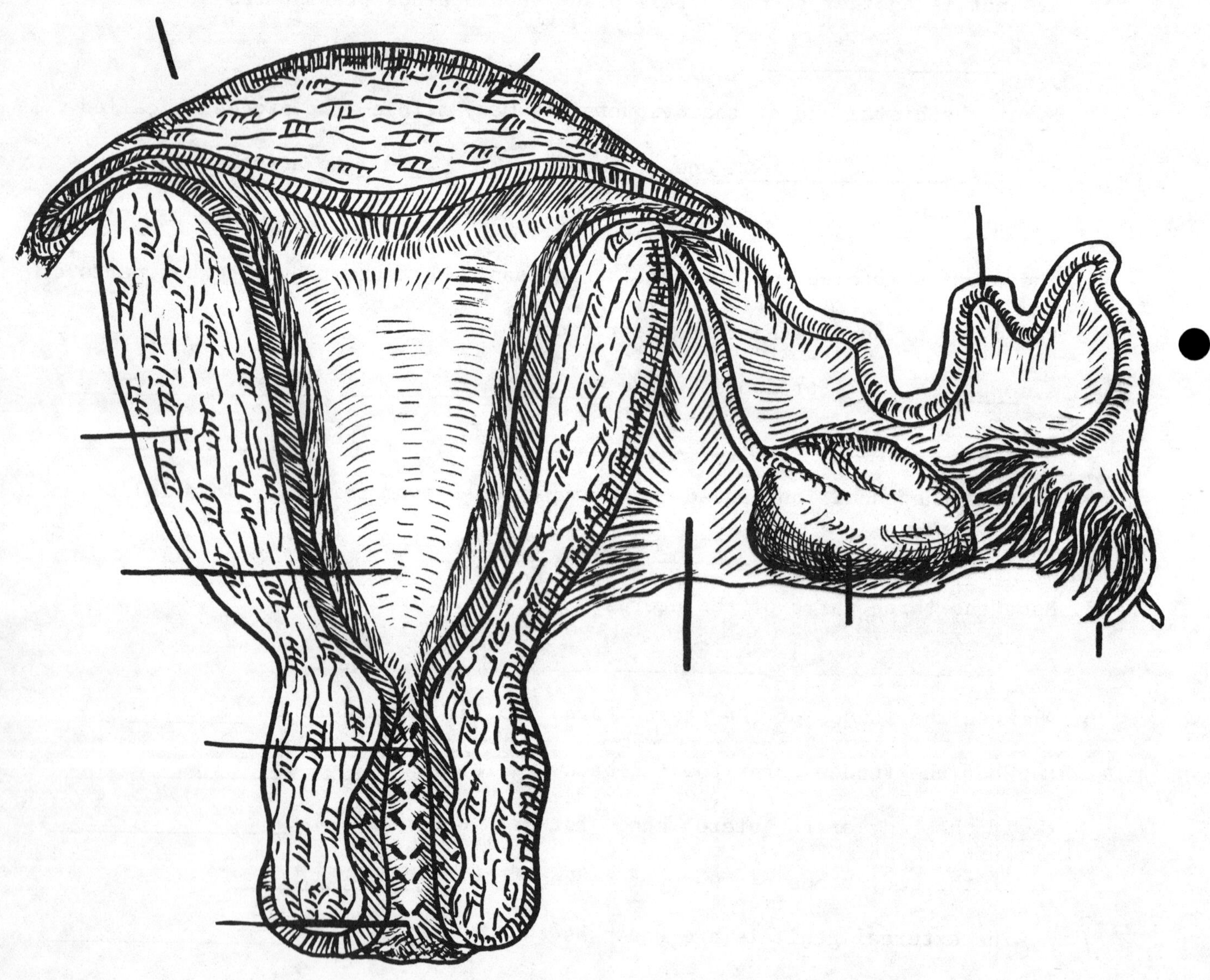

Using the drawing on page 219 for reference identify the various organs of the male reproductive system as indicated here. Also identify any other areas indicated.

The Male Pelvic Organs

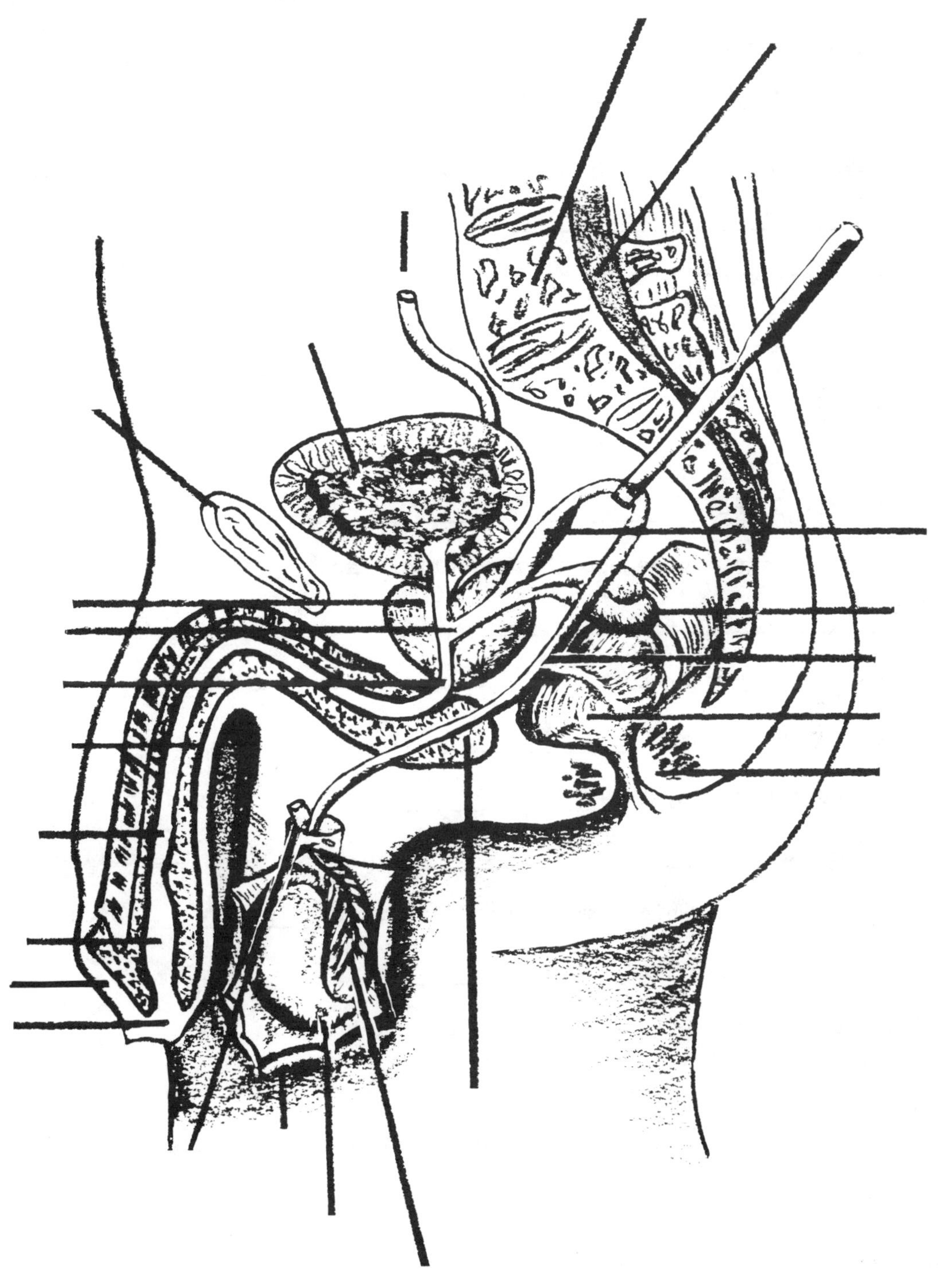

8. A. What is the perineum?

____

____

B. What perforates the perineum in the female? ____________________

9. A. In the male the ________________ is about eight inches long and passes through the ____________________ and then through the _____________ . The opening of the ________________ is known as the __________ ___________.

B. The coverings of the testes are 1. _________, 2. ____________ _________, 3. _____________ ________ 4. ____________ 5. _________________ and 6. __________ _____________

10. The excretory ducts are

A. _________________ B. ____________________ C. ______________________

11. The slight thickening of skin at the distal end of the penis is called the _________ __________. Also at the distal end the skin is folded doubly and is called the ____________ or _______________.

12. Name the urinary organs and the number of each.

A. _______________ B. _________________ C. ____________ D. ___________.

13. A. The outer layer or cortex of the kidney contains the _________________ and the functioning _________________.

B. The inner portion, the _________________, is arranged in conical masses called the ___________ ____________ which contain the collecting ______________ which empty into the minor ___________ which in turn empty into the major _______________.

14. A. In the male the urinary bladder lies in front of the ___________ above the ______________ gland.

B. In the female the urinary bladder lies in front of the ___________ and ______________.

15. The fundus of the bladder is triangular in shape with _________________ _____________ behind each corner of the base and the _____________ orifice at the apex in front. This triangular area is known as the ______________.

Refer to the illustrations on pages 221 and 222 when identifying the component parts of the urinary system shown on this page.

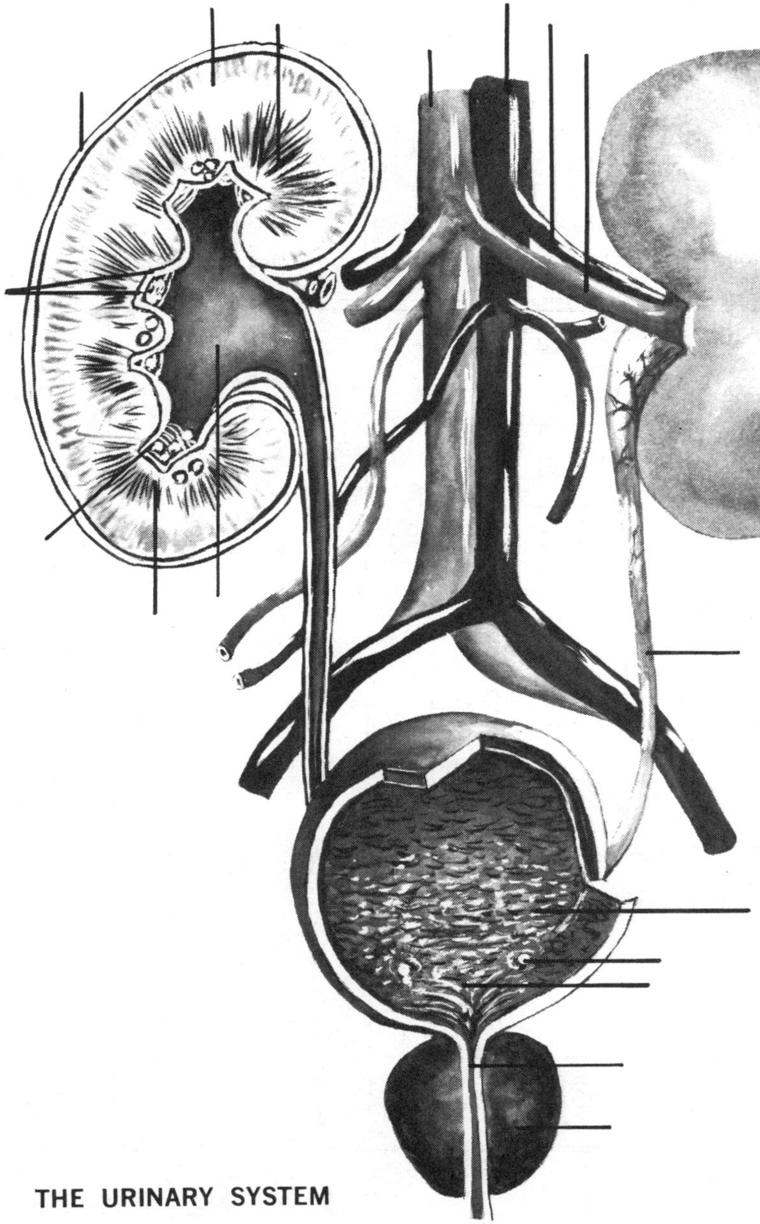

THE URINARY SYSTEM

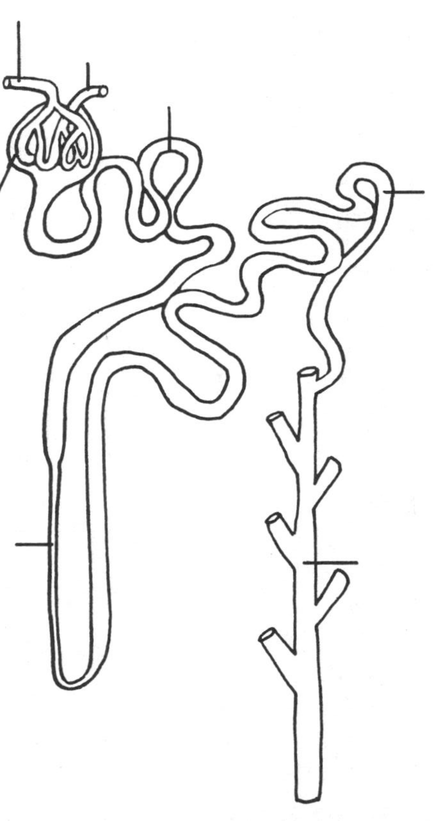

RENAL UNIT (NEPHRON)
OF THE CORTEX OF THE KIDNEY

16. List the infectious diseases of the female genital tract.

A. ______________________ G. ______________________

B. ______________________ H. ______________________

C. ______________________ I. ______________________

D. ______________________ J. ______________________

E. ______________________ K. ______________________

F. ______________________ L. ______________________

17. List the skin disorders of the vulva.

A. ______________________ D. ______________________

B. ______________________ E. ______________________

C. ______________________ F. ______________________

18. List the benign tumors of the vulva.

A. ______________________ G. ______________________

B. ______________________ H. ______________________

C. ______________________ I. ______________________

D. ______________________ J. ______________________

E. ______________________ K. ______________________

F. ______________________

19. Serous cysts include:

A. ______________________ D. ______________________

B. ______________________ E. ______________________

C. ______________________ F. ______________________

20. Pseudomucinous cysts include:

A. ______________________ B. ______________________

21. What are the two varieties of ovarian teratoma?

A. ______________________ B. ______________________

22. A. What are the three masculinizing tumors of the ovary?

1. ______________________ 2. ______________________

3. ______________________

22. B. These tumors cause defeminization manifested by

1. ______________________ 4. ______________________

2. ______________________ 5. ______________________

3. ______________________ 6. ______________________

C. Masculinization is evident in

1. ______________________ 4. ______________________

2. ______________________ 5. ______________________

3. ______________________ 6. ______________________

23. A. Benign tumors of the uterus are known as ______________. They are also called ____________, ______________ or ______________.

B. A highly malignant tumor of the uterus is ______________________.

24. When carcinoma occurs in the corpus it is usually an ______________.

25. A. Retention of water and salt in the body because of diminution in the output of urine is called ____________ ____________.

B. Diminution of plasma proteins is called ____________ __________.

26. A. There are three varieties of Bright's disease. They are:

1. the inflammatory type called ______________;

2. the degenerative type called ______________;

3. the type secondary to vascular disease called __________________.

B. Another type of Bright's disease is often called diffuse

________________________.

27. List the varieties of nephrosis.

A. __________ or ____________ D. __________________

B. ________________________ E. __________________

C. ________________________

28. Name the pus-producing germs which may infect the kidneys.

A. ________________________ C. ________________________

B. ________________________ D. ________________________

29. A. Stone in the kidney is known as ____________________.

    B. Stones block the passages through which urine flows and cause

    __________________________.

30. A. The commonest primary tumor of the kidney is ____________________.

    B. Give the two types of cystic disease of the kidneys.

    1. __________________________ 2. __________________________.

    C. The retention of urinary constituents within the body is called

    __________________.

31. Fill in the diagnosis or surgical procedure (whichever is missing) in the following:

    A. ____________________ or __________________ are performed for atresia of the hymen.

    B. Vulvectomy is performed for ____________________ and ________________.

    C. Injury to the vulva and perineum are corrected by

    ____________________________.

    D. For tense perineum in second stage labor an ______________ is performed and ____________________ is done for obstetrical laceration of the perineum.

    E. For relaxation of the vaginal musculature a ______________________ is performed.

32. A. What does D & C stand for? __________________________________

    B. What is the abbreviation for the word "abortion?" ____________

    C. Give the indications for cesarean section.

    1. __________________________ 4. ______________________________

    2. __________________________ ______________________________

    3. __________________________ 5. ______________________________

    __________________________ 6. ______________________________

32. D. For ruptured ectopic pregnancy a unilateral ________________ is performed.

E. For removal of ectopic pregnancy and repair of the fallopian tube a ________________ is performed.

F. For obstetrical laceration of the cervix ________________ is done.

33. What are some of the more common fetal presentations?

A. ________________ F. ________________

B. ________________ G. ________________ or

C. ________________ ________________

D. ________________ H. ________________ or

E. ________________ ________________

34. A maneuver used particularly as a method of diagnosis of pregnancy is ________________.

35. A. Give the types of version.

1. ____________ 6. ____________ 11. ____________

2. ____________ 7. ____________ 12. ____________

3. ____________ 8. ____________ 13. ____________

4. ____________ 9. ____________ 14. ____________

5. ____________ 10. ____________ 15. ____________

B. Removal of amniotic fluid is called ________________.

36. A. Uterine suspension is called ________________.

B. Hernial protrusion of the urinary bladder is called ________________.

C. Hernial protrusion of part of the rectum is called ________________.

D. What is meant by A & P repair? ________________.

E. What is it a repair of? ________________ and ________________

F. Removal of the uterus through the vagina is known as ________________ ________________

36. G. What are the indications for hysterectomy?

1. ______________ 4. ______________

2. ______________ 5. ______________

______________ ______________

3. ______________ 6. ______________

H. Total hysterectomy is called ______________. It is the removal of the ________ (________) and ________ (________) of the uterus.

I. Herniation of the bowel into the cul-de-sac is called ______________ and is corrected by a ______________ type of surgery

J. Removal of the oviducts and ovaries, either unilateral or bilateral, is called ______________ or ______________.

K. It is performed for

1. ______________ 3. ______________

______________ 4. ______________

2. ______________

L. Excision of an ovarian cyst is called ______________ and plastic surgery of the ovary for ovarian cyst is called ______________.

M. Elevating and fixing the fallopian tube and ovary to the broad ligament for obstructed tubes is called ______________.

N. Removal of the ovary is called ______________.

O. Plastic repair of a scarred fallopian tube is called ______________.

37. A. Surgical procedure performed for diffuse benign disease of the female breast is simple ______________. It is also performed in the male for chronic ______________ or for ______________.

B. For carcinoma of the breast ________ ________ is performed.

C. For depressed or ______________ nipple a ______________ is performed.

38. Give the types of incisions used in surgery on the kidneys.

A. ________________ C. ________________

B. ________________ D. ________________

39. Give the conditions for which nephrectomy is performed.

A. ________________ D. ________________

B. ________________ E. ________________

C. ________________

40. A. What is the term for floating kidney? ________________

B. What is the surgical procedure performed for this condition?

____

41. Give the name of the surgical procedure performed for each of these diagnoses.

A. for a dilated and scarred calyx ________________

B. when part of the kidney is destroyed by stone ________________

C. for traumatic injuries ________________

D. for renal calculi ________________ or ________________

E. in cases of tumors such as Wilm's tumor ________________ with ________________ and sometimes ________________

F. for calculi in the renal pelvis ________________

G. for stone in the ureter which cannot be extracted endoscopically

____

H. for stricture of the ureter ________________ and ________________

42. List the open surgical procedures performed on the bladder.

A. ________________ D. ________________

B. ________________ E. ________________

C. ________________ F. ________________

____

or ________________

43. A. List the various types of electrical procedures used for closed surgery on the bladder.

1. ______________________ 3. ______________________

2. ______________________ 4. ______________________

______________________ ______________________

______________________ ______________________

B. List the nonelectric instruments used in bladder surgery.

1. ______________________ 4. ______________________

2. ______________________ 5. ______________________

3. ______________________ 6. ______________________

44. A. Elusive ulcer is known as ____________ ulcer or ____________ ____________.

B. Bladder stones are removed by ____________ which is done with the visual or blind ____________.

C. What are the types of bladder tumors?

1. ______________________ 3. ______________________

2. ______________________ 4. ______________________

D. How are operations performed for bladder tumors? ____________

E. What corrective surgery is used for extrophy of the bladder?

____

45. A. What does BPH mean? ______________________

B. List the surgical procedures performed on the prostate.

1. ______________________

2. ______________________

3. ______________________ (   )

4. ______________________

C. What procedures are performed for carcinoma of the prostate?

____

46. Fill in the surgical procedure on each of the following

    A. for chronic recurrent epididymitis ______________________

    B. for varicocele ______________________

    C. for spermatocele ______________________

    D. for hydrocele in the young associated with hernia ______________________

       and ______________________

47. A. List the tumors of the testicle.

       1. ______________________ 4. ______________________

       2. ______________________ 5. ______________________

       3. ______________________

    B. What is the surgical procedure performed for tumors of the testicle?

       ____

    C. What is the term for undescended testicle? ______________________

    D. What procedures are performed to correct it?

       1. ______________ 2. ______________ 3. ______________

48. What procedure is performed on the male or female for urethral meatal stenosis? ______________________

49. A. Name two congenital abnormalities of the penis.

       1. ______________________ 2. ______________________

    B. Give the three diagnoses for which circumcision of the penis is performed.

       1. ______________ 2. ______________ 3. ______________

50. Refer to the index beginning on page 241 for the page and line number of the following words. Then write the English translation beneath each word component.

C O L P O / P E R I N E O / P L A S T Y

A R R H E N O / B L A S T / O M A

A D N E X / E C T O M Y

G L O M E R U L O / N E P H R / I T I S

H E R N I O / R R H A P H Y

E P I / D I D Y M / E C T O M Y

G Y N E C O / M A S T I A

H Y P O / P L A S I A

L E U K O / P L A K I A

I N T R O / I T U S

I N T R A / M U R A L

U R E T E R O / N E O / C Y S T O / S T O M Y

T R I C H O / M O N A S

V A R I C O / C E L E

U R / E M I A

T R I G O N E

S A L P I N G O -/ O O P H O R / E C T O M Y

P Y E L O / L I T H O / T O M Y

P R O C I D E N T I A

O R C H I O / P E X Y

CHAPTER X
THE SENSES
STUDY LESSON

1. A. What are the two layers of the skin?

   1. ________________, ________________ or ____________________

   2. ________________, ________________ or _____________

   B. What are the four layers of the epidermis?

   1. _________________________ 3. _______________________________

   2. _________________________ 4. _______________________________

   C. What are the two layers of the corium?

   1. ___________________ or _______________________

   2. _________________________

2. A. List the appendages of the skin.

   1. ______________ 2. _____________ 3. _________________________

   4. __________________ or _________________ and __________________

   B. What are the glands called which are found in the external auditory canal?

   ____

   C. What is the name of the substance these glands secrete? ________________

3. A. List the names of the primary lesions of the skin.

   1. _______________ 4. _______________ 7. _________ or _________

   2. _______________ 5. _______________ 8. ______________

   3. _______________ 6. _______________ 9. ______________

   B. List the names of the secondary lesions of the skin.

   1. ____________________ 4. _______________

   2. _____________ 5. _______________

   3. _____________

4. A. What is the term which applies to pink or red lesions which turn white on pressure? __________________

4. B. Give the terms which apply to the discolorations which are

1. macular in size ______________, for those

2. larger ______________, 3. for pinhead size ______________.

5. A. List the diseases which fall under the term of dermatitis.

1. ______________ 6. ______________

2. ______________ 7. ______________

3. ______________ 8. ______________

4. ______________ 9. ______________

5. ______________

B. Give the abnormalities of the skin concerned with discoloration resulting from other conditions in the body.

1. ______________ 3. ______________

2. ______________ 4. ______________ or ______________

6. A. List the various tumors which may affect the skin.

1. ______________ 4. ______________

2. ______________ 5. ______________

3. ______________

B. Pigmented moles may become malignant. What is the term for this type of tumor? ______________ ______________

7. A. Name the conditions caused by malfunction of the sebaceous (oil) glands.

1. ______________ 2. ______________ 3. ______________

B. What is the name of the vesicles which occur in prickly heat?

____

8. A. What is the term for baldness? ______________

B. Early, hereditary baldness is called ______________ ______________

C. Progressive baldness into middle age is called ______________ ______________

D. Baldness which occurs in patches is called ______________ ______________.

A. Excessive, abnormal or premature growth of hair is called

______________________.

B. Decreased growth of hair is called ______________________.

10. A. Overgrowth of the nails in size or thickness is called ______________.

B. Thinning or decrease of the size of nails is called ____________.

C. Inflammation of the nail bed is called ____________.

D. Inflammation of tissues adjacent to the nail is called ______________.

E. Loosening of the nail is called ________________.

11. A. Give the classification of skin grafts.

1. _______________

a. ___________________

b. _________________________

2. _________________________

a. ___________________

b. ___________________

B. Intermediate split-thickness grafts are called thick ____________ grafts.

C. Pedicle flaps may be ________ or _________.

D. Skin grafts taken from other individuals are called ________________.

12. A. List the three methods of cutting skin grafts.

1. _______________

2. ____

____

3. __________________

B. List the names of other types of tissue transplantation besides skin.

1. ______________ or __________________

2. _________________________

3. _____________________________

4. _________________________

5. _____________________

13. A. The surgical procedure for cleft lips is called ________________.

B. The procedures for cleft palate are called ____________________

and ____________________.

14. A. Give the names only of infections of the skin and subcutaneous tissues.

1. __________ or __________
2. ____________________
3. ____________________ (____________________)
4. ____________________
5. ____________________
6. ____________________ (________)
7. ____________________ (____________________)
8. ____________________

B. List the benign tumors of the skin and subcutaneous tissues.

1. ____________________
2. ____________________
3. ____________________
4. ____________________
5. ____________________
6. ____________________
7. ____________________
8. ____________________
9. ____________________

C. List the epithelial tumors:

1. ____________________
2. ____________________
3. ____________________
4. ____________________ or ____________________ (________)

D. What is the most malignant of all tumors? ____________________

E. Two of these are the most malignant. What are they?

1. ____________________
2. ____________________

15. What are the three common plastic procedures and why are they done?

A. ____

____

B. ____

C. ____

Refer to the illustrations on pages 246 and 258. Then write in the identifications indicated on these drawings.

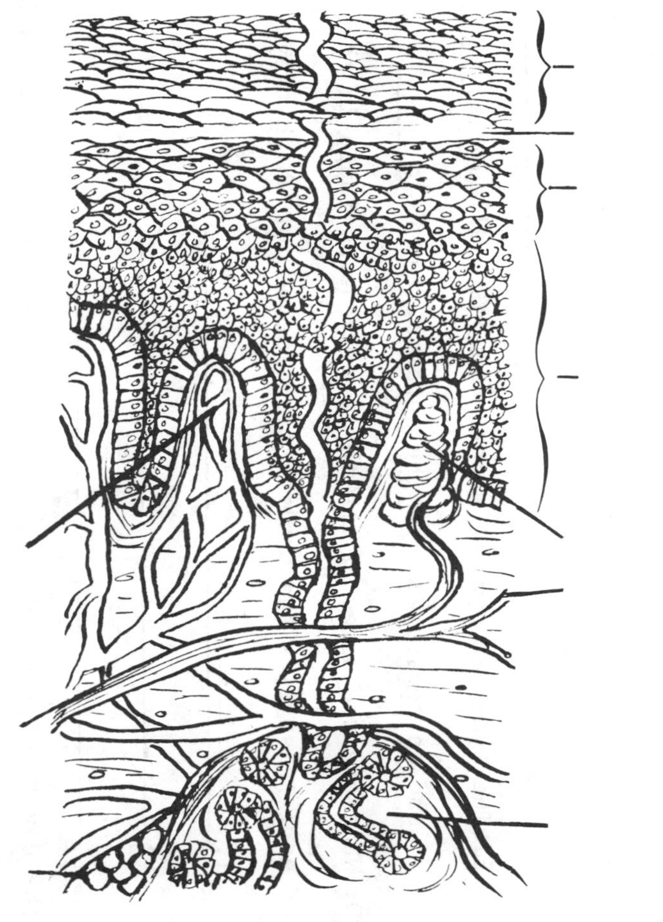

STRUCTURE OF THE SKIN (Touch)

THE TONGUE (Taste)

16. A. What are the four varieties of papillae which cover the tongue?

1. ____________ or ________________ 3. ____________________________

2. __________________________ 4. ____________________________

B. Where do the taste-buds occur?

1. ____________________________ 4. ____________________________

2. ____________________________ 5. ____________________________

3. ____________________________

17. A. What are the special nerves of the sense of smell? ____________________

____________.

B. What nerve furnishes the tactile sense for nasal perception of the sensations of cold, heat, pain, tickling, and tension or pressure?

_________________________ or __________________________________

18. A. List the parts which make up the auditory apparatus.

1. ____________________________ 3. ____________________________

2. ____________________________ 4. ____________________________

________________ ____________________

B. What is the external ear composed of?

1. ______________ or ___________ 2. ____________________________

C. 1. What separates the external auditory canal from the tympanic cavity?

__________________________ or ____________________(____________)

2. The tympanic cavity is more commonly called the ________________,

and is separated from the internal ear by a _______ _______ ______ ______.

D. What are the names of the three tiny bones found in the cavity of the middle ear? Also give the English translation for which they were named.

1. ________________ or ________________

2. ________________ or ________________

3. ________________ or ________________

19. The cavity of the middle ear is connected with the pharynx by the ______________

(______________)____________ .

20. The internal ear contains the ______________ __________________ which is made up of a series of oddly shaped cavities called the ________________, ________________, and the _____________________ ____________.

21. List the congenital malformations of the ear.

A. _____________ B. ______________ C. ______________ D. ____________.

22. What are some of the more common middle ear infections?

A. ____

B. ____

C. ____

23. List the tumors, benign and malignant, which may occur in the ear.

A. ____________________________ E. _________________________________

B. __________________________ or F. _________________________________

____________________________ G. _________________________________

C. ____________________________ H. _________________________________

D. ________ or _________________

24. A. Inflammation of the lining of the mastoid cells is ____________________.

B. Pathologic changes associated with middle ear disease are

___________________ and _________________________.

C. A complication which may occur in both acute and chronic otitis media is

______________ ____________________.

25. A. Inflammation of the labyrinth is called __________________________.

B. What are the two types of this inflammation?

1. ___________________________ 2. ________________________________

C. What are the causes of conduction hearing loss?

1. ___________________________ 3. ________________________________

2. ___________________________ 4. ________________________________

D. What conditions are caused by diseases of the inner ear?

1. ____

__________________2. _______________________ 3. _______________

Use the illustrations on pages 259 and 260 for reference to identify the areas indicated on these drawings.

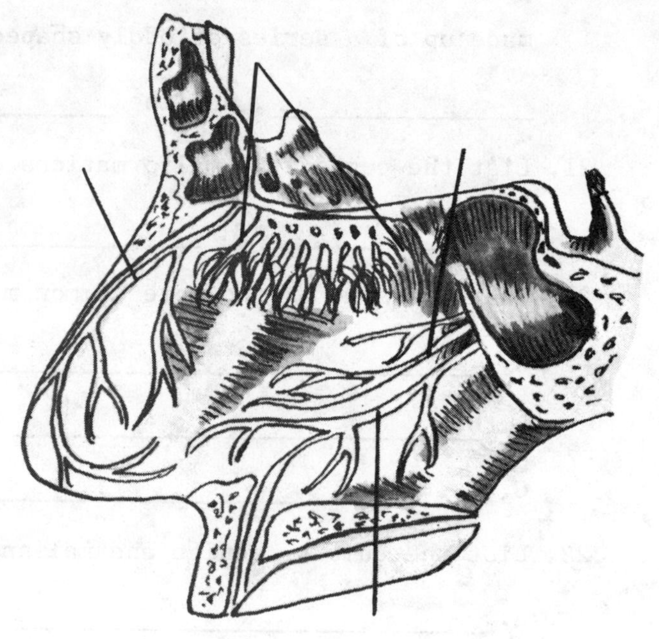

THE NOSE (Smell)

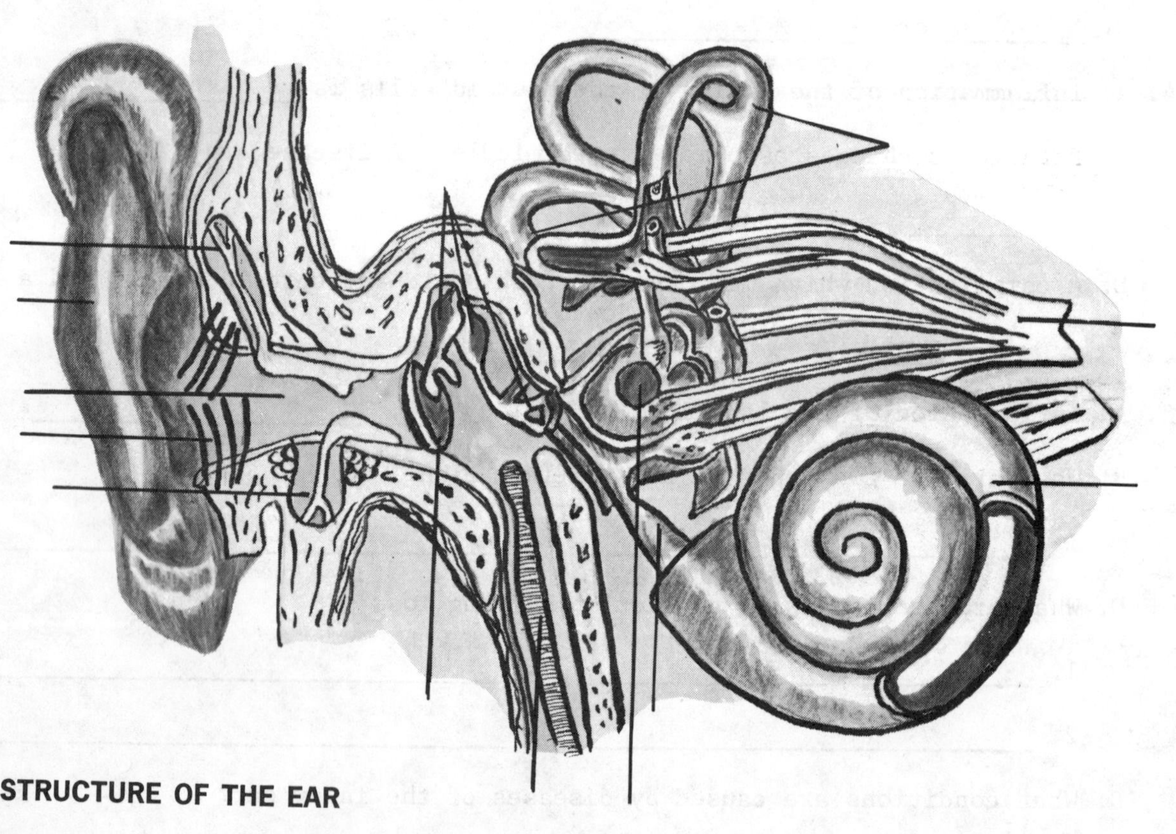

STRUCTURE OF THE EAR

26. A. Plastic repair of the ear is ____________________.

B. The procedure used for diagnostic purposes as well as for removal of foreign bodies or lesions in the external auditory canal is called ____________________.

C. What three procedures are performed for otitis media?

1. ____________________
2. ____________________
3. ____________________

D. Perforation or hole of the ear drum is repaired by ____________________.

27. What are the procedures performed for chronic suppurative otitis media?

A. ____________________ C. ____________________

B. ____________________ D. ____________________

____

28. Name the two procedures performed for otosclerosis.

A. ____________________ B. ____________________

29. A. What three types of mastoidectomy are performed for mastoiditis?

1. ____________ 2. ____________ 3. ____________

B. What recent procedure is performed for old, chronic cases of mastoiditis?

____

30. Name the tumors which may occur in the external auditory canal.

A. ____________________ D. ____________________

B. ____________________ E. ____________________

C. ____________________ F. ____________________

31. Surgical procedures used for various types of labyrinthitis are ____________ or ____________ ____________________ with or without ____________________.

32. A. What are the essential organs of the eye?

1. ____________ or the ____________ 2. ____________________

3. ____________________

32. B. What are the accessory organs?

1. ____________________ 4. ____________________

2. ____________________ 5. ____________________

3. ____________________ 6. ____________________

33. A. What is another term for the eyelids? ______________

B. What is the name of the small muscle that elevates the upper lid?

____

C. What is the name of the sphincter muscle around the eye?

____

D. The slit between the edges of the upper and lower lids is called the

____

E. At each end of this fissure are angles called the

______________________ or ____________________ and the

______________________ or ____________________

34. The sebaceous glands which open on the edge of each lid are called the

__________ or ____________________.

35. A. The lacrimal complex is composed of

1. ____________________ 3. ____________________

2. ____________________ 4. ____________________

B. Situated at the medial commissure is a small reddish body, the

______________________ or ______________.

36. A. Name the two groups of eye muscles.

1. ____________________ 2. ____________________

B. What cranial nerves innervate the eye?

1. ____________________ 4. ____________________

2. ____________________ 5. ____________________

3. ____________________

Refer to the illustrations on pages 265 and 267. Then identify the areas indicated on these drawings.

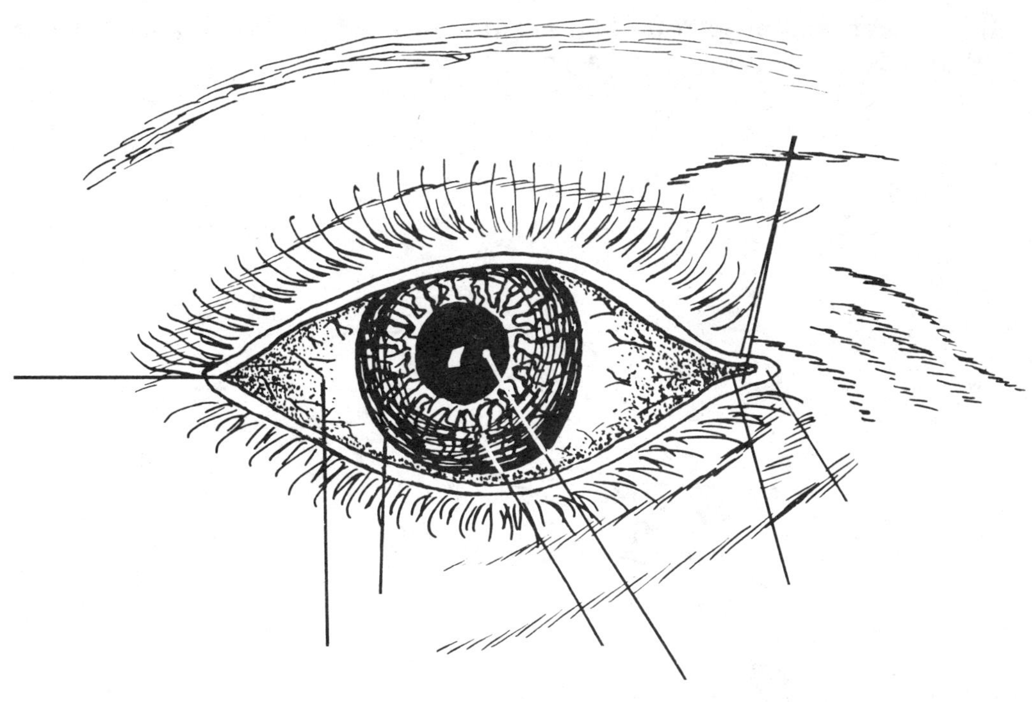

Front View of Right Eye

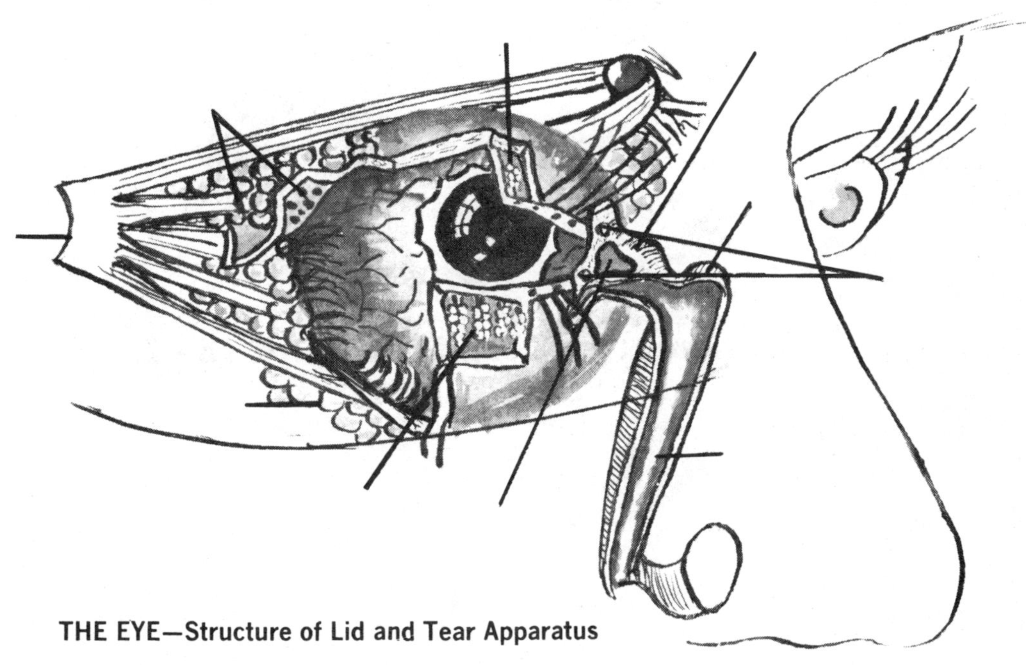

THE EYE—Structure of Lid and Tear Apparatus

The illustration on page 268 should be used for reference to identify the components, indicated here, which make up the eye.

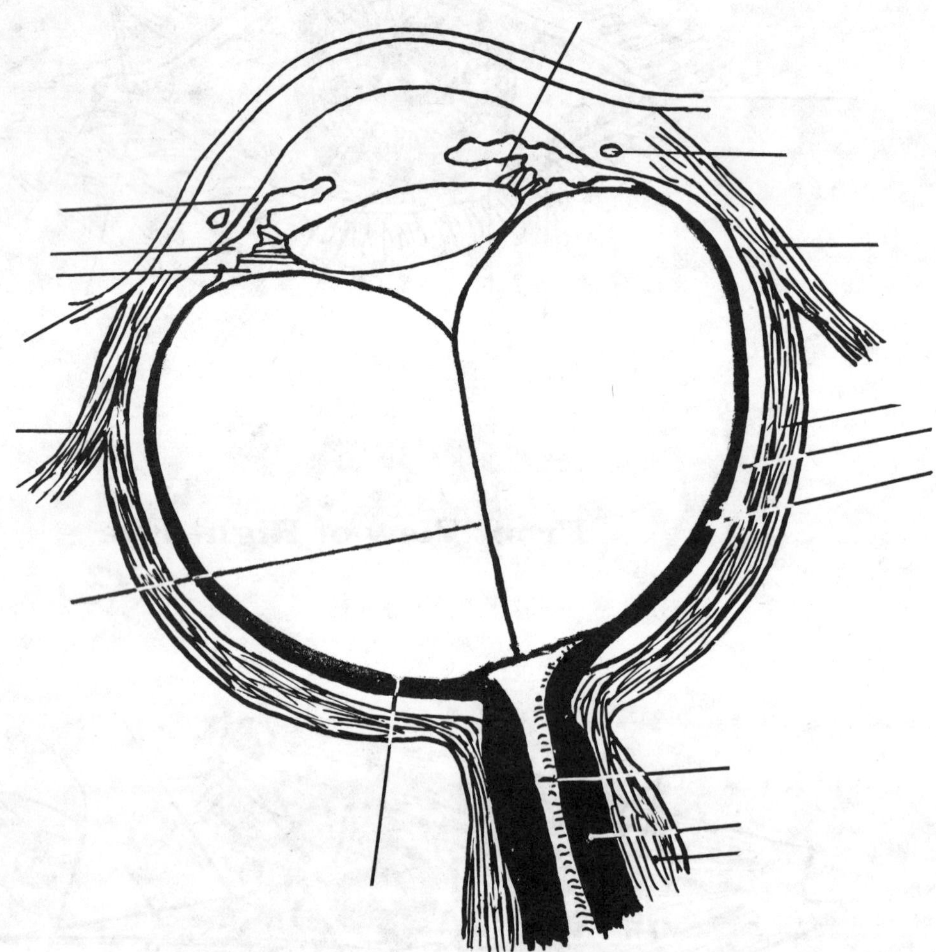

Schematic Cross Section of the Eye

37. A. What seven bones form the orbits?

1. ________ 4. ________ 6. ________

2. ________ 5. ________ 7. ________

3. ________

B. What are the contents of each orbit?

1. ________ 4. ________ 7. ________

2. ________ 5. ________ 8. ________

3. ________ 6. ________

C. The fascia bulbi is also known as the ________.

38. A. Name the three coats of the eyeball and what part of the eye each coat forms.

1. ________ which forms the ________.

2. ________ which forms the ________.

3. ________ which forms the ________

B. What are the three refracting media of the eyeball?

1. ________ 2. ________ 3. ________

C. What covers the posterior five-sixths of the eyeball?

________ or ________

D. What covers the anterior one-sixth of the eyeball? ________

E. What has the cornea been called? ________

F. What parts make up the ciliary body?

1. ________ 3. ________

2. ________

G. The circular, colored disk behind the cornea is called the ________.

The circular hole or ________ in its middle admits light into the eye chamber.

H. The two sets of muscles of the iris are the ________, ________ and the ________, ________.

39. A. The choroid, ciliary body and the iris make up the __________.

B. The inner, nervous coat of the eyeball is called the __________. It covers the back part of the eye as far as the _____ __________. In the center of the posterior part of the retina is the _________ _______ and in the center of this is the _______ ___________ which is the center of direct vision.

C. What is the principal refracting medium of the eye?

____

D. Four-fifths of the bulb of the eye is filled by the ___________________.

40. A. Normal vision is called _________________.

B. What are the terms which relate to the various abnormalities in vision?

1. _________________________ 4. ______________________________

2. _________________________ 5. ______________________________

3. _________________________

41. A. The disease characterized by increased tension or pressure within the eye is called _______________.

B. Opacity of the crystalline lens or of its capsule is known as __________.

C. The medical term for "cross-eyed" is _______________ or __________.

D. When the eyes turn inward it is ______________ ____________ or ______________.

E. When the eyes turn outward it is _______________ _____________ or ______________.

42. List the names of the congenital anomalies of the eyelids.

A. _____________________________ C. ________________________________

B. _____________________________ D. ________________________________

43. List the names of the common affections of the eyelids.

A. __________________ D. ___________________ F. _____________________

B. __________________ E. ___________________ G. _____________________

C. __________________

44. A. Give the benign tumors of the eyelids.

1. ____________ 3. ____________ 5. ____________

2. ____________ 4. ____________

B. What injuries are the eyelids subject to?

1. ____________ 4. ____________

2. ____________ 5. ____________

3. ____________ 6. ____________

45. A. Adhesion of the margins of the two lids is called ____________.

B. Contraction of the palpebral fissure at its outer canthus is called ____________.

C. A redundance of skin of the upper lid occasionally occurring in elderly persons is known as ____________.

D. A cicatricial attachment between the conjunctiva and the eyeball is known as ____________.

46. A. What are the three types of strabismus?

1. ____________ 2. ____________ 3. ____________

B. What procedures are used when the muscle is too strong?

1. ____________ 2. ____________ 3. ____________

C. What procedures are used if the muscle is too weak?

1. ____________ 2. ____________

47. A fan-shaped growth of conjunctiva and blood vessels progressing toward the cornea is called a ____________.

48. The procedure used to restore sight in eyes with impaired vision caused by opacity of the cornea is called ____________ ____________ or ____________. This procedure is also used for ____________ and corneal scars.

49. Removal of aqueous fluid for diagnostic and treatment purposes is called ____________ of the cornea or ____________.

50. A. List the names of the surgical procedures used to treat glaucoma.

1. ______ 3. ______ 5. ______

2. ______ 4. ______ 6. ______

B. The use of diathermy to reduce the production of aqueous fluid is called ______.

51. A. List the types of surgical procedures performed for cataract.

1. ______ or ______ 3. ______

2. ______ 4. ______

B. What is the name of the enzyme used in intracapsular extraction?

______ ______

52. Surgeries performed on the retina are called

A. ______ B. ______ C. ______

53. A. Removal of the eyeball is called ______.

B. Removal of all of the contents of the orbit is termed ______.

C. Removal of the contents of the eyeball but leaving the sclera is known as ______.

D. The last procedure is done on eyes which have been lost by infection such as ______.

54. Eversion of a various number of eyelashes is called ______.

Surgical procedure performed is ______.

55. A. Rolling in of the lid is ______. It occurs in two forms:

1. ______ and 2. ______.

B. What procedure is performed for the spastic type?

______

C. What procedures are performed for the cicatricial type?

1. ______ 2. ______

56. A. Rolling out of the lid is known as ______.

B. List the forms in which it occurs.

1. ______ 2. ______ 3. ______ 4. ______

56. C. List the surgical procedures used.

1. ______________________ 3. ______________________

2. ______________________

57. A. Adhesion of the lid to the globe is called ______________.

B. Surgical procedure is ______________ and sometimes ______________.

C. Adhesion of the margins of the lids is ______________. It is corrected by ______________ with ______________.

D. When the palpebral fissure appears to be contracted at the outer canthus it is called ______________. Surgical procedure is ______________.

58. A. Removal of the lacrimal sac is ______________.

B. Creation of a new opening between the tear sac and nose is called ______________.

C. Both procedures are performed for ______________.

59. What are the three procedures performed for orbital tumors?

A. ______________ C. ______________

B. ______________

60. Refer to the index beginning on page 279 for the page and line number of the following words. Then write the English translation beneath each word component.

C H O L E / S T E A T / O M A

H E M O / L Y M P H / A N G I / O M A

P A N / O P H T H A L M / I T I S

O N Y C H O / L Y S I S

A N K Y L O / B L E P H A R O N

P R E S B Y / O P I A

M A C R / O T I A

S E B A C E / O U S

T Y M P A N O / P L A S T Y

D A C R Y O / C Y S T O / R H I N O / S T O M Y

T A R S O / R R H A P H Y

R H Y T I D / E C T O M Y

S U D O R I / F E R O U S

S E B O / R R H E A

E P I / D E R M O / P H Y T / O S I S

P T E R Y G I U M

E X / C O R I / A T I O N

P A R A / C E N T E S I S

I R I D / E N / C L E I S I S

H Y P E R / T R I C H / O S I S